a LANGE Medical book

UNDERSTANDING TELEHEALTH

Karen Schulder Rheuban, MD
Professor of Pediatrics
Director, University of Virginia Center for Telehealth
University of Virginia Health System
Charlottesville, Virginia

Elizabeth A. Krupinski, PhD, FSIIM, FSPIE, FATA
Professor and Vice Chair of Research
Department of Radiology and Imaging Sciences
Emory University
Atlanta, Georgia

McGraw Hill Education

New York   Chicago   San Francisco   Athens   London   Madrid   Mexico City
Milan   New Delhi   Singapore   Sydney   Toronto

Understanding Telehealth

1 2 3 4 5 6 7 8 9 DSS 22 21 20 19 18 17

ISBN 978-1-259-83740-1
MHID 1-259-83740-8

NOTICE

Medicine is an ever-changing science. As new research and clinical experience broaden our knowledge, changes in treatment and drug therapy are required. The author and the publisher of this work have checked with sources believed to be reliable in their efforts to provide information that is complete and generally in accord with the standards accepted at the time of publication. However, in view of the possibility of human error or changes in medical sciences, neither the author nor the publisher nor any other party who has been involved in the preparation or publication of this work warrants that the information contained herein is in every respect accurate or complete, and they disclaim all responsibility for any errors or omissions or for the results obtained from use of the information contained in this work. Readers are encouraged to confirm the information contained herein with other sources. For example and in particular, readers are advised to check the product information sheet included in the package of each drug they plan to administer to be certain that the information contained in this work is accurate and that changes have not been made in the recommended dose or in the contraindications for administration. This recommendation is of particular importance in connection with new or infrequently used drugs.

This book was set in Minion Pro 10/12 by MPS Limited.
The editors were Amanda Fielding and Kim J. Davis.
The production supervisor was Richard Ruzycka.
Project management was provided by Gaurav Prabhu of MPS Limited.
The cover design was RANDOMATRIX.
RR Donnelley Shenzhen was printer and binder.

Library of Congress Cataloging-in-Publication Data

Names: Rheuban, Karen S., editor. | Krupinski, Elizabeth A., editor.
Title: Understanding telehealth / [edited by] Karen S. Rheuban, Elizabeth A. Krupinski.
Description: New York : McGraw-Hill Education, [2018] | Includes bibliographical references and index.
Identifiers: LCCN 2017012757| ISBN 9781259837401 (pbk. : alk. paper)
ISBN 1259837408 (pbk. : alk. paper) | ISBN 9781259837418 (ebook)
ISBN 1259837416 (ebook)
Subjects: | MESH: Telemedicine | United States
Classification: LCC R858 | NLM W 83 AA1 | DDC 610.285–dc23 LC record available at https://lccn.loc.gov/2017012757

McGraw-Hill Education Professional books are available at special quantity discounts to use as premiums and sales promotions, or for use in corporate training programs. To contact a representative, please visit the Contact Us pages at www.mhprofessional.com.

Contents

Contributors

Richard Alcorta, MD
State of Maryland, State Emergency Services; Medical Director, Maryland Institute for Emergency Medical Services Systems (MIEMSS), Baltimore, Maryland
Chapter 8. Adult Emergency and Critical Care Telehealth

Dale C. Alverson, MD, FAAP, FATA
Professor Emeritus of Pediatrics and Regents' Professor, Professor in Health Sciences Library and Informatics Center; Medical Director, Center for Telehealth, University of New Mexico Health Sciences Center; Chief Medical Informatics Officer, LCF Research, Albuquerque, New Mexico
Chapter 20. The Role of Telehealth in International Humanitarian Outreach

Gary Capistrant, MA
Chief Policy Officer, American Telemedicine Association, Washington, DC
Chapter 23. Medicare Coverage and Reimbursement Policies

Alison L. Curfman, MD
Department of Pediatrics, Washington University in St. Louis, St. Louis, Missouri
Chapter 13: Pediatric Emergency and Critical Care Telehealth

Rachel Dixon
Colorado Access, Denver, Colorado
Chapter 10. Telepsychiatry

Gary Gilbert, PhD, MS
Telemedicine and Advanced Technology Research Center, U.S. Army Medical Research and Materiel Command, Fort Detrick, Maryland
Chapter 19. Telehealth in the Department of Defense

Neil E. Herendeen, MD, MS
Director, Golisano Children's Hospital Pediatric Practice, University of Rochester Medical Center, Rochester, New York
Chapter 15. School and Childcare Center Telehealth

Jana Katz-Bell, MPH
Assistant Dean, Interprofessional Programs, UC Davis School of Medicine and Betty Irene Moore School of Nursing, Sacramento, California
Chapter 1. History of Telehealth

Elizabeth A. Krupinski, PhD
Professor and Vice Chair of Research, Department of Radiology and Imaging Sciences, Emory University, Atlanta, Georgia
Chapter 4. Supporting Seamless Delivery of Telehealth Solutions

Nathaniel M. Lacktman, JD, CCEP
Partner, Chair of Telemedicine and Virtual Care Practice, Foley & Lardner, LLP, Tampa, Florida
Chapter 24. Legal and Regulatory Issues

Charles Lappan, MPA, MBA
U.S. Army Office of the Surgeon General, Fort Sam Houston, Texas
Chapter 19. Telehealth in the Department of Defense

Ivy A. Lee, MD
Assistant Clinical Professor, Department of Medicine, UCLA Geffen School of Medicine; Director of Telemedicine, UCLA Olive View Medical Center, Pasadena Premier Dermatology, Pasadena, California
Chapter 9. Teledermatology

Michelle S. Lee, BA
Research Associate, Department of Health Care Policy, Harvard Medical School, Boston, Massachusetts
Chapter 18. The Dawn of Direct-to-Consumer Telehealth

Curtis Lowery, MD
Chairman and Professor, Department of Obstetrics and Gynecology, University of Arkansas for Medical Sciences, Little Rock, Arkansas
Chapter 6. High-Risk Obstetrics and Telehealth

James P. Marcin, MD, MPH
Department of Pediatrics, UC Davis School of Medicine, Sacramento, California
Chapter 13: Pediatric Emergency and Critical Care Telehealth

Ateev Mehrotra, MD, MPH
Associate Professor of Medicine and Health Policy, Harvard Medical School; Hospitalist, Beth Israel Deaconess Medical Center, Boston, Massachusetts
Chapter 18. The Dawn of Direct-to-Consumer Telehealth

Thomas S. Nesbitt, MD, MPH
Associate Vice Chancellor, Strategic Technologies & Alliances; Director, Center for Health and Technology; Professor, Family & Community Medicine, UC Davis Health System; Director, Health Initiative: Center for Technology Information Research in the Interest of Society, Sacramento, California
Chapter 1. History of Telehealth

Hon Pak, MD
Chief Medical Officer, 3M Health Information System, Silver Spring, Maryland
Chapter 9. Teledermatology

Ronald Poropatich, MD
Center for Military Medicine Research, University of Pittsburgh, Pittsburgh, Pennsylvania
Chapter 19. Telehealth in the Department of Defense

Jack Resneck, Jr., MD
Professor and Vice-Chair of Dermatology, University of California, San Francisco School of Medicine; Core Faculty, Institute for Health Policy Studies, University of California, San Francisco, San Francisco, California
Chapter 21. Patients, Their Physicians, and Telehealth

H. Neal Reynolds, MD
Associate Professor of Medicine, University of Maryland School of Medicine, Baltimore, Maryland
Chapter 8. Adult Emergency and Critical Care Telehealth

Karen Schulder Rheuban, MD
Professor of Pediatrics; Director, University of Virginia Center for Telehealth, University of Virginia Health System, Charlottesville, Virginia
Chapter 2. Workforce, Definitions, and Models
Chapter 3. Rural Health

Trevor G. Russell, BPhty, PhD
School of Health and Rehabilitation Sciences, The University of Queensland, St. Lucia, Brisbane, Queensland, Australia
Chapter 12. Rehabilitation

Craig Sable, MD
Associate Chief, Division of Cardiology; Director, Echocardiography and Telemedicine, Children's National Health System; Professor of Pediatrics, George Washington University School of Medicine, Washington, DC
Chapter 16. Telehealth in Pediatric Cardiology

Kristin Schleiter, JD, LLM
Senior Legislative Attorney, American Medical Association, Chicago, Illinois
Chapter 21. Patients, Their Physicians, and Telehealth

Lee H. Schwamm, MD
Professor of Neurology, Harvard Medical School; Director, Partners TeleStroke Center, Massachusetts General Hospital, Boston, Massachusetts
Chapter 5. Telestroke

Scott Shipman, MD, MPH
Director, Primary Care Initiatives and Workforce Analysis, Association of American Medical Colleges, Washington, DC
Chapter 2. Workforce, Definitions, and Models

Jay H. Shore, MD, MPH
Helen and Arthur E. Johnson Depression Center, University of Colorado School of Medicine, Anschutz Medical Campus; Colorado Access, Aurora, Colorado
Chapter 10. Telepsychiatry
Chapter 14. Child Telepsychiatry

Neal Sikka, MD
Associate Professor of Medicine, Department of Emergency Medicine, Chief of Section on Innovative Practice and Telehealth, Medical Faculty Associates, The George Washington University, Washington, DC
Chapter 8. Adult Emergency and Critical Care Telehealth

Nina J. Solenski, MD
Associate Professor of Neurology; Director, Stroke Telemedicine and Tele-education (STAT) Program, University of Virginia, Charlottesville, Virginia
Chapter 5. Telestroke

Andrew M. Southerland, MD, MSc
Assistant Professor of Neurology and Public Health Sciences, University of Virginia, Charlottesville, Virginia
Chapter 5. Telestroke

Deborah G. Theodoros, BSp Thy (Hons), PhD
School of Health and Rehabilitation Sciences, The University of Queensland, St. Lucia, Brisbane, Queensland, Australia
Chapter 12. Rehabilitation

Latoya S. Thomas
American Telemedicine Association, Washington, DC
Chapter 22. The State Policy Framework of Telehealth

Sylvia J. Trujillo, MPP, JD
Senior Washington Counsel, American Medical Association, Washington, DC
Chapter 21. Patients, Their Physicians, and Telehealth

Amy L. Tucker, MD, MHCM, FACC
Associate Professor of Medicine, Cardiovascular Division, University of Virginia Health System Charlottesville, Virginia
Chapter 11. Remote Patient Monitoring and Care Coordination

Lori Uscher-Pines, PhD, MSc
Policy Researcher, RAND Corporation, Arlington, Virginia
Chapter 18. The Dawn of Direct-to-Consumer Telehealth

Maryann Waugh, MEd
University of Colorado Anschutz Medical Campus, School of Medicine, Helen and Arthur E. Johnson Depression Center, Denver, Colorado
Chapter 10. Telepsychiatry
Chapter 14. Child Telepsychiatry

Kathleen A. Webster, MD, MBA, FAAP
Advocate Children's Hospital, Oak Lawn, Illinois
Chapter 17. Telehealth in Children with Special Needs

John D. Whited, MD, MHS
Associate Chief of Staff, Research and Development, Durham Veterans Affairs Health Care System; Associate Professor, Department of Medicine, Duke University School of Medicine, Durham, North Carolina
Chapter 9. Teledermatology

Katharine Hsu Wibberly, PhD
Director, Mid-Atlantic Telehealth Resource Center, Karen S. Rheuban Center for Telehealth, University of Virginia, Charlottesville, Virginia
Chapter 3. Rural Health

Peter Yellowlees, MD
Department of Psychiatry & Behavioral Sciences, University of California, Davis School of Medicine & Health System, Sacramento, California
Chapter 10. Telepsychiatry
Chapter 14. Child Telepsychiatry

Christine Y. Yoon
Chapter 7. Teleophthalmology

Alice Yang Zhang, MD
Johns Hopkins University, Baltimore, Maryland
Chapter 7. Teleophthalmology

Ingrid E. Zimmer-Galler, MD
Associate Professor of Ophthalmology, Wilmer Eye Institute; Director of Telemedicine, Johns Hopkins University, Baltimore, Maryland
Chapter 7. Teleophthalmology

Marc T. Zubrow, MD
Vice President of Telemedicine, University of Maryland Medical System; Associate Professor of Medicine, University of Maryland School of Medicine, Baltimore, Maryland
Chapter 8. Adult Emergency and Critical Care Telehealth

Preface

The digital transformation of health care, coupled with an expansion of broadband communications services and an increasing volume of empirical data, has driven innovation and greater adoption of telehealth across a broad range of clinical services, specialties, technologies, applications, and facilities, including the home.

Understanding Telehealth was written for a broad range of stakeholders, including physicians, nurses, and allied health professionals, both in practice and in training; health care executives; public health advocates; hospitals; clinics; payors; telecommunications and technology providers; health care advocates; researchers; and entrepreneurs.

Our goal is to advance the reader's understanding of the opportunities to integrate telehealth solutions to improve timely access to care, to mitigate acute and chronic illness, and to improve clinical outcomes, wherever possible, within the context of the medical home. A secondary goal is to encourage and promote further research in this growing field with respect to critically important topics such as quantifying clinical outcomes, assessing costs, and evaluating emerging technologies in order to leverage and pivot valid and reliable empirical evidence into policy changes that foster the seamless integration of these solutions into everyday clinical practice and general health care.

Addressing the challenges of workforce shortages and high rates of chronic illness requires a paradigm shift from the model of physician-centered care to models focused on patient-centered care using interdisciplinary teams, evidence-based medicine, and informatics in decision support, all enhanced by telehealth tools.

To help understand how telehealth can advance these objectives, we have included chapters that address a broad range of technologies, evidence-based clinical guidelines, and applications of telehealth across the health care continuum and among different patient populations. We have also summarized the legal and regulatory framework currently underpinning telehealth practice. We have provided clinical vignettes supporting the clinical chapters to remind readers that at the core of our efforts and of all of those engaged in telehealth are the patients and their families.

The editors are profoundly grateful to our chapter authors, each luminaries in their respective fields, and to our colleagues and families for their support of this effort and our work to advance telehealth across the disciplines.

Karen Schulder Rheuban
Elizabeth A. Krupinski
September 2017

Introduction

Understanding Telehealth comes at an opportune time in the continued evolution of the important role telehealth technology can play in enhancing access, supporting clinicians, and improving the patient experience. I applaud the authors for the breadth of topics and issues covered in this publication. It is reflective of the growth of clinical applications that are leveraging this technology to support health care delivery.

We certainly have a vested interest in this issue at the Federal Office of Rural Health Policy (FORHP) within the Health Resources and Services Administration (HRSA) of the U.S. Department of Health and Human Services. FORHP began supporting telehealth projects in the early 1990s as a way to improve access to health care services that were not available locally in rural communities. We have been joined in those efforts by a host of federal partners ranging from the Indian Health Service (IHS) to the Veterans Health Administration (VHA). FORHP's early efforts were focused mostly on supporting demonstration programs, and we were joined in this effort by similar projects funded by the Centers for Medicare & Medicaid Services (CMS, though then known as the Health Care Financing Administration). Our early efforts sought to inform broader policy issues related to reimbursement, safety, quality, and licensure.

Much has changed in the ensuing years. By the late 1990s, Congress had formally created the Office for the Advancement of Telehealth (OAT), which is located within FORHP, and authorized a range of telehealth programs within HRSA to support the development of telehealth network grants and a nationwide network of telehealth resource centers, as well as the Licensure and Portability Grant program. Around the same time, Medicare began covering a limited range of services that has been steadily growing. At the state level, 48 states and the District of Columbia now provide some form of Medicaid reimbursement for telehealth services.

Developments that are more recent include a 2012 HRSA-sponsored workshop, convened by the Institute of Medicine (IOM), to determine the role of telehealth in the rapidly changing U.S. health care system.[1] The meeting came at a critical time, with the health care system rapidly evolving from one that emphasizes volume to one that focuses on delivery of high-value care. Throughout the two-day IOM workshop, one common theme was that telehealth can facilitate access for patients to interact with their providers, which reduces barriers to receiving high-value care. This publication will pick up on that specific theme and many other issues raised by the IOM.

As *Understanding Telehealth* explores in more detail in the subsequent chapters, telehealth continues to deal with a number of long-standing policy issues such as licensure and reimbursement, as noted in Chapters 22–24. Clinicians and state and national licensing bodies continue to wrestle with the challenge of how to ease the regulatory burden of providers who deliver services across state lines via telehealth while still protecting patient safety. We have seen some progress in this area through the OAT Licensure and Portability Grant program, which has provided funding to the Federation of State Medical Boards and the Provincial Boards of Psychology to develop ways to address this challenge.

Payment for telehealth services has been evolving to reflect this movement toward value by providing payors opportunities to invest in telehealth capabilities outside the traditional fee-for-service payment. Medicare historically has paid for telehealth under limited circumstances, but the statutory authority is limited, as discussed in Chapter 23. Still, incremental progress has been made.

CMS has undertaken efforts to address reimbursement limitations through alternative payment models such as the recent Next Generation ACO Model, which offers greater flexibility for telehealth reimbursement.[2] The Medicare Access and CHIP Reauthorization Act of 2015 (MACRA) also includes incentives for clinicians to coordinate care using telehealth, because they could be "rewarded" for that activity[3] under the Improvement Activities category of the Merit-Based Incentive Payment System in the Quality Payment Program (QPP) that will assess clinicians' performance and adjust their payments.[4] A recent Medicaid Home Health Final Rule clarified that the Medicaid eligibility requirements for face-to-face encounters include telehealth.[5] Since 2012, the CMS Innovation Center has funded eight states with telehealth activities under its State Innovation Models (SIM) initiative[6] and 22 projects with a telehealth focus under its Health Care Innovation Awards (HCIA).[3,7]

Across HHS, there is increasing adoption of telehealth technology. For example, telehealth activities are woven into many of HRSA's programs beyond OAT. The Bureau of Health Workforce and the HIV/AIDS Bureaus support grant programs that rely on telehealth links to support training and education. The Bureau of Primary Health Care has seen an expanded use of telehealth in community health centers. The Maternal and Child Health Bureau intends to fund several telegenetics grants to serve children with special health needs.[8]

HHS' Office of the National Coordinator for Health IT (ONC) recently completed an assessment of the various telehealth activities funded by federal agencies, showing a broad range of these activities across the department.

HHS has made investments in telehealth in a number of its other agencies. For instance, the Agency for Healthcare Research and Quality (AHRQ) recently released an evidence map for telehealth that analyzed which applications showed the greatest promise for improving patient outcomes.[9] The National Institutes of Health (NIH) has supported a number of studies that develop, utilize, or evaluate a telehealth component to show how this technology can help address chronic disease.[10] Also, the Centers for Disease Control and Prevention (CDC) has supported efforts to address public health issues using telehealth, including an e-pathology program to link pathologists to public health providers.[11] The Substance Abuse and Mental Health Services Administration (SAMHSA) has invested in grants to support mental health care coordination through telehealth and other health information technology applications.[12] More recently, the IHS awarded a contract to expand its ability to provide telehealth services in the IHS Great Plains Area, representing frontier areas of the United States.[13]

As the number of federal programs involved in telehealth activities has grown, so has the need for identifying areas of collaboration and the ability to share information. Toward that end, HRSA established the Federal Telemedicine Working Group (FedTel) to summarize key telehealth activities and facilitate information sharing among participants in 26 agencies and departments throughout the federal government, not just HHS. The workgroup holds monthly conference calls and meets semiannually face to face.[14]

The increase in federal activity is not happening in isolation. There is growing interest in telehealth across a broad range of stakeholders. One study estimates that 58% of health care providers used some form of telehealth in 2015.[15] Towers Watson reported that 22% of large employers in 2014 covered telemedicine consultations and that more than 68% planned to do so by 2017.[16] In 2013, the market for telehealth-generated annual revenue was $9.6 billion, a 60% growth from 2012.[17]

Amidst all of this activity, it is clear that the field of telehealth is continually evolving and maturing. It is becoming an increasingly expected part of the health care delivery system and an essential tool for clinicians and patients. It is also important to note that delivering services through telehealth is no longer solely an issue to reach rural communities, as urban patients may also benefit from the flexibility of the technology to more efficiently deliver access and services. Fields like dermatology and mental health are well-established users of this technology.

With each passing year, however, more clinicians are finding ways to deliver these services via telehealth. This publication includes chapters that examine some of these emerging applications of the technology, including areas such as high-risk obstetrics, direct-to-consumer primary care, and pediatric cardiology, just to name a few.

This publication's chapters focusing on public policy highlight a range of ongoing policy issues that will need to be addressed. These issues range from ensuring access to robust and affordable broadband services as the backbone for telehealth to the need to find ways to balance the requirement to ensure quality and safety without the regulatory burden associated with licensure for clinicians who deliver telehealth services in multiple states.

Although policy issues such as reimbursement and licensure continue to pose challenges, other systemic changes in health care delivery may offer a path toward greater integration of this technology into the daily patient experience. The emerging emphasis on creating a value-driven health care system that focuses more on outcomes and quality and less on volume creates a unique opportunity to leverage telehealth technology.

The traditional fee-for-service payment structure has never been a particularly good fit for telehealth. New payment models focused on accountable care or global budgeting offer interesting new possibilities for telehealth because the emphasis is more on the outcome and less on the site of service.

Although this volume-to-value transition has begun, it is still in its early stages. This publication will help inform a growing effort to better understand how telehealth can fit into a value-based system. There is a need to expand the current evidence base for telehealth services. At FORHP, we have taken initial steps in this direction by focusing our TNGP funding not only on enhancing access, but also on gathering data as part of a broader research effort to compare outcomes for patients seen through telehealth compared to patients receiving similar services face to face. The previously mentioned AHRQ Telehealth Evidence Map will be an important tool to better inform future telehealth investments. The ensuing chapters cover these and many other issues and inform much of the current state of how clinicians are using this technology to enhance care for their patients.

REFERENCES

1. *The Role of Telehealth in an Evolving Health Care Environment - Workshop Summary.* November 20, 2012. http://www.nationalacademies.org/hmd/Reports/2012/The-Role-of-Telehealth-in-an-Evolving-Health-Care-Environment.aspx. Accessed December 14, 2016.

2. Centers for Medicare & Medicaid Services. *Next ACO Model.* https://innovation.cms.gov/initiatives/Next-Generation-ACO-Model/. Accessed December 14, 2016.

3. U.S. Department of Health and Human Services. *Report to Congress E-health and Telemedicine.* August 12, 2016. https://aspe.hhs.gov/sites/default/files/pdf/206751/TelemedicineE-HealthReport.pdf. Accessed December 14, 2016.

4. Centers for Medicare & Medicaid Services. *Quality Payment Program.* https://qpp.cms.gov/. Accessed December 14, 2016.

5. Centers for Medicare & Medicaid Services. *Face-to-Face Requirements for Home Health Services; Policy Changes and Clarifications Related to Home Health.* February 2, 2016. https://s3.amazonaws.com/public-inspection.federalregister.gov/2016-01585.pdf. Accessed December 14, 2016.

6. Centers for Medicare & Medicaid Services. *State Innovation Models Initiative.* https://innovation.cms.gov/initiatives/state-innovations/. Accessed December 14, 2016.

7. Centers for Medicare & Medicaid Services. *Health Care Innovations Awards.* https://innovation.cms.gov/initiatives/Health-Care-Innovation-Awards/. Accessed December 14, 2016.

8. *Maternal and Child Health Services Title V Block Grant Puerto Rico.* March 16, 2016. https://mchb.tvisdata.hrsa.gov/uploadedfiles/2016/submittedFiles/printVersion/PR_TitleV_PrintVersion.pdf. Accessed December 14, 2016.

9. Agency for Health Care Research and Quality. *Telehealth: Mapping the Evidence for Patient Outcomes From Systematic Reviews.* Technical Brief Number 26. https://www.effectivehealthcare.ahrq.gov/ehc/products/624/2254/telehealth-report-160630.pdf. Accessed December 14, 2016.

10. U.S. National Library of Medicine. *Telehealth and Telemedicine.* https://lhncbc.nlm.nih.gov/project/telehealth-and-telemedicine. Accessed December 14, 2016.

11. Centers for Disease Control. *Infectious Diseases Pathology Branch.* https://www.cdc.gov/ncezid/dhcpp/idpb/epathology/index.html. Accessed December 14, 2016.

12. Substance Abuse and Mental Health Services Administration. *SAMHSA's Efforts in Health Information Technology.* http://www.samhsa.gov/health-information-technology/samhsas-efforts. Accessed December 14, 2016.

13. Indian Health Service. *Indian Health Service Awards $6.8 Million Telemedicine Services Contract to Avera Health.* September 20, 2016. https://www.ihs.gov/newsroom/pressreleases/2016pressreleases/indian-health-service-awards-6-8-million-telemedicine-services-contract-to-avera-health/. Accessed December 15, 2016.

14. Doarn C, Pruitt S, Jacobs J, et al. *Federal Efforts to Define and Advance Telehealth: A Work in Progress.* May 1, 2014. https://www.ncbi.nlm.nih.gov/pmc/articles/PMC4011485/. Accessed December 15, 2016.

15. HIMSS Analytics. *The Healthcare Information and Management Systems Society. 2015 Telemedicine Study.* September 2015. http://www.himssanalytics.org/research/essentials-brief-telemedicine-study.

16. Tower Watson. *Current Telemedicine Technology Could Mean Big Savings.* August 11, 2014. http://www.towerswatson.com/en-US/Press/2014/08/current-telemedicine-technology-could-mean-big-savings. Accessed December 15, 2016.

17. Drobac K. 2015: *Another Unstoppable Year for Telehealth.* Published March 24, 2015. http://www.connectwithcare.org/2015-another-unstoppable-year-telehealth/. Accessed December 15, 2016.

Background

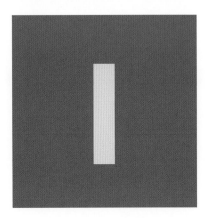

History of Telehealth

Thomas S. Nesbitt, MD, MPH and Jana Katz-Bell, MPH

Since early human history and throughout many cultures, accessing a healer or someone with "expert health knowledge" was considered beneficial in alleviating maladies. Healers such as shamans, priests, and medicine men or women are known to have been part of prehistoric cultures. These healers normally required communication with and ideally visualization of the patient in order to diagnose and treat.[1] In many cultures, over time, healers became known as physicians; the first acknowledged physician, an Egyptian named Imhotep, lived during the 27th century BCE.[1] By 420 BCE medicine began to develop standards, with Hippocrates credited for initiating the age of "rational medicine." That era was characterized by the development of the idea that diseases have natural causes and the origination of the concept of ethics in medicine, perpetuated as the Hippocratic Oath. The Asclepion Temples that the Greeks erected became some of the world's first health centers.[2] People (pilgrims) traveled great distances to these temples to seek medical advice, prognosis, and healing.[2,3] In approximately 300 BCE in India, specific structures were constructed for health care, with basic sanitization standards.[4] Around 100 BCE, the Romans erected buildings called valetudinarians for the care of sick slaves, gladiators, and soldiers.[3] With the fall of the Roman, Greek, and Egyptian civilizations came a decline in the formal study and practice of medicine in these cultures.[5]

Medical care improved in the early Middle Ages (6th to 10th century CE), when an infirmary became an established part of nearly every monastery, under the influence of the Benedictine Order. Also during that time the first medical schools were opened. Quite possibly the earliest, reported to have developed out of a monastery dispensary, was the Schola Medica Salernitana at Salerno in southern Italy.[6] During the late Middle Ages (beyond the 10th century) monastic infirmaries continued to expand, and public hospitals were opened, financed by city authorities, the church, and private sources. Specialized institutions, including leper houses, also originated at this time.[7]

Health care evolved over time, from a largely nonscientific discipline involving home remedies and traveling doctors, to one encompassing vast amounts of scientific knowledge, increasingly reliant on technology, technical expertise, and complex systems of care. The work of Benjamin Franklin and Dr. Thomas Bond led to the establishment of Pennsylvania Hospital, which upon its opening in 1751 became the first hospital in the continental United States.[8] This was followed by New York Hospital, which was chartered in 1771. During the 1800s, significant advancements began to occur, including the development of the stethoscope, antiseptic surgery, anesthesia, germ theory, and vaccines. During this time, Johns Hopkins and other academic centers were built. However, despite the development of formal hospitals, physicians generally performed medical care in the homes of their patients, a practice that continued throughout that century.[9] As the equipment and treatments became more sophisticated and cumbersome, physicians opened offices or treated patients in hospitals. Only 40% of physician encounters were conducted via house call by 1930. By 1950, house calls decreased to 10% of visits, and to less than 1% by 1980.[9,10]

The shift in site of care delivery from the home to clinics and hospitals was also partially the result of the growth of third-party payers and increasing liability concerns.[11] However, throughout the history of health care, obstacles have impeded consistent access to the right expertise, at the right time, and in the right place for those in need. Hence, a desire emerged to make expertise more widely available through distance communications.

HISTORY OF DISTANCE COMMUNICATION TECHNOLOGY

Communication and the exchange of information have been important to humans throughout time. Early forms of communication included runners in mountain villages, fires, beacons, smoke signals, communication drums, horns, and reflective devices.[3] For instance, one form of early communication involved the "heliograph"—sending messages by reflecting the sun with a mirror or other shiny surface toward the intended recipient. The Greeks are believed to have used polished shields to signal their fellow soldiers as far back as 405 BCE.[12] Later, the Roman emperor Tiberius used light reflection to signal orders to the mainland from his "Villa Jovis" on the Isle of Capri.[13] Although often slow and limited to relatively small distances, these forms of communication served a functional purpose within the geographic boundaries of the people of those times.

The concept was modernized in the early 1800s, when Gauss developed the heliotrope for surveying land. Reflected sunlight continued to be used for communications into the late 1800s, notably by the United States military in Arizona and New Mexico.[14] In France, also in the 1800s, a more sophisticated optical line-of-sight method of communications was developed using a series of towers that held large horizontal beams with smaller connected pieces that could be configured into various shapes associated with a code. This was referred to as an optical telegraph.[15] Around 1867, Aldis signal lamps used light to communicate using a code between towns on land and ships at sea, as well as between land and sea.[16]

The electronic age of communication began with the electrical telegraph. Although numerous scientists throughout Europe and Russia experimented with electromagnetic telecommunications in the 1800s, Samuel Morse is credited with bringing the telegraph to scale because of a standard code for communications. He made his first transmission in January 1838, across 2 miles of wire near Morristown, New Jersey.[17] In 1844, he sent a message from the Capitol in Washington to Baltimore, after which commercial telegraphy began to scale quickly in America. Over the next 10 to 15 years lines linked most of the major cities on the East Coast. The transcontinental telegraph was connected on October 24, 1861.[18] The golden age of the telegraph was cut short with Alexander Graham Bell's invention of the telephone in 1876, with the direct dial phone patented just 13 years later.[19,20] Wireless communications, innovated in the late 1800s, began to mature in the early 1900s. By 1912 two-way radio communication was available on ships. Two-way radio transmission expanded to police units, throughout the military, and eventually to outer space in the early 1960s.

In 1927, Philo Farnsworth demonstrated a television transmission in his laboratory in San Francisco. However, it took 20 years for commercial television to begin.[21] Although the first color television signals were broadcast in 1954, more than a decade passed before television stations began broadcasting prime-time shows in color.

The mid-1960s also saw the beginnings of broadband technology linking computers. It was then that Massachusetts Institute of Technology (MIT) and Dartmouth College linked up with speeds of up to 50 Kbps. Before the end of the decade, this network was expanded to include institutions on the West Coast with higher bandwidth. In 1969, ARPANET (Advanced Research Project Agency Network) was funded by the Advanced Research Projects Agency (ARPA) of the United States Department of Defense. This was one of the first wide-area packet-switching networks, the first to use Transmission Control Protocol and Internet Protocol (TCP/IP), and represents the beginning of today's Internet.[14] By the mid-1980s, a network of universities across the country had attained data transfer speeds of up to 1.544 Mbps (T1); however, households and private businesses did not begin Internet use until the 1990s, primarily with dial-up modems with speeds of only 56 Kbps. In 2016, competition for home and small business customers was significant, with service providers advertising speeds of up to 100 Mbps.

Despite this, a "digital divide" still places rural and some urban intercity areas at a disadvantage.

One of the most significant changes to communications in the late 20th and early 21st centuries was the rapid development and expansion of wireless communications and cellular-based technologies. Martin Cooper, a Motorola engineer, reportedly made the first cell phone call on April 3, 1973.[22] A decade would pass before mobile phones were sold commercially. In 1983, mobile phones cost $4,000 and used a 1G analog network. The next generation of mobile phones, introduced in the 1990s, communicated on a 2G digital network. At the turn of the 21st century, the advancement to 3G networks enabled support of multimedia and Internet access, which quickly gave way to 4G, allowing for relatively high-quality interactive video from handheld devices.[23]

HISTORY OF COMMUNICATIONS OVER DISTANCE FOR HEALTH

Communications over distance for health purposes also has a long history. Signal flags flew on ships and over ports to indicate outbreaks of various contagious diseases. Aboriginal peoples of Australia carried "message sticks" to communicate news of death and disease to distant tribal gatherings.[3] Consulting by written correspondence was common from the mid-1600s through the 1700s, sometimes because of the lack of local access to physicians in some areas, or sometimes to obtain an opinion from a famous physician.[24] Also in the 17th century, distance diagnostic medicine occurred with patients sending urine samples to distant physicians who provided diagnoses based on uroscopy[25] and dispatched "prescription-by-post" and thorough instructions on recommended treatment.[26]

The first use of electronic communication for health purposes in the United States occurred during the American Civil War. The Union Army used the telegraph to communicate casualty reports, coordinate patient transport, and request medical supplies.[14] Evidence shows that the newly constructed telegraph was used in Australia in 1874 in the care of a wounded person and to connect a dying man with his wife 2,000 kilometers away.[27] Five years later, in 1879, a report in *The Lancet* described a telephone call between a mother and a physician to determine whether a baby had croup. In that report, the physician listened to the baby's cough through the phone.[28] In 1905, Willem Einthoven demonstrated the transmission of heart sounds from a hospital to his laboratory using the telephone. He called it a "telecardiogram."[14] Five years later, two New York cardiologists reported the remote transmission of electrocardiograms (ECGs) for diagnosing "hypertrophy and arrhythmias."[29]

In 1910, Sidney Brown, an engineer in England, made improvements to the telephone that led him to state that it was now possible to accurately listen to the sounds of a stethoscope that a patient held in place miles away and "to arrive at a correct diagnosis."[30]

In the 1920s, Haukeland Hospital (now Haukeland University Hospital) in Norway began using two-way radio communications with ships to consult with physicians and to direct treatment.[14] Similar services developed in other countries during the next decade. Police reportedly began using mobile two-way radios in 1923 in Victoria, Australia, to communicate. By 1925, the theoretical concept of the "radio doctor" providing distance care using audio and video was described in an often-cited article in *Science and Invention* magazine (Figure 1-1).[31]

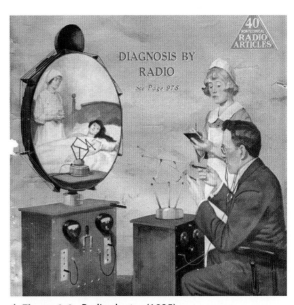

▲ **Figure 1-1.** Radio doctor (1925).

TELEHEALTH 1940–1990

The five-decade period from 1940 to 1990 was a time during which conceptualization of new ideas and innovative experimentation proliferated. In some cases, the technology had to be developed, and the lack of a telecommunication infrastructure limited the scale of projects. However, some landmark projects were developed by the pioneers of the field. During this time, the vocabulary that we use today was just being invented. In fact, the idea of technology-assisted distance diagnosis was captured with the term *telognosis*, which appeared in the medical literature in 1950 in reference to the 1948 transmission of radiologic images by telephone between West Chester and Philadelphia, Pennsylvania.[32] This model of "teleradiology" was replicated more formally in Montreal at Jean-Talon Hospital in the 1950s.[33,34] In 1959, the transmission of fluoroscopy images was reported to also have occurred in Canada.[35] Radiology has been a pioneering specialty in telemedicine, particularly in developing standards of practice, described in a later chapter.

The first widely reported use of interactive video communications for health care in the United States occurred at the University of Nebraska, where clinicians transmitted neurological examinations across campus to medical students in 1959.[36,37] Several years later, a 112-mile, closed-circuit, two-television link was established between the university and Norfolk State Hospital for psychiatric and neurologic consultations.[38]

During the 1960s, numerous accounts of wireless transmission of ECGs, cardiac monitoring, and even X-ray images were reported.[39] Although not normally discussed as telemedicine, the critical ability for first responders to send cardiac monitoring information to responding emergency physicians who were en route was accomplished in Miami in 1967 using voice radio channels.[40]

In 1968, a seminal telemedicine project was established involving Massachusetts General Hospital (MGH) and Logan Airport. Staffed by nurses, the "medical station" at the airport was linked via microwave relay to MGH as a means of providing primary and emergency services to travelers and airport staff.[41] The telemedicine efforts at the MGH continued two years later with a telepsychiatry link with the Veterans Administration Hospital in Bedford, Massachusetts, that remained in service into the 1980s.[42]

Multiple hospitals in two states, Vermont and New Hampshire, participated in another important project during this time period. This network, called INTERACT, involved a combination of telemedicine, remote education, and administration.[14] It is important not only because it encompassed multiple states and multiple services, but also because it attracted significant federal funding from multiple agencies. The Health Care Technology Division of the Department of Health, Education and Welfare (now the Department of Health and Human Services) and the National Science Foundation funded several other notable telemedicine demonstration projects during this time period.[14]

The National Aeronautics and Space Administration (NASA) played a major role in the development of telemedicine. NASA had an obvious need to assess the health of astronauts while in space, beginning with the Mercury program in the early 1960s. As part of the process to test and refine protocols using satellite-based telemedicine, NASA and Lockheed partnered in a project through which medical services were made available to the Papago Indians in Arizona. The program, named STARPAHC (Space Technology Applied to Rural Papago Advanced Health Care), lasted until the late 1970s.[38] Satellite communication opened up telemedicine opportunities for large rural areas. In 1972, NASA's Applications Technology Satellite (ATS-1) began providing telecommunications access for health care between numerous smaller communities in Alaska and larger hospitals.[43] The success of this program resulted in a significant expansion over the next several years.

In the mid-1970s Memorial University of Newfoundland began working in the area of telehealth, with 30 projects undertaken over 20 years. This Newfoundland program notably has been cited as the only pre-1986 program that survived into the 1990s.[44] In 1984, the Australian government set up the Q-network via satellite. A pilot program called the North-West Telemedicine Project delivered health care to five remote towns in the Northern Territory. A 1989 publication on this program described improvement in quality of health care and discussed how it reduced some health care costs.[45]

Although several university programs began serious planning efforts toward the end of the 1980s, reports of telemedicine consultations were modest during this time, as evidenced by the scarcity of literature on the subject during this decade. However, one noteworthy project quickly developed following the massive Soviet Armenian earthquake that occurred December 7, 1988. Just five days later, NASA, as part of the U.S./USSR working Group on Space Biology, made an offer to the USSR to provide humanitarian aid to the region. The project, designated as the U.S.-USSR Telemedicine Space Bridge to Armenia and Ufa, began in March 1989, with consultations by physicians from four U.S. medical centers: University of Utah/LDS Hospital, University of Texas, Maryland Institute for Emergency Medical Service Systems, and Uniformed Services University of the Health Sciences. According to the final project report, "Intelsat and Comsat donated free access to uplink and satellite transponders, and the Soviet Union donated the downlink channels".[46]

TELEHEALTH 1990–2000

Following the early exploration into telemedicine through notable projects in Nebraska, Massachusetts, and Vermont-New Hampshire,[14] the 1990s came to be regarded as the "developmental years" of telemedicine. This was the decade during which many large state and system projects emerged, telecommunications evolved to the point that it was more available and affordable, and passage of state and federal legislation propelled the field forward by recognizing telemedicine as a reimbursable mode of care provision.

Investment in telehealth from a state and system level began in the early 1990s and rapidly expanded during this decade. What differentiated this time period from the early years of telehealth was the emergence of large hub-and-spoke networks in contrast to the customarily project-based approaches of the prior decade. Programs in the 1990s began to involve dozens of "spokes" (patient sites) linking to one or several large specialty or acute care health care organizations.

Several of the noteworthy programs of the early 1990s were subsidized by legislative appropriations or by funds related to telecommunications mergers. Most programs were launched with a focus on improving specialty access to outpatient services and health professions education. Because of the role of academic health centers in providing safety net access, they were frequently in leadership positions with these systems during this decade; programs in the early part of this

decade emerged largely in response to inadequacies in health care access in rural areas.

In the early part of this decade, equipment was extremely expensive; videoconferencing systems enhanced with scopes cost upwards of $100K. Early in this decade there were no dominant technology providers of telehealth units—programs repurposed videoconferencing systems for clinical use. Telecommunications options likewise were limited to using telephone circuit-switched networks. Integrated Services Digital Network (ISDN) lines became the norm for video connectivity because it required high bandwidth. This combined multiple 128 Kbit ISDN Basic Rate Interface (BRI) lines for each video call known as bonding. Where ISDN was not available, programs installed dedicated point-to-point circuits such as T1 (1.544 Mbit) and fractional T1 lines for a hefty price. A defining feature in this decade was the first ratified standard enabling videoconferencing capabilities over packet-switched networks, which are still widely used in business and the Internet today. In November 1996 the International Telecommunications Union (ITU) published H.323, which, after its adoption in the late 1990s and early 2000s, became a crucial milestone for telemedicine and interoperability between providers. That said, adoption of this standard introduced an operational barrier, as firewalls during this decade were not H.323-aware, requiring participating organizations to modify their firewalls to allow videoconferencing to function. Although the H.323 standard offered many benefits over ISDN, such as using the Internet for a fixed cost, which introduced an unlimited amount of connections globally, ISDN remained the more reliable option during this decade.

The launch of telemedicine programs was frequently a result of grant funding during this decade. The federal government was one source of funds, and during this decade the Office for the Advancement of Telehealth (then called the Office for Rural Healthcare) was established and administered a grant program. This office, in the Federal Office of Rural Health Policy (FORHP), was created in 1987 to advise the secretary of the U.S. Department of Health and Human Services on health care issues affecting rural communities.[47] The U.S. Department of Agriculture also distributed grants and loans that supported telehealth and distance education via the Rural Utilities Services program.

In 1993 the American Telemedicine Association was launched with an inaugural meeting of 250 people in Albuquerque, New Mexico. Early programs typically established novel collaborations with the goal of sustaining the field (and thus their individual programs). Health systems that were customary competitors formed telehealth alliances during this decade, typically with the goal of overcoming barriers and advancing a legislative and regulatory agenda necessary to support telehealth. Other alliances formed to share access to telecommunication infrastructure.

Recognizing that reimbursement was a fundamental requirement of sustainability, many of the alliances focused on state legislation. For example, in California a coalition of academic health centers, health systems, technology vendors, and policy staffers developed a policy road map in 1994–1995 that resulted in State Senator Mike Thompson (now U.S. Representative Mike Thompson) sponsoring the Telemedicine Development Act of 1996. This legislation redefined the requirement of "face-to-face" for a health care encounter and required the state's Medicaid system to implement a reimbursement policy.[48] Partner legislation passed that same session required the California Medical Board to address licensure as it related to telehealth. These two statutes became model language that other states adopted to advance telehealth reimbursement.[49] The first organization dedicated to address policy issues was launched in this decade: the Center for Telemedicine Law, now called the Robert J. Waters Center for Telemedicine and eHealth Law.

On the national level, organizations began to coordinate demands for Medicare reimbursement, without which programs would struggle financially. The expansion of Medicare reimbursement began when Congress passed the Balanced Budget Act of 1997 (BBA), which mandated Medicare reimbursements for telehealth care and funding for telehealth demonstration projects. Even though this first federal law had significant restrictions, its enactment was important because it recognized telemedicine as a mechanism to provide care to geographically isolated people. Reimbursement was limited to enrollees living in medically underserved rural regions, to specific providers, and to billing codes selected by the Centers for Medicare and Medicaid Services (CMS). The first version of this reimbursement also required splitting fees between specialists and primary care providers, which was unprecedented given overarching policies that strictly prohibit referral arrangements with any perceived or real collusion between providers. Despite the imperfections in the legislation, the telemedicine community celebrated this important milestone in the emergence of the field as the result of a broad, grassroots coalition of telehealth providers.[50]

The Veterans Health Administration (VHA) was in a period of internal reorganization during this decade, with a significant emphasis on the electronic health record and on local innovation, with the goal of providing access to entitled veterans. During this decade, telehealth pilots emerged in a number of clinical areas around the country in a "grassroots" model. Between 1994 and 2004 VHA staff members published about 80 peer-reviewed journal articles, contributing to the evidence base for telehealth. The positive findings of a Kaiser Permanente home telehealth (HT) study corroborated the VHA's strategy of piloting HT and developing an associated care coordination model.[51]

Correctional health organizations began to explore telehealth as a delivery strategy during this decade. Although Florida was the first to experiment with telemedicine in prison, introducing it in state penitentiaries in the late 1980s, Texas became best known for the use of telehealth in penal institutions and began using telehealth to care for its prison population in the early 1990s. Given that transporting inmates for health care is expensive—the cost of security personnel—and presents a community safety risk, telemedicine became a strategy of interest by county, state, and federal correctional organizations.

▶ Georgia

Recognized for its pioneering program in the field of telehealth, Georgia enacted legislation in 1992 to establish a statewide network led by the Medical College of Georgia and the state's Department of Administrative Services. Funding for the launch of the program came from a settlement with the Southern Bell telecommunications company related to an "overearnings" program was proposed as a means to help counteract escalating health care expenses and disparities in access. Starting with a pilot program in 1991 at Dodge County Hospital (which predated the legislation), the network grew to include an academic hub, "secondary" specialty services hubs, correctional sites, and ambulatory care sites. Georgia's operational and clinical training and consultation influenced the design and implementation of many programs in the 1990s.[52]

Texas

In 1993, the Texas legislature established a correctional managed care plan that incorporated telemedicine and an operational strategy to respond to escalating health care costs and to obstacles that impeded services for remote prisons, despite the constitutional requirement to provide health care to inmates. The University of Texas Medical Branch (UTMB) in Galveston, which together with Texas Tech Health Sciences, was capitated for inmate health services, implemented a hub-and-spoke telemedicine model providing a broad spectrum of specialty services.[53] As an early adopter of telemedicine, UTMB overcame the challenges of the 1990s, including expensive equipment and installation of telecommunications infrastructure, and remains a leader in correctional/prison telemedicine. Texas continues to have the nation's largest prison population, currently 153,000 inmates. However, per-prisoner medical care expenditures in Texas are approximately 60% of the national average; a UTMB correctional-managed care administrator attributes those cost savings to efficiencies achieved through telemedicine.[54]

Alaska

Alaska's significant barriers in terms of geography, weather, and isolation stimulated early adoption of telecommunications to overcome health care access barriers. Dating back to the 1920s, when telephone and telegraph were used to direct the distribution and administration of diphtheria antitoxin to the most remote regions of the state, the state has been an innovator in the use of telemedicine. In 1996, the National Library of Medicine funded a test project using telemedicine to address the high prevalence of otitis media. Two years later, an unprecedented coalition of federal agencies (Department of Defense, Office for the Advancement of Telehealth, the Department of Health and Human Services, the Indian Health Services, and the Department of Veterans Affairs) appropriated

funds to establish a broad telehealth network called the Alaska Federal Health Care Access Network (AFHCAN). The 235 AFHCAN sites are associated with diverse partners, including Alaska Native organizations, public health offices, and military and Veterans Affairs sites.[14]

Arizona

Leveraging early experience in telemedicine (as described earlier in this chapter, including STARPAHC, NASA, and experience at Massachusetts General Hospital), leaders in the state of Arizona engaged in the early 1990s in establishment of the Arizona Rural Telemedicine Network, subsequently renamed the Arizona Telemedicine Network. Launched as a project encompassing rural sites, a correctional facility, and a hospital on an Indian reservation, the program now has status as a statewide enterprise. Utilizing a membership model that offers organizations flexible options for engagement, the network provides telecommunications infrastructure, training, distance education programming, research and program assessment, and "open forum" telemedicine consultations. This notable program from the early days of telehealth, developed through a collaboration of public and private organizations, has integrated research with education and practice, and has solidified diverse funding sources consisting of membership fees, state and university support, and grants.[55]

TELEHEALTH 2000–2010

This decade was characterized by a maturation of the field in both outpatient and inpatient telehealth, as well as a renewed interest in and broadening of services to the home. By the end of the first decade of the new millennium, telehealth outpatient services included nearly every conceivable outpatient clinical service. Programs existed in all 50 U.S. states and around the world, and programs were actively expanding services, specialties, and the number of sites being served.

Inpatient and emergency telehealth experienced significant expansion during this decade, driven in part by teleneurology and tele-intensive care (tele-ICU). Neurologists started exploring telehealth strategies in the end of the 1990s, and the field expanded significantly during the first decade of the new millennium. The Food and Drug Administration (FDA) approved the use of intravenous tissue plasminogen activator (tPA) in patients with acute ischemic stroke in 1996; however, initial safety concerns led to low utilization. As the evidence base for the safety and effectiveness of tPA grew, its underutilization became a concern.[56] Researchers demonstrated that telestroke services could increase the use of tPA[57,58]; that prompted national professional organizations to actively promote telemedicine as a valid response to the disparity in geographic distribution of stroke neurologists and with a goal to increase the appropriate use of tPA.[58] For this application telehealth became not just a strategy to expand access or to avoid patient travel, but additionally was regarded as an essential tool enabling hospitals lacking a stroke neurologist to meet standards of care.[58,59]

Another area of telemedicine that expanded significantly during this decade was tele-ICU. Although examples of remote consultations to intensive care units existed in previous decades, a new comprehensive model emerged with a command center staffed by intensivists, critical nurses, and other staff, with capacity for protocol-driven remote monitoring with "smart alarms" combined with interactive video conferencing.[60] In 2000, Sentara Healthcare in Virginia became the first to implement this approach. Although the literature was somewhat mixed on mortality outcomes and cost effectiveness, studies generally viewed this approach favorably.[61] By 2010, more than 5,000 intensive care unit beds in nearly 250 hospitals were being covered via tele-ICU.[62]

Pediatrics is another field that led the expansion in emergency care and inpatient telehealth models of care. Given that children's services are largely regionalized and concentrated in urban areas, several notable children's hospitals developed programs in this field supporting various services, including neonatal telemedicine, services to the home for ventilator-dependent children, and emergency consultation for ill and injured children.[63] Notable examples include the University of California Davis pediatric emergency medicine network, comprising 28 remote facilities—research about which has demonstrated improved outcomes, few medication errors, and decreased costs of care.[63,64,65] The applicability of telehealth technology to neonatal intensive care is demonstrated by the Antenatal and Neonatal Guidelines Education and Learning System (ANGELS) program in Arkansas, developed in 2003. This program, which developed practice-based guidelines and is supported by weekly tele-education conferences and 24/7 telemedicine consultations, has demonstrated more appropriate utilization of neonatal intensive care unit (NICU) services in the state.[66]

In chronic disease management and home care, the VHA emerged as a leader during this decade. Studying early outcomes in 2005 and 2008, VA researchers showed promising results related to patient satisfaction, quality measures, improved adherence to treatments, and hospital bed day and emergency room use at reasonable costs.[67,68] Telehealth became a core strategy for the VHA, a system bearing total responsibility for the health of its patients, without the complication of third-party payment.

Those working in telemedicine continued to increase their national voice through participation in various organizations. By 2010, the membership of the American Telemedicine Association had grown to around 3,100 U.S. and international members from diverse organizations: industry, academic organizations, and commercial provider groups.

This was also the decade during which the Internet and e-commerce exploded and changed the world economy and culture. As people began to conduct more of their banking, shopping, and communicating with friends and family online, there was a growing expectation that health care should be as easily accessible. Naturally, telehealth evolved rapidly as well, forever changing how providers and patients would interact and deliver care. Dramatic improvements in Internet service speeds and affordability occurred concurrently with the advent of telecommunications options capable of delivering health care services for many organizations, as well as to the home. That said, extensive regions of the country were bypassed in the broadband revolution. In response, the Federal Communications Commission (FCC) released a call for pilot programs in 2007 to install broadband to advance access to health services in rural areas. This program was a recognition that the subsidy program operated by the FCC for more than a decade was not optimized, because fundamental infrastructure was lacking in much of the United States. Sixty-nine awards totaling $417 million over 3 years were granted to programs that greatly expanded access to broadband in underserved regions of the United States and thereby enabled more widespread use of telehealth and health information exchanges.[69]

The American Recovery and Reinvestment Act of 2009 (ARRA) had far-reaching implications in a number of fields, including health care. Notably, $19 billion was earmarked for health information technology (HIT) and further implementation of electronic health records (EHR). Although telehealth was not directly included in the adoption incentives related to EHR, the overarching focus on HIT and EHR advanced the thinking and implementation of technology-enabled models of care. The ARRA funding did include a number of options leveraged by telehealth programs for development and expansion. During this decade, as a result of the ARRA funding, the nation saw the implementation of telehealth programs related to disaster preparedness with the National Telecommunications & Information Administration's BroadbandUSA (formerly the Broadband Technology Opportunities Program, BTOP).

The federal government also played a role in this field through the Office for the Advancement of Telehealth (OAT), which oversaw grant programs funding a number of clinical telehealth networks, as well as resource centers located throughout the United States. These regional resource centers, in collaboration with a national resource center focused on policy, served to provide local organizations with much-needed information and technical assistance to launch and sustain programs. OAT funded two national resource centers to support programs throughout the nation with technical assistance and policy issues. In addition to the programs under OAT, the federal government made awards through the National Institutes of Health (NIH) and the National Library of Medicine (NLM) to advance scholarship in the area of telehealth related to efficacy, effectiveness, and quality.

Policy advancements supported the evolution of telehealth. By 2010, California and 10 other states had enacted some form of health insurance coverage mandate for telemedicine. Five states (Colorado, Hawaii, Kentucky, Oklahoma, and Texas) have since adopted telemedicine statutes similar to California's that in some way prohibit the requirement of face-to-face contact for reimbursement. Five states (Georgia,

Louisiana, Maine, New Hampshire, and Oregon) have stronger requirements; among them, three (Louisiana, New Hampshire, and Oregon) mandate coverage for telemedicine for any service that would be covered in person. Thirty-six states had adopted telemedicine statutes or policies for coverage of telemedicine in Medicaid, five other states are considering doing so, and Florida covers telemedicine under the terms of a federal Medicaid waiver.[70]

This decade marked a movement in the field signaling that telehealth plays a role in the delivery of health care services in this nation. The models of care that were observed during this time frame were predominantly services that emulated traditional in-person care translated over technology. Examples revealed an emerging shift to new models of care that didn't "look" like in-person care. But much of that innovation was yet to come in the most recent decade.

TELEHEALTH TODAY

Development and innovation in telehealth continues at an exponential rate. The pioneers in this field likely would be amazed at the state of telehealth in the current decade. Telehealth has truly become mainstream in many areas of health care and has been increasingly accepted as a legitimate and, in some cases, the preferred method of care delivery. This is reflected in the growing evidence base in the peer-reviewed literature. A search of PubMed from 2010 to 2016 using the keywords "telemedicine" and "telehealth" reveals more than 11,000 papers published. In 2016, *Time* magazine, in its issue on "240 reasons to celebrate America," cited telemedicine as one of those reasons. That article noted that health care organizations are investing heavily in digital health, exemplified by the VHA and the 700,000 vets who were treated in 2015 using a technology-enabled modality of care.[71] In addition, 46% of health care providers answering a Healthcare Information and Management Systems Society (HIMSS) survey stated that in their practice they used multiple telemedicine technologies, by far the most popular of which is two-way video messaging.[72]

State and federal policy changes, although slow, are removing barriers to a seamlessly functioning technology-enabled health care system. One of the barriers that telemedicine providers encounter is the requirement for them to undergo the privileging process at every health care organization for which they hope to provide services. To resolve this problem, CMS, the federal agency that administers Medicare, Medicaid, and the state Children's Health Insurance Program, in July 2011 issued a rule authorizing the proxy credentialing of providers: "Hospitals and CAHs (Critical Access Hospitals) may rely, when granting telemedicine privileges, upon the privileging decisions of a distant-site hospital or telemedicine entity with which they have a written agreement that meets Medicare requirements." Policy issues related to reimbursement have also moved forward significantly. This has historically been one of the most cumbersome barriers to the advancement of telemedicine. As of August 2016, 48 state Medicaid programs and the District of Columbia were reimbursing for live video telehealth, with 12 state Medicaid programs offering some reimbursement for store-and-forward, not counting states that reimbursed only for teleradiology. Remote patient monitoring was reimbursed by 19 state Medicaid programs by late 2016.[73]

The telecommunications infrastructure, once an unwieldy barrier, is rapidly improving as well, with Internet access speeds of 10 Mbps or greater available in 99% of the United States. In addition, 98% of Americans live in areas with 4G LTE service for mobile devices that support video. As the processing speeds of computers and mobile devices have increased to the point where they now support high-quality video, and with increasing cloud-based video conferencing options, the threshold for doing telehealth is much lower than in years past.

The incoming generation of health care providers has grown up in a digital world in which the difference between in-person and distance communication is less significant. They are willing and expect that some of the care they provide can be conducted via telecommunication technology. Although their world and the world of the sick are radically different from the early healers and patients, the benefit of facilitating a connection between them is not. Those early visionaries in the many fields that contributed to the current state of telehealth have already clearly improved the lives of many people. We are only just beginning to realize the full potential of this growing area of health science.

REFERENCES

1. Reiling J. ed. JAMA 100 years ago. *JAMA* 2009;302(7):807.
2. Risse GB. *Mending Bodies, Saving Souls: A History of Hospitals.* Oxford, UK: Oxford University Press; 1990.
3. Martin S. *A Short History of Disease: From the Black Death to Ebola.* Harpenden, UK: Oldcastle Books; 2015.
4. Finley JH. ed. *Nelson's Perpetual Loose-Leaf Encyclopaedia.* Vol VI. New York: The Trow Press; 1909:265A.
5. Porter R. *The Greatest Benefit to Mankind. A Medical History of Humanity.* New York: W.W. Norton & Company; 1997:106–134.
6. Packard FR. History of the School of Salernum. In: *The School of Salernum* – The English version by Sir John Harrington. New York: Augustus M. Kelley Publishers; 1970:11–12.
7. Cilliers L, Retief FP. The evolution of the hospital from antiquity to the end of the middle ages. *Curationis* 2002;25(4):60–66.
8. Penn Medicine. *History of Pennsylvania Hospital.* 2016. http://www.uphs.upenn.edu/paharc/features/creation.html.
9. Star P. *The Social Transformation of American Medicine.* New York: Basic Books; 1982.
10. Driscoll CE. Is there a doctor in the house? *Am Acad Home Care Physicians Newslett* 1991;3:7–8.
11. Leff B, Burton JR. Acute medical care in the home. *J Am Geriatri Soc* 1996;44(5):603–605.
12. Xenophon: Hellenica, trans. H. Dakyns, Project Gutenberg, 1998. http://www.gutenberg.org/etext/1174.
13. Holzmann G, Pehrson B. *The Early History of Data Networks.* Hoboken, NJ, Wiley-IEEE Computer Society Press; 1994. http://people.deas.harvard.edu/~jones/cscie129/papers/Early_History_of_Data_Networks/Chapter_1.pdf.
14. Bashshur RL, Shannon GW. History of technological foundations of telemedicine. In: *History of Telemedicine: Evolution, Context, and Transformation.* New Rochelle, NY: Mary Ann Liebert, Inc., 2009:25–76.
15. Dilhac J. The telegraph of Claude Chappe — An optical telecommunication network for the XVIIIth century. Paper presented at the 2001 IEEE Conference on the History of Telecommunications, 2001; Newfoundland, Canada.
16. Sterling CH, ed. *Military Communications: From Ancient Times to the 21st Century.* Santa Barbara, CA: ABC-CLIO; 2008:17.
17. Manning MJ, Wyatt CR. Mexican-American war. In: Manning MJ, Wyatt CR, eds. *Encyclopedia of Media and*

Propaganda in Wartime America. Santa Barbara, CA: ABC-CLIO, LLC; 2011:285.

18. History.com. Western Union completes first transcontinental telegraph line. 2009. http://www.history.com/this-day-in-history/western-union-completes-the-first-transcontinental-telegraph-line.

19. Gastil J. *Political Communication and Deliberation*. Thousand Oaks, CA: SAGE Publications; 2008:47.

20. Peterson JK. Electromagnetic surveillance; radio. In: *Understanding Surveillance Technologies: Spy Devices, Privacy, History & Applications*. 2nd ed. Boca Raton, FL: Auerbach Publications; 2007:307.

21. Abramson A. Commercial operations (1946-1955). In: *Electronic Motion Pictures: A History of the Television Camera*. Berkeley and Los Angeles, CA: University of California Press; 1955:116.

22. National Geographic Society (U.S.), Diamond J. Modern age. In: *1000 Events that Shaped the World*. National Geographic Books; 2008:375.

23. Dixon P. Cellular phones. In: Dixon P, ed. *Surveillance in America: An Encyclopedia of History, Politics, and the Law*, Santa Barbara: ABC-CLIO, LLC, 2016:62.

24. Louis-Courvoisier M, Mauron A. 'He found me very well; for me, I was still feeling sick': The strange worlds of physicians and patients in the 18th and 21st centuries. *Med Humanit* 2002;28(1):9–13.

25. Fine L. Circle of urine glasses: art of uroscopy. *Am J Nephrol* 1986;6(4):307–311.

26. Wild W. Doctor-patient correspondence in eighteenth-century Britain: a change in rhetoric and relationship. *Stud Eighteenth Century Culture* 2000;29:47–64.

27. Eikelboom RH. The telegraph and the beginnings of telemedicine in Australia. *Stud Health Technol Inform* 2012;182:67–72.

28. Aronson S. The Lancet on the telephone, 1876–1975. *Med Hist* 1977;21(1):69–87.

29. James W, Williams H. The electrocardiogram in clinical medicine. *Am J Med Sci* 1910;140:408–421, 644–669.

30. Bashshur RL, Shannon GW, Smith BR. The empirical foundations of telemedicine interventions for chronic disease management. *Telemed J E Health* 2014;20(9):769–800.

31. Gernsbeck H. Radio teledactyl. *Sci Invent* February 1925.

32. Gershon-Cohen J, Cooley AG. Telognosis. *Radiology* 1950;55(4):582–587.

33. Allen A. Teleradiology I. Introduction. *Telemed Today* 1996;4(1):24.

34. Allen A, Allen D. Teleradiology 1994. *Telemed Today* 1994b;2(3):14–23.

35. Jutra A. Teleroentgen diagnosis by means of videotape recording. *Am J Roentgenol Radium Ther Nucl Med* 1959;82:1099–1102.

36. Benschoter RA, Garetz C, Smith P. The use of closed circuit TV and videotape in the training of social group workers. *Social Work Education Reporter* 1967;15(1):18–20.

37. Wittson CL, Benschoter RA. Two-way television: helping the medical center reach out. *Am J Psychiatry* 1972;129(5):136–139.

38. Institute of Medicine Committee on Evaluating Clinical Applications of Telemedicine. Evolution and current applications of telemedicine. In: Field MJ, ed. *Telemedicine: A Guide to Assessing Telecommunications in Health Care*. Washington, DC: National Academy Press; 1996:36.

39. Monnier AJ, Wright IS, Lenegre J, et al. Ship-to-shore radio transmission of electrocardiograms and X-ray images. *JAMA* 1965;193(12):144–145.

40. Nagel EL, Hirschman JC, Mayer PW, et al. Telemetry of physiologic data: an aid to fire-rescue personnel in a metropolitan area. *South Med J* 1968;61:598–601.

41. Murphy RL Jr, Bird KT. Telediagnosis: a new community health resource. Observations on the feasibility of telediagnosis based on 1000 patient transactions. *Am J Public Health* 1974;64(2):113–119.

42. Crump WJ, Pfeil T. Telemedicine primer: an introduction to the technology and an overview of the literature. *Arch Fam Med* 1995;4(9):796–803.

43. Hudson HE, Parker EB. Medical communication in Alaska by satellite. *N Engl J Med* 1973;289:1351–1356.

44. Perednia DA, Allen A. Telemedicine technology and clinical applications. *JAMA* 1995;273(6):483–487.

45. Watson DS. Telemedicine. *Med J Aust* 1989;151:62–71.

46. Third Joint Working Group on Space Biology and Medicine. US – USSR Telemedicine Consultation Spacebridge to Armenia and Ufa: Final Project Report. NASA, 1991. https://ntrs.nasa.gov/search.jsp?R=19940007337.

47. Marquette University. *Brief History of Telehealth*. http://www.eng.mu.edu/wintersj/rehab/rehab167/mod1/tele/history.htm.

48. California Telehealth Resource Center. *California Telehealth Legislation History*. 2013. http://www.caltrc.org/legislation_reg/california-legislation/.

49. Preston B, Powers P, Kwong MW. *Advancing California's Leadership in Telehealth Policy*. 2011. http://cchpca.org/sites/default/files/resources/Telehealth%20Model%20Statute%20Report%202-11.pdf.

50. Center for Telehealth & eHealth Law. *Medicare Reimbursement*. 2014. http://ctel.org/expertise/reimbursement/medicare-reimbursement/.

51. Darkins A. The growth of telehealth services in the Veterans Health Administration between 1994 and 2014: a study in the diffusion of innovation. *Telemed J E Health* 2014;20(9):761–768.

52. Adams LN, Grigsby RK. The Georgia State Telemedicine Program: initiation, design, and plans. *Telemed J* 1995;1(3):227–235.

53. Brecht RM, Gray CL, Peterson C, et al. The University of Texas Medical Branch—Texas Department of Criminal Justice Telemedicine Project: findings from the first year of operation. *Telemed J* 1996;2(1):25–35.

54. Ollove M. State prisons turn to telemedicine to improve health and save money. Pew Charitable Trusts paper. January 21, 2016. http://www.pewtrusts.org/en/research-and-analysis/blogs/stateline/2016/01/21/state-prisons-turn-to-telemedicine-to-improve.

55. Krupinski EA, Weinstein RS. Telemedicine in an academic center—The Arizona Telemedicine Program. *Telemedicine J E Health* 2013;19(5):349–356.

56. Zivin JA. Acute stroke therapy with tissue plasminogen activator (tPA) since it was approved by the U.S. Food and Drug Administration (FDA). *Ann Neurol* 2009;66(1):6–10.

57. Meyer BC, Raman R, Hemmen T, et al. Efficacy of site-independent telemedicine in the STRokE DOC trial: a randomized, blinded, prospective study. *Lancet Neurol* 2008;7(9):787–795.

58. Schwamm LH, Holloway RG, Amarenco P, et al. on behalf of the American Heart Association Stroke Council and the Interdisciplinary Council on Peripheral Vascular Disease. A review of the evidence for the use of telemedicine within stroke systems of care: a scientific statement from the American Heart Association/American Stroke Association. *Stroke* 2009;40(7):2616–2634.

59. Akbik F, Hirsch JA, Chandra RV, et al. Telestroke: the promise and the challenge. Part one: growth and current practice. *Neurointerv Surg* 2016:1–6.

60. Lilly CM, Cody S, Zhao H, et al. Hospital mortality, length of stay, and preventable complications among critically ill patients before and after tele-ICU reengineering of critical care processes. *JAMA* 2011;305(21): 2175–2183.

61. Wilcox ME, Adhikari N. The effect of telemedicine in critically ill patients: systematic review and meta-analysis. *Crit Care.* 2012;16(4):R127.

62. Kumar S, Merchant S, Reynolds R. Tele-ICU: efficacy and cost-effectiveness of remotely managing critical care. *Perspect Health Inf Manag* 2013;Spring:1–13.

63. Ellenby MS, Marcin JP. The role of telemedicine in pediatric critical care. *Crit Care Clin* 2015;31(2):275–290.

64. Yang NH, Dharmar M, Yoo BK, et al. Economic evaluation of pediatric telemedicine consultations to rural emergency departments. *Med Decis Making* 2015;35(6):773–783.

65. Committee on Pediatric Workforce. The use of telemedicine to address access and physician workforce shortages. *Pediatrics* 2015;136(1):202–209.

66. Bronstein JM, Ounpraseuth S, Jonkman J, et al. Improving perinatal regionalization for preterm deliveries in a Medicaid covered population: initial impact of Arkansas ANGELS intervention. *Health Serv Res* 2011;46(4):1082–1103.

67. Schofield RS, Kline SE, Schmalfuss CM, et al. Early outcomes of a care coordination-enhanced telehome care program for elderly veterans with chronic heart failure. *Telemed J E Health* 2005;11(1):20–27.

68. Darkins A, Ryan P, Kobb R, et al. Care coordination/home telehealth: the systematic implementation of health informatics, home telehealth, and disease management to support the care of veteran patients with chronic conditions. *Telemed J E Health* 2008;14(10):1118–1127.

69. Federal Communications Commission. *The FCC's Rural Health Care Pilot Program: Consumer Guide.* Washington, DC: FCC; 2016. https://transition.fcc.gov/cgb/consumerfacts/RuralHealthProgram.pdf.

70. Kelch D. Staying connected – a progress report: reimbursement under the Telemedicine Development Act of 1996, Center for Connected Health Policy, March 2010. http://cchpca.org/sites/default/files/resources/Staying_Connected_CA_Telemedicine_Development_Act.pdf.

71. *Time* Magazine. 240 reasons to celebrate America right now. July 11/July 18, 2016.

72. HIMSS Analytics. *2016 Telemedicine Study.* April 2016. http://www.himssanalytics.org/research/himss-analytics-essentials-brief-2016-telemedicine-study.

73. Center for Connected Health Policy. *State Telehealth Laws and Medicaid Program Policies,* August 2016. http://cchpca.org/sites/default/files/resources/50%20STATE%20COMPLETE%20REPORT%20PASSWORD%20AUG%202016_1.pdf.

Workforce, Definitions, and Models*

Karen Schulder Rheuban, MD and Scott Shipman, MD, MPH

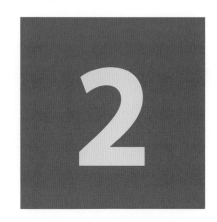

Appropriate access to high-quality care is a priority for patients and policy makers alike. Though many social and economic factors influence access to care, one important domain that affects timely access is the adequacy of the health care workforce supply. When the capacity of the workforce enables patient needs to be met, capacity is adequate. When the capacity of the workforce is insufficient, access to care will be suboptimal. Increases in workforce capacity can be achieved in one or more of the following ways: increase the workforce supply (eg, the number of physicians being trained), reduce attrition of the workforce (eg, physician retirement or shifting to nonclinical roles), train others to take over some aspects of the work effort (eg, physician assistants, nurse practitioners, and others who serve a substitution role for traditionally physician-centric activities), and increase efficiency/reduce waste (eg, reduce time spent on documentation and use the time gained on direct patient care) (Table 2-1).

The evolving needs of patients, coupled with new models of reimbursement and care delivery in the United States, are driving significant change in the health care workforce of the 21st century. New health professional and paraprofessional roles are emerging, and traditional roles are being reimagined as the concept of team-based care becomes increasingly standard to high-quality, high-value care delivery. Care innovations such

as telehealth accentuate the need for new skills and new roles in the health care workforce.

For several years, concerns have mounted about the adequacy of the supply of physicians in practice, particularly in light of the aging of the U.S. population, with its greater burden of chronic diseases. The Association of American Medical Colleges projects a physician shortage ranging between 61,700 and 94,700 by the year 2025.[1] Workforce projections have historically been imprecise in predicting physician shortages or surpluses. However, a 20-year cap on the number of residency positions funded through the Medicare program (the principal funder of graduate medical education) and an aging workforce in many areas of the country create a context for concern. In particular, concerns are widespread about a shortage of primary care physicians among numerous professional organizations and the federal government. The Health Resources and Services Administration (HRSA) estimates that there were just over 215,000 full-time–equivalent primary care physicians in 2013 and projects 11% growth in supply by 2025. However, HRSA predicts that demand for primary care services will grow by 17% in this same time span.[2]

There has been tremendous growth in the number of advanced practice providers, namely physician assistants and advanced practice nurses, which will help to offset the projected shortage of physicians. Indeed, by 2025 the supply of physician assistants is projected to increase by 50%, an estimate that does not take into account ongoing growth in the number of PA training programs opening across the country.[3] Similarly, the supply of advanced practice nurses graduating

* Dr. Rheuban has a financial interest in Tytocare, LLC, for which she serves as a member of the advisory board. The terms of this arrangement have been reviewed and approved by the University of Virginia.

Table 2-1. U.S. Healthcare Workforce Supply and Projected Growth Through 2025

	Current supply (in FTE)	Projected supply (FTE) in 2025 (increase relative to current supply)	Is projected supply adequate to meet projected demand?
Physicians (MD, DO)			
Primary care	216,580	239,460 (11%)	No
Nonprimary care	498,800	602,700 (21%)	No
Advance practice nurses (APN, NP)			
Primary care	57,330	110,540 (93%)	Yes
Nonprimary care	126,900	306,000 (141%)	*
Physician assistants (PA)			
Primary care	33,390	58,770 (76%)	Yes
Nonprimary care	52,500	109,300 (108%)	*
Nurses (RN)	2,897,000	3,849,000 (33%)	Yes

*HRSA projections of nonprimary care supply did not assess adequacy. AAMC projects shortages of physician supply in both primary care and nonprimary care. FTE, full-time equivalents.

Sources: IHS, Inc. *The Complexities of Physician Supply and Demand 2016 Update: Projections from 2014 to 2025*. Washington, DC; 2016. Accessed at https://www.aamc.org/data/workforce/reports/439206/physicianshortageandprojections.html.
U.S. Department of Health and Human Services, Health Resources and Services Administration, National Center for Health Workforce Analysis. *National and Regional Projections of Supply and Demand for Primary Care Practitioners: 2013-2025*. Rockville, MD U.S. Department of Health and Human Services; 2016.
U.S. Department of Health and Human Services, Health Resources and Services Administration, National Center for Health Workforce Analysis. *Highlights From the 2012 National Sample Survey of Nurse Practitioners*. Rockville, Maryland: U.S. Department of Health and Human Services; 2014.
U.S. Department of Health and Human Services, Health Resources and Services Administration, National Center for Health Workforce Analysis. *Projecting the Supply of Non-Primary Care Specialty and Subspecialty Clinicians: 2010-2025*. Rockville, MD: Department of Health and Human Services; 2014. Accessed at https://bhw.hrsa.gov/sites/default/files/bhw/nchwa/projections/clinicalspecialties.pdf.
U.S. Department of Health and Human Services, Health Resources and Services Administration, National Center for Health Workforce Analysis. *The Future of the Nursing Workforce: National- and State-Level Projections, 2012-2025*. Rockville, MD: Department of Health and Human Services; 2014.

annually more than doubled between 2002 and 2012, with ongoing growth in supply anticipated.[4]

Separate from the advanced practice nursing workforce, the nursing workforce has undergone substantial growth, doubling the number of diploma RN graduates from 68,000 to 150,000 annually between 2001 and 2013. The growth of the nursing workforce in the past decade has completely mitigated previous projections of a severe nursing shortage. Indeed, workforce planners now project that the supply of nurses will meet or exceed demand through 2025.[5]

There are, of course, numerous additional roles that are essential to delivering the full complement of health care services. Traditional personnel, ranging from doctoral-trained pharmacists to certificate-level medical assistants, are adapting into new roles, often with a more direct hand in delivering care to patients. Pharmacists, for instance, actively participate in medication management, adherence, and safety oversight in both inpatient and ambulatory clinical settings. Using care protocols and templates, medical assistants are serving a diverse set of roles in the ambulatory setting, from initiating patient visits by collecting relevant history, scribing for the physician in the electronic medical record, and finally closing visits by ensuring that patients understand the plan of care and scheduling follow-ups as needed. A similar diffusion of roles and settings of work is underway for many allied health professionals, such physical therapists and dietitians. New roles have also emerged, including health coaches, community health workers, and nurse care coordinators. Many of these positions have been created in an effort to target population health improvement, often by focusing on those individuals with more complex health and/or social needs.

As roles emerge and evolve to meet the needs of patients and the realities of an increasingly complex delivery system, it can be difficult to project adequate workforce capacity accurately. However, one certainty in this time of rapid change in delivery is the need for all health care professionals to have a high degree of adaptability and a willingness to work effectively in teams, including a high level of communication and coordination. New technologies can facilitate communication and coordination, but to do so they must be harnessed through concerted efforts by health professionals and information technology professionals to be an asset rather than a barrier.

Overall estimates of health care workforce supply can obscure areas of particular need. A prime example is in behavioral and mental health services, including services for substance use disorders. A wide range of health care professionals serves the behavioral and mental health needs of the population, including (but not limited to) psychiatrists; clinical, counseling, and school psychologists; substance abuse and behavioral disorder counselors; mental health and substance abuse social workers; mental health counselors; and school counselors. HRSA projects a substantial shortage of *all* of these behavioral and mental health professionals in the coming years.[6]

The geographic distribution of the workforce has been a persistent problem for access to care that has defied solution to date, despite widespread recognition by health workforce planners and researchers. Years of research have demonstrated that in the midst of overall growth in the health care workforce, there are tremendous variations in the local and regional supply of physicians and other clinicians. Furthermore, physicians entering the workforce disproportionately tend to settle in areas that are already well populated by their peers.[7] This leaves many rural and inner-city communities without the physicians and other clinicians they need. This problem persists despite national efforts such as the National Health Service Corps, which specifically targets workforce development for underserved areas through incentives such as scholarships and loan repayment programs for those who practice in needed fields within such regions. Many states offer similar incentives to attract

providers to underserved communities. Even when a small town has an adequate supply of primary care providers, it may not be able to support subspecialists due to its limited size. The result is an urban–rural maldistribution of specialists, which presents a significant burden on patients when the services of a subspecialist are required, particularly in regions with long distances to drive or geographic barriers (such as mountain ranges) that make travel difficult and risky at certain times of the year.

Thus, health care in the contemporary digital era has experienced a transformation driven by need, workforce shortages, consumer demand and engagement, innovations in technology, expansions of broadband communications services, and innovative "connected health" care delivery models.[8,9] Advancements in state and federal public policy, coupled with greater engagement by providers, payers, employers, and consumers, have led to new paradigms of care enhanced by telemedicine. Not a specialty in and of itself, telemedicine and telehealth offer tools to address the significant challenges of access, quality, and cost—the "triple aim" articulated by the Institute for Healthcare Innovation.[10,11]

The American Telemedicine Association (ATA) defines *telemedicine* as "the use of medical information exchanged from one site to another via electronic communications to improve a patient's clinical health status."[12] *Telehealth* generally refers to a broad range of health-related services across a wide range of disciplines supported by telecommunications technology that includes telemedicine, as well as health-related distance learning, remote patient monitoring, call centers, consumer-facing virtual and e-health applications, and other services that enhance health but do not necessarily represent the delivery of clinical care.

A number of definitions of telemedicine and telehealth are used by both federal and state agencies.[13] HRSA, home to the federal Office for the Advancement of Telehealth (OAT), defines telehealth as "[t]he use of electronic information and telecommunications technologies to support long-distance clinical healthcare, patient and professional health-related education, public health and health administration."[14] State definitions vary and often include definitions in code, such as that of California: "The mode of delivering health care services and public health via information and communication technologies to facilitate the diagnosis, consultation, treatment, education, care management, and self-management of a patient's health care while the patient is at the originating site and the health care provider is at a distant site. Telehealth facilitates patient self-management and caregiver support for patients and includes synchronous interactions and asynchronous store and forward transfers."[15] Virginia code specifically defines telemedicine as "the use of electronic technology or media, including live inter-active audio or video (IAV), for the purpose of diag-nosing or treating a patient or consulting with other healthcare providers regarding a patient's diagnosis or treatment."[16]

Telemedicine includes a growing variety of applica-tions and services using two-way videoconferencing, either with or without the use of peripheral devices, store and forward asynchronous technologies, mobile and wireless tools through which clinical care is pro-vided, and hybrids between these three options. There is considerable overlap in care delivery models pro-vided through mobile (m-health) technologies using high-speed and lower-bandwidth telecommunications networks.

Examples of telehealth-related services include a) video-based specialty and primary care consultations and follow-up visits, with or without the use of periph-eral devices appropriate to the patient's condition; b) store and forward services—the asynchronous trans-fer of patient images and data for interpretation by the clinician not necessarily in the presence of the patient (eg, teledermatology, teleophthalmology); c) hybrid models of (a) and (b) to support patient care, includ-ing electronic intensive care unit (ICU) care models; d) remote patient monitoring, including the collection and transfer of biometric data to a monitoring facil-ity or agency (eg, daily weight, heart rate, blood pres-sure, blood sugar, oximetry, electrocardiogram [ECG], gait); e) mobile health services that support the earlier models; f) patient and provider health education; and g) e-consults between providers.[17,18] These models will be addressed in subsequent chapters.

Live-interactive (synchronous) face-to-face tele-medicine connections are provided over secure high-definition endpoints and/or other video technologies and include provider-to-patient encounters, provider-to-provider video-based consultations, group case management discussions (such as tumor boards or case conferences), and provider-to-patient educational pro-grams. A broad range of digital peripheral devices (eg, specialty cameras, electronic stethoscopes, otoscopes) can support clinical encounters with the goal of rep-licating in-person care. It should be noted that some teleconsultants are providing services using security options that are less than ideal (eg, Skype, FaceTime) and these are not recommended or approved by the majority of health care systems.

Store and forward (asynchronous) services include (but are not limited to) radiographic and patho-logic studies, photos, patient data, and video clips of patient examinations. These services may maximize provider efficiency when sufficient data are provided to support the clinical service requested to render a diagnosis. Peripheral devices may also support the acquisition of clinically relevant data for store and forward encounters.

Remote patient monitoring utilizes digital tech-nologies to collect and transmit patient data (eg, ECGs) to providers for assessment and follow-up care, for chronic disease management, postacute hos-pitalization readmissions prevention, and many other applications. Although not always, most of these devices are approved (cleared) by the Food and Drug Administration (FDA) and are devices typically used during face-to-face encounters but have been adapted for remote data collection and transmission. They are generally prescribed by a provider for patient use for both short- and long-term data collection periods.

Mobile health (m-health) technologies blend the earlier services when acquired via mobile devices, including smart phones, and sensing devices (eg, FitBit) facilitated by application software downloaded onto mobile devices (apps). Peripheral devices can also be used to acquire images and data through mobile tech-nologies. Although not always, the majority of these data collection devices and apps are not FDA approved/cleared, and the provider may choose whether or not to accept such data for use in patient care.

E-consults include secure electronic communi-cations between providers (such as primary care to specialist) or between providers and patients where permitted by applicable statute and regulation. Such platforms can improve care coordination, enhance timely access to specialty care, and potentially lower the cost of care through improved case management.

TELEHEALTH MODELS OF CARE

Models of telehealth-supported care are as diverse as health care in general. These include the model of connecting tertiary and quaternary health care facilities (academic or otherwise) to other facilities in a hub-and-spoke model to provide specialty care services. Other models include "networks of networks," as has been developed in the provincewide "Ontario Telehealth Network" driven, in some cases, by governmental or quasigovernmental entities leveraging regional or statewide investments in broadband communications services and health information exchanges. Consortia models have been developed that include contracting to enhance collaboration between academic providers and other entities, both within and beyond state borders (eg, prison telemedicine). Payer- and employer-driven models have been developed in the urgent care/primary care direct-to-consumer market. Private telemedicine specialty care companies offer contracted services across multiple states to provide services such as telestroke, telepsychiatry, remote monitoring, and other services.

Specialty consultations and follow-up visits have long represented the traditional model of telemedicine. Nearly all clinical medical specialties have applicability and contributions to the evidence base for telehealth across the continuum from prenatal care to end-of-life care, including acute care and chronic disease management. Specialties such as critical care, emergency services, pediatrics, psychiatry, radiology, neurology, surgery, primary care, dermatology, ophthalmology, cardiology, obstetrics, pulmonology, pediatric subspecialties, neurosurgery, gastroenterology, infectious diseases, orthopedics, endocrinology, plastic surgery, pathology, genetics, and rehabilitation have made significant contributions to the evidence base for telemedicine. In addition, other nonphysician disciplines fully engaged in telehealth include nursing, dentistry, pharmacy, behavioral health, physical and occupational therapy, speech and language services, and home health. These care models can be accomplished using either synchronous or asynchronous telemedicine technologies, the outcomes of which have been documented in the peer-reviewed literature.[19-23] The Standards and Guidelines group of the ATA and many of the specialty societies have developed policies and guidelines surrounding many of these clinical models of telehealth-facilitated care.[24,25]

Direct-to-consumer platforms and services represent a broad range of care delivery models and platforms primarily designed to provide convenient acute care consultations for low-acuity conditions either within the framework of a health care system or medical home, or through the use of appropriately licensed and credentialed providers, in many cases external to the patient's medical home. Consumer and employer demand for convenient access has driven investments in these care delivery models and platforms, driven by the proliferation of smart phones.[26] Clinical outcomes, prescribing rates, utilization rates, and financial metrics in direct-to-consumer platforms are undergoing analysis.[27,28] The ATA has developed urgent care/primary care guidelines that specifically address direct-to-consumer models of care.[29]

Standards and Guidelines: The ATA, along with many of the national specialty societies, has developed standards and guidelines and model policies for telemedicine practice.[25] Currently published standards and guidelines include the following:

- **American Telemedicine Association**
  - Dermatology Practice Guidelines 2016
  - Practice Guidelines for Live, On-Demand Primary and Urgent Care
  - Clinical Guidelines for Telepathology
  - Guidelines for TeleICU Operations
  - Core Operational Guidelines for Telehealth Services Involving Provider–Patient Interactions
  - A Lexicon of Assessment and Outcome Measures for Telemental Health
  - Practice Guidelines for Video-Based Online Mental Health Services
  - Quick Guide to Store-Forward and Live-Interactive Teledermatology for Referring Providers
  - Expert Consensus Recommendations for Video-conferencing-Based Telepresenting
  - Telehealth Practice Recommendations for Diabetic Retinopathy
  - A Blueprint for Telerehabilitation Guidelines
  - Practice Guidelines for Videoconferencing-Based Telemental Health
  - Evidence-Based Practice for Telemental Health
  - Teleburn Guidelines

- Practice Guidelines for Telemental Health with Children and Adolescents
- Practice Guidelines for Telestroke
- Operating Procedures for Pediatric Telehealth

Position papers have also been published by a number of specialty societies and advocacy organizations. Many of these will be addressed in clinical specialty-specific chapters of this book. Some of the key ones include:

- American Medical Association
  - American Medical Association Report of the Council on Medical Service: coverage of and payment for telemedicine[30]
  - Guidance for Ethical Practice in Telemedicine[31]
- American College of Physicians
  - Policy Recommendations to Guide the Use of Telemedicine in Primary Care Settings: An American College of Physicians Position Paper Recommendations for the Use of Telemedicine in Primary Care Settings[32]
- American Academy of Family Practice Robert Graham Center
  - Family Physicians and Telehealth: Findings from a National Survey[33]
- American Academy of Pediatrics
  - The Use of Telemedicine to Address Access and Physician Workforce Shortages[34]
- Federation of State Medical Boards
  - Model Policy for the Appropriate Use of Telemedicine Technologies in the Practice of Medicine: Report of the State Medical Boards' Appropriate Regulation of Telemedicine (SMART) Workgroup[35]
- American Psychological Association
  - Guidelines for the Practice of Telepsychology[36]
- American Academy of Ambulatory Care Nursing
  - Scope and Standards of Practice for Telehealth Nursing[37]

TECHNOLOGIES

Telecommunications technologies provide the communications infrastructure over which telehealth solutions are driven that enable a range of connected care options. Video-based services, store and forward services, and mobile technologies all require sufficient bandwidth to transfer images and data in a timely fashion. Broadband networks provide the foundation for telehealth solutions and can be wired or wireless, fixed or mobile, satellite, or terrestrial-fixed networks. Network availability and performance are more challenging for mobile services than for fixed broadband and relate, in part, to spectrum availability. Transitioning from 3G to 4G (LTE) networks provides improved broadband performance. Greater demand and innovation have led to both federal and private investments in broadband services.

Videoconferencing: In simple terms, a videoconference is a meeting that connects two parties at a distance, allowing the participants to see and hear one another in real time. This can be accomplished with a camera, microphone, speakers, and either a software program that encodes and decodes the stream (CODEC) or a software program (a "bridge") that manages the exchange between participants. "Point-to-point" videoconferencing connects one party with another, whereas "multipoint" video calls require central software/hardware programs ("MCU" or multipoint control unit) that can control and manage participants joining at different communications protocols and connection speeds, converting those protocols to a common language, thereby ensuring a functional connection. Communications protocols may include H.323 (Integrated Services Digital Network [ISDN]), H. 264 (Internet Protocol [IP]), and SIP (Session Initiation Protocol) in addition to other proprietary audio-video compression protocols.

Bandwidth: Bandwidth represents the rate of data transfer measured in bits per second (bps) and ranges from low-bandwidth kilobits per second (Kbps) to high-bandwidth service in the ranges of millions of bits per second (megabits per second or Mbps) or gigabits per second (Gbps). Different telemedicine applications require a range of bandwidth, from text messaging at <1000 bps, to a phone call at 5600 bps (56 kbps), to standard-definition video at 1 megabit/sec (1 Mbps), to high-definition video at 4 megabits/sec (4 Mbps). Within a network, the ultimate bandwidth for the video connection is limited to the bandwidth of the lowest bandwidth of the end user. Other factors affecting performance include level and type of compression used, packet loss, latency, and jitter. The National Broadband Plan commissioned by the

Federal Communications Commission established aspirational goals for bandwidth allocated for a wide range of health care connections.[38] The commission articulated the progress toward that goal in 2016.[39]

Mobile medical applications are software applications and devices that leverage the portability offered by mobile technologies. Some target health and wellness, some capture and incorporate biometric data, and others facilitate the delivery of care to patients. The FDA has formally defined a mobile platform as "commercial off-the-shelf computing platforms, with or without wireless connectivity that are handheld in nature." The FDA has defined a mobile application as a "software application that can be executed (run) on a mobile platform (i.e., a handheld commercial off-the-shelf computing platform, with or without wireless connectivity), or a web-based software application that is tailored to a mobile platform but is executed on a server." The FDA has provided guidance that a "mobile medical app is a mobile app that meets the definition of device in section 201(h) of the Federal Food, Drug and Cosmetic Act and either is intended to be used as an accessory to a regulated medical device or, to transform a mobile platform into a regulated medical device."[40] The FDA considers the intended use of the mobile app as to whether it meets the definition of a "device." If an app is intended for use in performing a function for diagnosis or treatment, it is considered a device regardless of the platform on which it runs. There are more non–FDA-approved apps than approved, and many are freely downloadable for consumer use. Users (providers and patients) need to be cautious with these apps, however, as they are not often validated or tested for reliability.

Electronic medical record (EMR) integration/ health information exchange (HIE): The exchange of patient medical information provided via telemedicine is optimized when integrated into a patient's medical record and is most easily exchanged between providers when documentation conforms to other standards for electronic records, such as HL7 (Health Level 7). Some telehealth providers have utilized EMR vendors that have integrated telehealth solutions into their platform (including video services, scheduling, documentation, and billing) that can be exchanged between providers, both within and external to the provider's system, and others have utilized cloud-based solutions to effect and document the telemedicine encounter. Standards and guidelines developed by the ATA and many of the specialty advocacy organizations call for documentation of the encounter within a medical record and, where appropriate and with the patient's consent, shared with the patient's referring provider/medical home.[25]

Peripheral devices: Telemedicine devices and applications that support patient encounters beyond a video-based service alone to allow the clinician to comport to the standard of in-person care include electronic stethoscopes, otoscopes, ophthalmoscopes, dermascopes, colposcopes, spirometers, electronic scales, glucometers, sphygmomanometers, electrocardiograms, thermometers, and a range of other digitally configured integrated examination tools. Interoperability of devices plays an important role. The Continua Health Alliance is an industry collaborative advocacy organization designed to advance and support standards of interoperability of devices, sensors, and other connected health tools.[41] FDA guidance indicates that when performing a function for diagnosis or treatment, any device, regardless of the platform on which it runs, is regulated as a medical device, and as such is subject to regulation. "The FDA also encourages mobile medical app manufacturers to search FDA's public databases, such as the 'Product Classification' database and the '510(k) Premarket Notification' database, to determine the level of regulation for a given device and for the most up-to-date information about the relevant regulatory requirements."[40]

WORKFORCE IMPLICATIONS OF TELEHEALTH

The spread of innovations in telehealth is likely to have a direct impact on patients' access to care for some services and an indirect impact on access through its net effect on workforce capacity. Many pioneers in telehealth established their programs specifically as a means to improve access to care for isolated, rural populations.[42] Using technology to establish a "virtual visit" between the patient and provider dramatically improves access and serves as an efficient use of time in contrast to the alternative need to travel, sometimes for hours, for a brief encounter with a clinician. As modern technology makes virtual connections increasingly straightforward and as broadband service becomes more widely available, such services are likely to expand. As such, telehealth services may be among the most promising solutions to the vexing access challenges of geographic and specialty workforce maldistribution.

Limited research has systematically explored the net impact of telehealth services on patient utilization of health care services and on physician productivity. Part of the reason for the dearth of evidence is the complexity of the interventions. Telehealth modalities are rarely employed strictly as a means of workforce enhancement, but rather as part of larger efforts to improve quality and access, to reduce costs, and/or to expand outreach. There are clear scenarios where the adoption of a telehealth delivery model improves efficiency in care delivery, such as switching to virtual visits through video technology rather than a traveling clinic where a clinician and associated staff travel hours to see patients in an outlying community. Interventions such as these can predictably enhance workforce capacity.

When telehealth modalities create an opportunity to shift utilization from high-cost centers to lower-cost centers, there may or may not be a net decrease in workforce requirements. For instance, remote monitoring and virtual visit technology enables some care to be shifted from the hospital to the home. This shifts services to a different set of health care professionals, but may require more, less, or the same person-hours of service from the health care workforce. There are also situations in which telehealth can increase demand for services. For instance, due to poor access at baseline to mental health services, patients have been found to have an increase in the use of the services of mental health providers once access is enabled through telehealth. Although telehealth in this case demands more of the workforce, the resultant increased use of services may be fully appropriate and lead to improved patient health and better outcomes of care.

Finally, adoption of telehealth services requires personnel with the appropriate skills to ensure that quality standards of care are maintained. This requires that health care workers who interface with the telehealth technologies have the knowledge and skills needed to use the modalities as intended, in a patient-centric way that overcomes any potential barriers to communication and connection between patient and provider. High-quality telehealth services require clinicians and support staff alike to be competent in the specific skills of their professional role. As telehealth services spread and become a standard approach to meeting patients' health care needs, these skills will no longer be relevant only to a select few in the health care workforce, but instead are likely to be a requirement for much of the health care workforce. Significant efforts across many professional organizations and accrediting bodies will be required to provide the training needed to develop these skills for the current workforce, as well as the health care professionals in training.

CONCLUSION

Telehealth is an essential tool to address the significant challenges of access to high-quality care, regardless of patient location. Telehealth tools and models of care delivery have been demonstrated to favorably affect both acute and chronic illnesses, reduce disparities, mitigate workforce shortages, improve population health, and lower the cost of care. In the digital era, it is imperative to advance evidence-based care delivery models and promulgate policies that foster high-quality, sustainable telehealth solutions that empower patients, providers, and payers to adopt 21st-century models of care.

REFERENCES

1. *AAMC Workforce Statement 2016.* https://www.aamc.org/data/workforce/reports/439206/physicianshortageandprojections.html.

2. U.S. Department of Health and Human Services, Health Resources and Services Administration, National Center for Health Workforce Analysis. *National and Regional Projections of Supply and Demand for Primary Care Practitioners: 2013-2025.* Rockville, MD: U.S. Department of Health and Human Services; 2016.

3. Hooker RS, Muchow AN. Supply of physician assistants: 2013-2026. *JAAPA* 2014;27(3):39–45.

4. U.S. Department of Health and Human Services, Health Resources and Services Administration, National Center for Health Workforce Analysis. *Highlights From the 2012 National Sample Survey of Nurse Practitioners.* Rockville, MD: U.S. Department of Health and Human Services; 2014.

5. U.S. Department of Health and Human Services, Health Resources and Services Administration, National Center

for Health Workforce Analysis. *The Future of the Nursing Workforce: National- and State-Level Projections, 2012-2025*. Rockville, MD, U.S. Department of Health and Human Services; 2014.

6. Health Resources and Services Administration/National Center for Health Workforce Analysis, Substance Abuse and Mental Health Services Administration/Office of Policy, Planning, and Innovation. *National Projections of Supply and Demand for Behavioral Health Practitioners: 2013-2025*. Rockville, MD: U.S. Department of Health and Human Services; 2015.

7. Goodman DC, Robertson RG. Accelerating physician workforce transformation through competitive graduate medical education funding. *Health Aff (Millwood)* 2013;32(11):1887–1892.

8. Iglehart JK. Connected health: emerging disruptive technologies. *Health Aff (Millwood)* 2014;33(2):190.

9. Institute of Medicine, Committee on the Future of Rural Health Care. *Quality through Collaboration: The Future of Rural Health Care*. Washington, DC: National Academies Press; 2004.

10. Institute for Healthcare Innovation. http://www.ihi.org/engage/initiatives/tripleaim/pages/default.aspx.

11. Lustig TA, Board on Health Care Services, Institute of Medicine. *The Role of Telehealth in an Evolving Health Care Environment: Workshop Summary*. Washington, DC: National Academies Press; 2012.

12. American Telemedicine Association Definition of Telemedicine. http://www.americantelemed.org/main/the-source/ata-wiki.

13. Doarn CR, Pruitt S, Jacobs J, et al. Federal efforts to define and advance telehealth—a work in progress. *Telemed J E Health* 2014;20(5):409–418.

14. HRSA Telehealth. http://www.hrsa.gov/healthit/toolbox/RuralHealthITtoolbox/Telehealth/whatistelehealth.html.

15. California Code Definition of Telehealth. http://leginfo.legislature.ca.gov/faces/codes_displaySection.xhtml?lawCode=BPC&sectionNum=2290.5.

16. Virginia Code Definition of Telehealth. http://law.lis.virginia.gov/vacode/title38.2/chapter34/section38.2-3418.16/.

17. American Telemedicine Association Glossary. http://thesource.americantelemed.org/resources/telemedicine-glossary.

18. Kvedar J, Coye M, Everett W. Connected health: a review of technologies and strategies to improve patient care with telemedicine and telehealth. *Health Aff (Millwood)* 2014;33(2):194–199.

19. Darkins A, Ryan P, Kobb R, et al. Care coordination/home telehealth: the systematic implementation of health informatics, home telehealth, and disease management to support the care of veteran patients with chronic conditions. *Telemed J E Health* 2008;14(10):1118–1126.

20. Dimmick SL, Mustaleski C, Burgiss SG, et al. A case study of benefits and potential savings in rural home telemedicine. *Home Healthc Nurse* 2000;18(2):124–135.

21. Bashshur RL, Shannon GW, Smith BR, et al. The empirical foundations of telemedicine interventions for chronic disease management. *Telemed J E Health* 2014;20(9):769–800.

22. Grabowski D, O'Malley A. Use of telemedicine can reduce hospitalizations of nursing home residents and generate savings for Medicare. *Health Aff (Millwood)* 2014;33(2):244–250.

23. Agency for Healthcare Research and Quality. *Effective Health Care Program*. https://effectivehealthcare.ahrq.gov/ehc/products/624/2254/telehealth-report-160630.pdf. Rockville, MD: Agency for Healthcare Research and Quality; 2016.

24. Krupinski EA, Bernard J. Standards and guidelines in telemedicine and telehealth. *Healthcare (Basel)* 2014;2(1):74–93.

25. American Telemedicine Association. *Practice Guidelines*. http://hub.americantelemed.org/resources/telemedicine-practice-guidelines.

26. U.S. Smartphone Use in 2015. http://www.pewinternet.org/2015/04/01/us-smartphone-use-in-2015/.

27. Uscher-Pines L, Mulcahy A, Cowling D, et al. Access and quality of care in direct-to-consumer telemedicine. *Telemedicine J E Health* 2015;22 (4):282–287.

28. Uscher-Pines L, Mulcahy A, Cowling D, et al. Antibiotic prescribing for acute respiratory infections in direct-to-consumer telemedicine visits. *JAMA Intern Med* 2015;175(7):1234–1235.

29. Gough F, Budhrani S, Cohn E, et al. ATA practice guidelines for live, on-demand primary and urgent care. *Telemed J E Health* 2015;21(3):233–241.

30. American Medical Association. *Report of the Council on Medical Service: Coverage of and Payment for Telemedicine. CMS Report 7-A-14*. Washington, DC: AMA; 2014.

31. American Medical Association, Report of the Council on Judicial and Ethical Affairs, Guidance for Ethical Practice in Telemedicine, 2016. https://www.ama-assn.org/sites/default/files/media-browser/i16-ceja-reports.pdf.

32. Daniel H, Sulmasy LS. Health and public policy committee of the American College of Physicians. Policy recommendations to guide the use of telemedicine in primary care settings: an American College of Physicians position paper. *Ann Intern Med* 2015;163(10):787–789.

33. American Academy of Family Physicians. *Physicians and Telehealth*. http://www.graham-center.org/content/dam/rgc/documents/publications-reports/reports/RGC%202015%20Telehealth%20Report.pdf.

34. Committee on Pediatric Workforce, Marcin JP, Rimsza ME, Moskowitz WB. The use of telemedicine to address access and physician workforce shortages. *Pediatrics* 2015;136(1):202–209.

35. Federation of State Medical Boards. *Model Policy for the Appropriate Use of Telemedicine Technologies in the Practice of Medicine*; April 2014. http://www.fsmb.org/Media/Default/PDF/FSMB/Advocacy/FSMB_Telemedicine_Policy.pdf.

36. American Psychological Association. *Guidelines for the Practice of Telepsychology*. http://www.apa.org/practice/guidelines/telepsychology.aspx.

37. American Academy of Ambulatory Care Nursing. *Scope and Standards of Practice for Telehealth Nursing*. 5th ed. Pittman, NJ: American Academy of Ambulatory Care Nursing; 2011.

38. Federal Communications Commission. Chapter 10: Healthcare. In: *The National Broadband Plan: Connecting America*. Washington, DC: Federal Communications Commission; 2011:197–222.

39. Federal Communications Commission. *2016 Broadband Progress Report*. https://www.fcc.gov/reports-research/reports/broadband-progress-reports/2016-broadband-progress-report.

40. U.S. Food & Drug Administration. *Medical Devices*. http://www.fda.gov/MedicalDevices/DigitalHealth/MobileMedicalApplications/default.htm.

41. Continua Health Alliance. http://www.pchalliance.org/continua.

42. Simpatico TA. Videoconferencing in mental health care: barriers, opportunities, and principles for program development. In: Reid WH, Silver SB, eds. *Handbook of Mental Health Administration and Management*. New York: Psychology Press; 2003;386.

Rural Health

Katharine Hsu Wibberly, PhD and
Karen Schulder Rheuban, MD

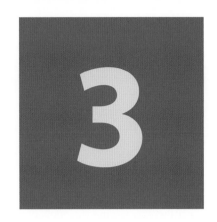

RURAL HEALTH DISPARITIES

Rural Americans experience significant health disparities, including higher incidence of disease and disability, increased mortality rates, and lower life expectancies as compared to the general population. Heart disease is the leading cause of death in the United States for both men and women.[1] However, when comparing rural–urban disparities in heart disease, Knudson, Meit, and Popat found:

- For adults 20 years and older, patterns of ischemic heart disease (IHD) death rates for men and women were highest in the nation's most rural counties.

- For both men and women, residents of the most rural counties had the highest age-adjusted prevalence of obesity.

- Nationwide, physical inactivity during leisure time was most common for men and women in rural counties when compared to urban counties.[2]

Life expectancy at birth is one of the most frequently used indicators of health status. Singh and Siahpush examined trends in rural–urban disparities for all-cause and cause-specific mortality in the United States between 1969 and 2009.[3] Key findings included:

- Mortality risks for both males and females and for blacks and whites have been increasingly higher in nonmetropolitan than metropolitan areas, particularly since 1990.

- Disparities widened over time; excess mortality from all causes combined and from several major causes of death in nonmetropolitan areas was greater in 2005–2009 than in 1990–1992.

- Causes of death contributing most to the increasing rural–urban disparity and higher rural mortality include heart disease, unintentional injuries, chronic obstructive pulmonary disease (COPD), lung cancer, stroke, suicide, diabetes, nephritis, pneumonia/influenza, cirrhosis, and Alzheimer disease.[3] In fact, one-third of all motor vehicle accidents occur in rural areas, but two-thirds of motor vehicle deaths occur on rural roads. Rural residents are also nearly twice as likely as urban residents to die from unintentional injuries other than motor vehicle accidents.[4]

PLACE MATTERS

According to the Federal Office of Rural Health Policy definition of rural, approximately 61 million people (about 20% of the population in the United States) live and work in rural areas. Where a person lives can determine their health status, health risks, and health outcomes. The interplay between six key factors that make up "place" is referred to as the social determinants of health. These include:

- Economic stability

- Education

- Food

- Neighborhood and physical/built environment

- Social and community context

- Health care

Rural Americans face significant challenges in all six factors.

Economic Stability

The economy in rural areas has suffered significantly from the decline in both agricultural and manufacturing jobs. Although rural employment growth increased a percentage point in 2014 after stagnating for 2 years, the number remains below what it was in 2007.[5] According to the U.S. Department of Agriculture (USDA) Economic Research Service:

- The rural poverty rate in 2014 was an estimated 18.1%, whereas the urban rate was 15.1%.
- Poverty rates for rural children underwent the largest increase during the 2007–2009 recession, rising from 21.9% in 2007 to 24.2% in 2009, and continued to increase at the start of the recovery reaching 25.2% in 2014.[6]

Education

One of the key predictors of childhood poverty is parental educational attainment. The educational attainment of people living in rural areas has improved markedly over time, with increases in high school completion rates and in the proportion of residents who have completed at least some college. The proportion of rural adults with a 4-year college degree or more increased by 4 percentage points between 2000 and 2014, and the proportion without a high school diploma or equivalent, such as a GED (General Education Diploma), declined by 9 percentage points. However, the share of the adult population with a 4-year college degree remains far lower in rural areas than in urban ones, and this gap has grown over time.

Food

Food insecurity refers to the state of being without reliable access to a sufficient quantity of affordable, nutritious food. According to the USDA, "vehicle access is perhaps the most important determinant of whether or not a family can access affordable and nutritious food."[7] Households with fewer resources are considerably less likely to have and use their own vehicle for regular food shopping than households with more resources.[7] Fifteen percent of rural households are food insecure,[8] and 50% of counties with the highest rates of food insecurity (those in the top 10%) are in rural areas. Rural areas also account for 64% of counties with the highest rates of *child* food insecurity.[9]

Neighborhood and Physical/Built Environment

As has already been noted, vehicle access affects food security. Transportation is a central issue for rural communities. Population density is one of the most important factors in transportation planning, as the smaller the population, the smaller the tax base for funding public transportation systems. On top of that, rural areas typically also face challenges of distance, terrain, and weather. The smaller tax base also affects the availability and affordability of parks and recreational activities, including public parks, green spaces, recreational facilities, and publicly subsidized organized youth and adult sports.

An ever-increasingly significant determinant of rural health is access to broadband. Access to broadband is becoming more and more essential for health care, including applications like telemedicine, remote patient monitoring, mobile health, and electronic health records. However, rural areas that have much to gain from these applications are also the ones with the least reliable and most expensive access. The Federal Communications Commission (FCC) 2016 Broadband Progress Report noted that although 10% of all Americans (34 million people) lack access to 25 Mbps/3 Mbps service, 39% of rural Americans (23 million people) lack access to 25 Mbps/3 Mbps service. The availability of fixed terrestrial services in rural America continues to lag behind urban America at all speeds: 20% lack access even to service at 4 Mbps/1 Mbps, down only 1% from 2011, and 31% lack access to 10 Mbps/1 Mbps, down only 4% from 2011.[10] The Connect2Health[FCC] Task Force's Mapping Broadband Health in America tool allows users to visualize, overlay, and analyze broadband and health data at the national, state, and county levels. This sample map (see Figure 3-1) developed by the FCC shows the power of the mapping tool to identify clusters and potentially convene public–private partnerships and private-sector collaborations and focus policy efforts. The five states in purple—Indiana, Louisiana, Mississippi, Missouri,

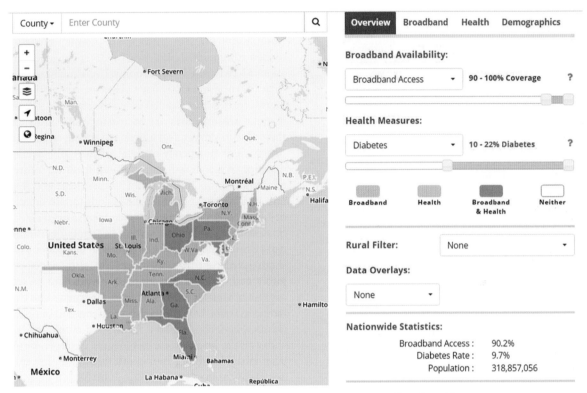

▲ **Figure 3-1.** Sample Map from FCC Connect2Health Task Force Mapping Broadband Health in America.

and Oklahoma—experience incidences of chronic disease above the national average. At the same time, fixed broadband access percentages in rural areas are, on average, below 50%, and in some cases far below.

▶ Social and Community Context

Within the community and cultural context, rural residents tend to value self-reliance and independence. In part, as a reflection of this, rural residents are more likely to own guns for hunting, protection, or self-defense. Rural children are approximately three times more likely to die by firearm compared to children in urban areas. A study published in *JAMA Pediatrics*[11] analyzed suicides among people aged 10 to 24 between 1996 and 2010 and found that rates were nearly doubled in rural areas compared to urban areas. Although this gap existed in 1996 at the beginning of the data set, it widened over the course of this time period. The

most common causes of death were firearm (51.1%), hanging and suffocation (33.9%), and poison (7.9%). Although there is no direct correlation between gun ownership and suicide or mental illness, gun owners are more likely to die if they do become suicidal.

RURAL HEALTH CARE

Rural Americans clearly face a large number of social determinants that contribute to poor health status, increased risks, and less-than-optimal outcomes. However, they also face significant challenges with their actual health care infrastructure, creating challenges with access to quality health care.

▶ Health Insurance

According to the Institute of Medicine, access to health care means having "the timely use of personal health services to achieve the best health outcomes."[12] Health insurance facilitates entry into the health care system. Those without insurance or with inadequate coverage are less likely to receive care. As noted earlier in the chapter, economic instability is one of the challenges faced by rural Americans. Compared to those in metropolitan areas, rural populations have lower incomes, making it more difficult to afford health insurance coverage. Additionally, workers in rural areas are less likely to have employer-sponsored health insurance. According the Henry J. Kaiser Family Foundation, "among workers, those in rural areas are more likely to work in blue collar jobs (jobs outside of managerial, business, and financial occupations) than workers in metropolitan areas (71% versus 63%). Blue-collar workers tend to earn less and have fewer overall benefits than white-collar workers. Half of all rural workers work in 'Low ESI industries,' or industries in which less than 80% of workers are covered by employer-sponsored insurance coverage."[13] Further exacerbating this issue, rural individuals are also more likely to live in states that have chosen not to adopt Medicaid expansion.

▶ Workforce

Nationally, the country is experiencing a health care workforce shortage. Rural communities are even more challenged. In the United States, 2,157 health professional shortage areas (HPSAs) are rural, compared to 910 urban. Rural communities frequently have difficulty attracting and retaining health care providers due to competition from urban facilities and practices who are able to offer better compensation and/or working conditions. By 2030, the proportion of Americans who are over 65 years old will be one in five, compared to one in eight today. The lack of an adequate workforce is magnified in rural areas because the elderly population is growing more rapidly in rural than in urban areas. The demand for services increases as the population ages. Among the aging population in rural areas are also the health care providers themselves, many of whom are expected to reach retirement age in the next 5 years. The loss of a single provider in a rural community could have potentially devastating effects in some rural communities.

▶ Hospitals

Rural hospitals are typically the economic foundation of their communities, with every $1.00 spent generating about $2.20 for the local economy. Unfortunately, more than 75 rural hospitals have closed since 2010—and many more may be headed down the same path. Rural hospital closure rates are increasing nationally, and these closures may affect access to basic inpatient, outpatient, and emergency medical services. The average distance of the closed rural hospital from the nearest remaining hospital is around 15 miles. Research findings indicate that 8% of rural hospitals (approximately 180) were at high risk of financial distress in 2013.[14]

A number of factors affect a hospital's decision to close or suspend operations, including low patient volume, declining inpatient utilization, and inadequate payer mix. Rural hospitals are typically not as well resourced as larger regional or urban hospitals and thus have been unable to make enhancements and improvements to its physical plant. As a result, rural residents with private insurance tend to travel to larger, newer hospitals outside the community, weakening the rural hospital's payer mix. In addition, small rural hospitals typically are not able to attract specialty care providers, thus forcing patients to travel to larger regional hospitals when their conditions require the services of a specialist or subspecialist. These factors combined put many small rural hospitals, which were already operating on very thin margins, at significant financial risk.

The closure of a rural hospital creates a major barrier to care, including emergency care. In addition, many physicians and other providers leave communities immediately following a rural hospital closure. Rural hospital closures also exacerbate gaps in access to specialty care.[15]

▶ Emergency Medical Services

Timely access to emergency care is a major issue for rural residents. Response times by emergency medical personnel and transport times via ambulance to hospitals are notably greater than in urban areas due to geographic barriers, including distance, terrain, and weather conditions. In addition, the majority of emergency medical services (EMS) first responders in rural areas are volunteers, making recruiting, training, and retaining a qualified EMS workforce particularly challenging. Although relying on an unpaid volunteer workforce is more cost effective for underresourced rural areas, it creates challenges in maintaining "24/7" coverage because the volunteers also have other jobs. These other commitments also make it hard for volunteers to keep up with their training requirements.

Rural residents face significant issues with their health care infrastructure. Although continued efforts to increase access to quality health care and transform the health care delivery system in rural areas are critically important, improving population health in rural areas will also require broader approaches that address the social, economic, and environmental social determinants of health.

RURAL INNOVATION

> *Necessity ... the mother of invention.*
> —Plato

Despite the many challenges faced by the residents of rural areas, many new models of care first took root in rural America. These include lay health promoters, community health workers, and community paramedicine. In fact, many of the earliest use cases for telehealth arose in rural America. The National Advisory Committee on Rural Health and Human Services issued a Policy Brief[16] to examine alternatives for the provision of emergency care and ancillary services in light of the recent surge in rural hospital closures. In the brief, the committee assesses four policy options, including the Frontier Extended Stay Clinic model and the rural Free-Standing Emergency Department model.

A recent Assistant Secretary for Planning and Evaluation (ASPE) Issue Brief[17] on rural hospital participation and performance in value-based purchasing and other delivery system reform initiatives concluded with the following:

> *Rural hospitals provide care and other services for the 59 million Americans living in rural areas, but statutory differences in payment structures and low patient volumes mean that most rural hospitals are not subject to payment incentives resulting from current mandatory hospital-based delivery system reform programs. However, rural hospitals*

> *and communities are increasingly represented in other initiatives, such as the Medicare Shared Savings Program, and have many strengths that lend themselves particularly well to the type of coordination and cooperation that delivery system reform hopes to promote.*

As our nation transitions from volume-based payment models to value-based care, rural communities indeed may have an advantage over more populous metropolitan areas. Smaller population sizes, the emphasis of rural health care professionals on building personal relationships with patients and their families, and the many telehealth-enabled collaborative care models that already exist in rural communities create a solid foundation on which to build.

REFERENCES

1. Centers for Heart Disease. *Heart Disease Facts.* http://www.cdc.gov/heartdisease/facts.htm. Accessed August 10, 2015.

2. Knudson A, Meit M, Popat S. Rural-urban disparities in heart disease policy brief #1 from the 2014 update of the Rural-Urban Chartbook. Rural Health Reform Policy Research Center. https://www.ruralhealthresearch.org/publications/974. Accessed October 2014.

3. Singh GK, Siahpush M. Widening rural-urban disparities in all-cause mortality. *J Urban Health* 2014; 91(2):272–292.

4. Goins RT, Williams KA, Carter MW, Spencer M, Solovieva T. Perceived barriers to health care access among rural older adults: a qualitative study. *J Rural Health* 2005;21(3):206–213.

5. USDA. *Rural America at a Glance 2015 Edition. Economic Research Service. Economic Information Bulletin 145.* Revised January 2016. Washington, DC: USDA.

6. Proctor BD, Semega JL, Kollar MA. *Income and Poverty in the United States: 2015.* http://www.census.gov/library/publications/2016/demo/p60-256.html. Accessed September 13, 2016.

7. Access to Affordable and Nutritious Food: Measuring and Understanding Food Deserts and Their Consequences. Report to Congress. USDA Economic Research Service. Washington, DC. June 2009.

8. Coleman-Jensen A, Rabbitt M, Gregory C, Singh A. *Household Food Security in the United States in 2015.* Table 2. http://www.ers.usda.gov/publications/pubdetails/?pubid=79760. Accessed September 7, 2016.

9. Gundersen C, Dewey A, Crumbaugh A, Kato M, Engelhard E. *Map the Meal Gap 2016: Food Insecurity and Child Food Insecurity Estimates at the County Level*. http://map.feedingamerica.org/county/2014/overall. Accessed October 3, 2016.

10. Federal Communications Commission. *2016 Broadband Progress Report*. https://www.fcc.gov/reports-research/reports/broadband-progress-reports/2016-broadband-progress-report. Accessed January 29, 2016.

11. Fontanella CA, Hiance-Steelsmith DL, Phillips GS, et al. *Widening Rural-Urban Disparities in Youth Suicides, United States, 1996-2010*. http://jamanetwork.com/journals/jamapediatrics/article-abstract/2195006. Accessed May 2015.

12. Institute of Medicine, Committee on Monitoring Access to Personal Health Care Services. *Access to Health Care in America*. Washington, DC: National Academy Press; 1993.

13. Newkirk V, Damico A. *The Affordable Care Act and Insurance Coverage in Rural Areas Issue Brief*. http://kff.org/uninsured/issue-brief/the-affordable-care-act-and-insurance-coverage-in-rural-areas/. Accessed May 29, 2014.

14. Kaufman B, Pink G, Holmes M. *Prediction of Financial Distress among Rural Hospitals. NC Rural Health Research Program Findings Brief*. https://www.ruralhealthresearch.org/alerts/106?utm_source=alert&utm_medium=email&utm_campaign=20160201northcarolina. Accessed October 18, 2016.

15. Wishner J, Solleveid P, Rudowitz R, Paradise J, Antonisse L. *Issue Brief: A Look at Rural Hospital Closures and Implications for Access to Care: Three Case Studies*. http://kff.org/report-section/a-look-at-rural-hospital-closures-and-implications-for-access-to-care-three-case-studies-issue-brief/. Accessed July 7, 2016.

16. National Advisory Committee on Rural Health and Human Services. Alternative Models to Preserving Access to Emergency Care. Policy Brief, July 2016. https://www.ruralhealthinfo.org/webinars/emergency-care-models-and-opioid-misuse. Accessed September 29, 2016.

17. Joynt KE, Nguyen N, Samson LW, Snyder JE, Lechner A, Ogunwumiju O. ASPE Issue Brief: Rural Hospital Participation and Performance in Value-Based Purchasing and Other Delivery System Reform Initiatives. https://aspe.hhs.gov/pdf-report/rural-hospital-participation-and-performance-value-based-purchasing-and-other-delivery-system-reform-initiatives. Accessed October 19, 2016.

Supporting Seamless Delivery of Telehealth Solutions

Elizabeth A. Krupinski, PhD

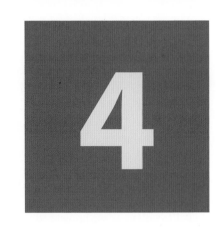

INTRODUCTION

Telemedicine has a fairly long and rich history when one considers its roots both in the context of medicine and communication.[1] Recent evidence clearly supports the use of telemedicine in a wide variety of clinical specialties in terms of feasibility, satisfaction, cost effectiveness, and clinical outcomes.[2-7] The success of telemedicine is evidenced by the recent rapidity with which it has become a commercial enterprise that provides services "on demand" to patients outside of the traditional health care enterprise.[8-10] The American Telemedicine Association (ATA) actually has an accreditation program that "recognizes organizations providing online, real-time patient health services that comply with operational, clinical and consumer-related standards. The program promotes patient safety, transparency of operations and adherence to all relevant laws and regulations."[11]

Clearly telemedicine is here to stay, but it does and will take many forms just as traditional health care always has. Many factors contribute to the success of individual programs, of which many are discussed in the other chapters in this book, especially as they relate to individual clinical specialties. Common to the success of all enterprises, from academic to commercial endeavors, is the degree to which telemedicine becomes integrated into the existing system in order to effectively and efficiently deliver telehealth solutions. Again, many factors affect the successful integration of new delivery modes into established systems, but this chapter deals with two: leveraging common points between new and existing technologies and health care environments, and optimizing the environment within which telemedicine is practiced from a human factors perspective. To address the first point, we provide an overview of perhaps the most successful telemedicine application: teleradiology. Afterward we provide a review of some of the more common human factors issues that should be considered during the planning, implementation, and operation of telemedicine services.

TELERADIOLOGY

Teleradiology is unique among telemedicine applications in that it grew out of the evolution of the specialty itself. Radiology by its nature is probably the most technology-dependent clinical specialty in existence and thus had an advantage over nearly all other specialties by having technology, technical support, practice procedures and knowledge, and research programs in place even before the "tele" option arose. Yet even with this infrastructure, radiology faced (and still faces) challenges when it came to convincing users that it was at least as good as traditional film-based radiology in terms of quality, diagnostic accuracy, cost, and utility.

Teleradiology has its origins in the development of digital radiography. For over 80 years patient care depended on film-based radiology, but these images had to be physically transported throughout a hospital, between hospitals, and between cities. This was very labor intensive and often involved radiologists doing "windshield" duty, driving from small town to small town to interpret batches of cases that had been acquired over the previous week or even month, delaying interpretation and thus treatment. Film-based radiology was also subject to lost or misplaced images.[12,13]

In the 1970s, the idea of an electronic-based imaging system replacing all X-ray film took root. Research with video-based and other digital detector systems primarily being conducted at the University of Arizona and the University of Wisconsin[14,15] led to the first digital subtraction angiogram being successfully performed and reported in 1977 followed by other digital imaging applications.[16-18] All of these early efforts led to digital radiology as we know it today and made direct transmission of digitally acquired images possible for teleradiology.[19]

From an integration point of view, it is very difficult to distinguish teleradiology from radiology today, as from the perspective of the radiologist, the majority of the workflow is very much the same. Before digital radiography, images were acquired and viewed on pieces of film that were put on a lightbox for viewing and interpretation. Digital imaging changed this dramatically. Although printed to film in the early days, it soon became obvious that digital images are most effectively displayed on digital/electronic computer monitors. This led to increased interacting between image and viewer as radiologists could now use window/level techniques to adjust the contrast of images, use zoom/pan (instead of a magnifying glass and hot light) to view fine image details at high resolution, and use image processing and image analysis tools to extract more information from the images and render more accurate decisions. Once digital images were introduced, computer-aided detection and diagnosis tools were rapidly developed and are becoming commonplace in many radiology applications such as breast and lung screening.[20]

In this transition from film to the digital world, however, issues arose that affected integration and acceptance of the new technologies—very much in the same ways that new technologies for other telemedical applications face integration challenges. In the transition, film images were the gold standard against which digital was judged due to its higher resolution and rendition of fine details required for interpretation (in fact, film is still technically better than digital in this respect). Complicating the transition to digital display

was the fact that electronic displays in the 1980s and early to mid-1990s were basically inadequate in terms of resolution and contrast. As a result of the mismatch between high-quality, high-resolution digital images and low-quality, low-resolution displays, significant developments in medical-grade display technology were started in the late 1980s and actually continue to today as new display technologies are developed.

The first displays used for digital radiographs were cathode ray tubes (CRTs),[21-23] and issues such as luminance and even the type of phosphor in the display faceplate were variable and less than ideal. Today liquid crystal displays (LCDs) and variants (organic light-emitting diodes, or OLEDs) are the norm in most radiology reading rooms.[24,25] As with telemedicine in general, the quality of images is the deciding factor on whether users (radiologists) are satisfied with the information presented to them clinically.[26,27]

Some of the key display parameters that have guided the development of these displays are directly related to the perceptual requirements of the radiologists and the digital nature of the images, and the complex nature of the anatomic structures and lesions in those images.[28] All of these factors are also important in telemedicine displays, including luminance (or brightness) and contrast,[29,30] viewing angle,[31,32] calibration methods,[33,34] and, more recently, the use of color and commercial off-the-shelf displays instead of more expensive medical-grade monochrome and color displays.[35-37] It is important to note that much of this foundational research on display optimization has been incorporated into the major practice guidelines for the practice of digital radiology and teleradiology.[38-40] Today even laptops, iPads, and smart phones are being considered for use, especially in teleradiology for viewing images[41-44] and capturing images.[45-47] Many of the recommendations in these guidelines are directly applicable to telemedicine applications and should be referenced as feasible when designing a telemedicine work area.

Another key aspect of integration that helped advance teleradiology was the development and use of the DICOM (Digital Imaging and Communications in Medicine) standard.[48,49] In fact, the DICOM standard is used today in many telemedicine applications as a tool for formatting, transmitting, and archiving visible light and other images (eg, ophthalmology, pathology, dermatology). The development of technical standards to optimize interoperability across platforms and institutions was fundamental to teleradiology, and the lessons learned in radiology are readily transferable to telemedicine in general.

Through joint efforts of the American College of Radiology (ACR) and the National Electrical Manufacturers Association (NEMA), DICOM was developed in 1993. DICOM is an internationally accepted standard for medical images and metadata (now extending beyond radiology to visible light and other images used in telemedicine) with respect to handling, storing, printing, and transmitting image and other medical record information. It includes standards for file format and network communications. For example, the communication protocol uses Transmission Control Protocol/Internet Protocol (TCP/IP) for system communications enabling system interoperability or the exchange of image and patient data in a standard format so that images acquired on a device from one vendor can be viewed on any workstation.

The display used in teleradiology is obviously critical for efficient and accurate diagnoses, and the same is true in any telemedicine application. Two DICOM standards are important when considering displays: the Grayscale Presentation State Standard (GSPS) and the Grayscale Standard Display Function (GSDF). These are not only important for teleradiology but also for any other tele-application in which radiographic images would be viewed—for example, telestroke, teleorthopedics, telesurgery, and telecardiology, to name a few. GSPS is a data object associated with an image specifying how it should be presented on any DICOM-compliant viewer. It includes features such as customized look-up tables (LUTs), text overlay, and zoom/pan. The GSDF addresses the issue of having multiple displays from multiple vendors, each with different luminance ranges, white points, and minimum and maximum luminance settings. Standardization was required because the same image would look very different depending on the display it was viewed on. The GSDF maximizes the perceptibility of information and promotes consistency of presentation across different displays. As a calibration tool, it is based on the concept of perceptual linearity across grayscale values, so changes in image pixel values across a grayscale range are perceived as having similar contrast.

A similar display standard does not exist for telemedicine or for color medical images in general, whether for telemedicine or standard clinical uses. This has been the topic of a number of papers, with a recent consensus report[50] being the most relevant to telemedicine. It is noted in this consensus report that areas that would benefit the most from consistency and standardization of color would be digital microscopy, telemedicine, medical photography (eg, ophthalmic, dental photography), and display calibration. It provides overviews of some of the most critical color applications (including telemedicine) and then notes that a variety of important organizations are addressing this issue, including DICOM, American Association of Physicists in Medicine (AAPM), International Color Consortium (ICC), International Commission on Illumination (CIE), International Engineering Consortium (IEC), Video Electronics Standards Association (VESA), International Committee for Display Metrology (ICDM), and the American College of Radiology (ACR). It does provide reference to some methods available for calibrating color displays.

At the heart of any radiology or teleradiology enterprise is its Picture Archiving and Communications System, or PACS. A PACS is usually composed of various digital acquisition imaging systems (eg, computed radiography/digital radiography [CR/DR], magnetic resonance imaging [MRI], computed tomography [CT]), a secure network for transmitting images from those devices to workstations (onsite or offsite as with teleradiology), archives (onsite, offsite, or cloud based) to store and retrieve images and related data, and viewing terminals (eg, workstations, mobile devices). Increasingly, PACS systems that were traditionally limited to radiology departments and their images are becoming enterprise-wide transmission and archiving systems that many departments use not only for routine images but also for those used in telemedicine practices.[51] Images from devices such as digital cameras, endoscopes, digital slit cameras (ophthalmology), digital otoscopes, and many other devices are being stored in and retrieved from PACS systems (often using a DICOM wrapper).

As with telemedicine in general, the main drivers for teleradiology were the need for after-hours (~5:00 p.m. to 8:00 a.m., weekends and holidays) coverage for urgent and emergent radiologic studies[19,52] and the need for subspecialist or expert reads. Even in its more advanced stage of acceptance and integration, however, there is still considerable debate in the radiology community regarding its use, regulation, and commoditization,[53-63] with many of the same concerns being raised in many other clinical specialties using telemedicine. It is clear and evidence supports its role, and with appropriate care[63] and consideration, one can select an appropriate teleradiology or any other telemedicine provider.

On the regulatory side, telemedicine may someday soon follow the path of teleradiology in some aspects. For example, how well teleradiology has been integrated into general radiology practice is demonstrated by the ACR Teleradiology Guidelines and its history. The ACR Standard for Teleradiology was first issued in 1994 and was revised in 1996, 1998, and 2002. In 2007 the ACR sunset it, as everyday digital practice could not be differentiated from teleradiology. Recently released white papers on teleradiology practice from the ACR and the European Society of Radiology summarize the pros and cons of teleradiology and comment on best practices.[64-66] With respect to licensing, the ACR position is that physicians who interpret images originating from another state must be licensed and credentialed at the site of origin of the images and in the state they are doing the interpretation.[67,68] Telemedicine has a number of practice guidelines as well (many from the ATA), and some of them have been updated over the years much like the ACR guidelines—and in many cases deal with similar issues: quality, process and procedures, legal and regulatory, safety, and privacy and security. It will be interesting to track these guidelines to see when and if they, too, sunset at some point in time!

INTEGRATION FROM THE HUMAN FACTORS PERSPECTIVE

The key thing to remember in any telemedicine enterprise is that although technology is integral to telemedicine, telemedicine is *not* about the technology, but rather about the people. Integration of technology obviously has its own challenges (in general a good Information Technology [IT] department can solve practically anything), but many would say it is the integration of people into the telemedicine environment that is the main challenge. In many cases, taking care of some rather basic and often commonsense variables makes this integration easier, as the users then do not

have to worry about all the "peripheral" aspects and can concentrate on the consultation. For example, one early consideration is the patients likely to be seen and what types of consultations will take place. A clinic for geriatric patients needs to account for their vision, hearing, and mobility challenges in the room design; pediatric rooms need to include toys or books to entertain the kids while they are waiting for consultations to start; and telesurgery clinics needs to position cameras and other equipment around the existing surgical equipment and tools. Even radiology room design was important in the transition from film to digital. With film, the film alternators or lightboxes used to face each other (with radiologists looking at the images and their backs toward each other). This was replicated with the move to digital and teleradiology, but it was quickly realized that it would not work because the monitors facing each other across the rooms produced reflections and glare that interfered with image quality and the interpretation process! Rooms had to be redesigned to address this, often using walls and other room separators to isolate workstations from each other (also isolating radiologists to some extent from each other).

Where the consult room is located is important.[69] In the early days (and now) there were stories about how janitor closets and other spare (but inappropriate) rooms were converted into telemedicine rooms simply because they were there and unused (and often remained unused for telemedicine, as they were inconvenient to get to or simply too small or poorly designed for effective use). A room near the outpatient check-in area of a hospital or clinic will likely have a wide variety of cases referred to telemedicine simply by proximity and familiarity. If it is situated in a pediatric wing, it will attract pediatric cases but likely not adult cases. One easy solution is to have a dedicated telemedicine room with portable equipment that is easy to deploy and move to where the patient is located. This is quite easy with teledermatology (especially store-forward) as the key piece of equipment is a digital camera and dedicated task lighting. Transporting a cardiology patient to the telemedicine clinic may be less feasible, but portable electrocardiogram (ECG) devices can be taken to the patient. Synchronous real-time (RT) services are increasingly portable using tablets, smart phones, and roaming robots. These portable devices are very useful with elderly and disabled patients.

It is useful to plan the layout of a room in advance of using it for telemedicine. Measure it and draw a floor plan, including locations of features such as doors and windows, HVAC (heating, ventilation, air conditioning) vents, electricity and plumbing fixtures, telecommunications lines, lighting fixtures, and so on. It often helps to act out clinical scenarios so equipment and furniture needs and locations are anticipated and space accounted for. Telerehabilitation consults, for example, may need to evaluate patient gait and ability to navigate between locations by having them walk from one end of a room to the other, so the room has to be long enough and free of obstacles to avoid tripping or falling; have enough room to accommodate walkers and other assistive devices; and the videoteleconferencing (VTC) equipment has to be situated properly and flexible enough to move the camera as the patient walks.

The arrangement of telemedicine equipment (eg, carts, cameras, docking stations, peripherals) should be considered. Rooms (even revamped closets!) should not be too crowded with lots of wires hanging loose or running along the floor without being taped down or secured. Provider and patients, especially those with mobility or stability issues and using a cane, walker, or wheelchair, should not have to worry about tripping over things, bumping into equipment, and injuring themselves.

In radiology, standard ergonomic concerns with workstations such as monitor height, monitor distance, mouse placement, and task lighting have been of concern since going digital,[25] and many of the human factors and ergonomic considerations addressed for teleradiology transfer directly to telemedicine. The ambient environment needs to be considered. In some areas (both rural and urban), dirt or dust blowing in from the outside can ruin equipment and cause problems for patients and clinicians (eg, telepulmonology clinics where patients already have respiratory problems). Using dust filters for the air system helps. Controlling temperature is important as telemedicine rooms have lots of electronic equipment that can generate extra heat. Even short amounts of time in a small hot room can exacerbate symptoms of ill and stressed patients. Fans and dehumidifiers can help with these conditions (or heaters in large or cold rooms).

Lighting is very critical, and lots of options are available. There are obviously differences for teleradiology and other specialties, but again teleradiology serves as a model. For example, all of the technical practice guidelines[38–40] for digital practice include statements about ambient lighting (should be 25 to 45 lux in most cases) as it affects the quality of the images displayed on the workstation monitors and thus diagnostic performance. The same types of considerations hold for telemedicine. When there are no patients (eg, reviewing store-forward images or charts), standard office lighting for computer environments can be used, but brighter lights may be needed when a patient is present.

A single lighting system may not suffice. The lighting should be adjusted as appropriate during exams or when images are being acquired. Some key points to consider include:

- Artificial "natural" light is preferred
- A range of 3200 to 4000 K is recommended as it is a warm, white light
- Avoid colored lighting (eg, yellow)
- Fluorescent is preferred
  - Usually 3500 K low-end "home" use, but commercially can get white light 5000 K
  - Dedicated fixtures (indirect wash fluorescent fixtures) are available specifically for videoconferencing and are available in cool white to reduce ambient heating
- When acquiring digital photos, the room should be well lit (150 foot-candles) using light white light, fluorescent daylight, or full-spectrum bulbs instead of incandescent bulbs
- For RT, the best lighting is 300 to 500 lux and angled away from the participants to avoid shadows
  - Place and aim fixtures to achieve vertical illumination on subject 35 to 40 degrees above horizontal
- Avoid traditional downlighting, as it creates facial shadows
- If only one light source is used, place it as close as possible in the same direction as the camera, but in back of the camera
- Multiple frontal light sources are recommended as this improves the "3-D" effect
- Backlighting helps the body stand out from the background

- Use desk lamps as task lighting and fill lighting to compensate for poor lighting conditions
- Avoid reflecting/glare surfaces in the field of view
  - Avoid white doctor's coats as they create reflections

The background is important as well:

- The recommended wall color is light blue, but only one or two walls
  - The color temperature (physical measurement in degrees Kelvin comparable to hue) should not affect the appearance of the skin
  - Use flat latex blue paint rather than gloss or semi-gloss to avoid glare and reflections
- Avoid clutter and distracting details or objects in the background

Display (monitor) options vary considerably, but some factors to consider include:

- Large monitor screens (≥50 inches) are useful in the clinic setting, but smaller monitors also work well
- HD (high-definition) cameras and displays are readily available at a reasonable cost
- Traditional desktop displays and mobile devices are very useful for reviewing store-and-forward (SF) data
- If viewing radiographic images, adequate spatial and contrast resolution is required

- It is not necessary to use a medical-grade radiology display, but it should be properly calibrated for reading radiographic images (DICOM GSDF)
- Calibrate color displays as feasible
  - Standards regarding what type of calibration should be performed do not exist, but there are some easy methods to at least standardize the appearance of color images[50]
- When using multiple displays, it is important to angle them optimally to avoid strain on the neck, back, and shoulders (Figure 4-1)
- Audio and cameras are critical factors as well, whether separate or integrated systems
- Speaker and microphone capabilities and placement need to accommodate all types of users
  - Some patients, like the elderly, are soft spoken or have trouble projecting, so microphones should be placed close to them
  - With mobile devices, move the device close to the speaker (if the same device serves as the camera, this can be a problem)
  - Speakers may need to be placed closer or the volume turned up to compensate for hearing loss/difficulties

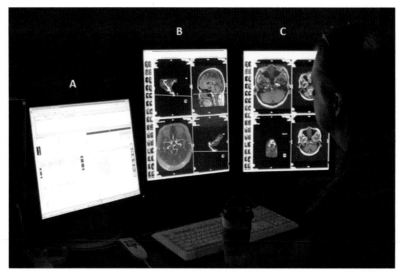

▲ **Figure 4-1.** Example of a typical teleradiology workstation with multiple monitors (A = standard display to access the radiology information system [RIS] and reporting system; B and C = medical-grade monitors for viewing images).

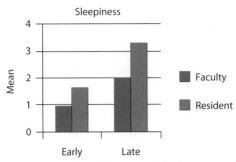

▲ Figure 4-2. Data from[75] the Swedish Occupational Fatigue Inventory (SOFI) to assess physical symptoms of stress and fatigue (sleepiness in this case) as a function of radiologists and radiology residents viewing images early or late in the day.

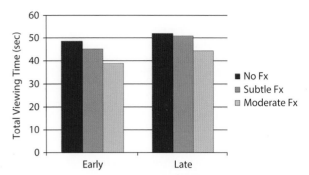

▲ Figure 4-3. Figure from an unpublished study by Krupinski showing how it takes longer to fixate (land the eyes on) fractures in X-ray images as a function of time of day.

- Cameras with as high a quality as possible should be secured on a stable platform to avoid wobbling and shaking
  - Tablets and phones may need stands to stabilize them
- Cameras should be placed at eye level with the face clearly visible to the other person

Workstations are abundant in traditional practice, as well as telemedicine, by virtue of increased use of electronic health records and simply everyday computer use. Care should be taken, however, because concerns arise as use increases. Radiology in particular has seen an increase in computer-related injuries and concerns about increased stress and fatigue (Figure 4-2) the more digital it has become[70-71]. There has also been an increase in the awareness of fatigue in the digital environment and its impact on diagnostic accuracy and efficiency.[72-76]

For example, it can take longer to find abnormalities like fractures in X-ray images the later in the day a radiologist reads them (Figure 4-3). Adhering to guidelines for good ergonomic computer use can help.[77] Using the 20-20-20 rule can help as well: every 20 minutes of working at a computer display, look 20 feet away for 20 seconds. Getting up every now and then helps as well, given recent concerns about sedentary behavior due to computer use in medicine.[78]

CONCLUSIONS

Telemedicine is fundamentally just a tool to improve the delivery of health care services, but it still requires attention to a number of details if it is going to be integrated efficiently and effectively into an existing or even a new telehealth practice. Teleradiology serves as a model of some of the issues and challenges that can arise when making the transition from traditional to technology-based modes of delivery. Adherence to guidelines regarding technology optimization, environment design, human factors, and ergonomics can readily facilitate the transition and reduce resistance and stress, making the experience beneficial and pleasant for patients and providers alike.

REFERENCES

1. Bashshur RL, Shannon GW. *History of Telemedicine.* New Rochelle, NY: Mary Ann Liebert, Inc.; 2009.

2. Bashshur RL, Shannon GW, Tejasvi T, et al. The empirical foundations of teledermatology: a review of the research evidence. *Telemed J E Health* 2015;21:953–979.

3. Bashshur RL, Shannon GW, Smith BR, et al. The empirical evidence for the telemedicine intervention in diabetes management. *Telemed J E Health* 2015;21:321–354.

4. Bashshur RL, Shannon GW, Smith BR, et al. The empirical foundations of telemedicine interventions for chronic disease management. *Telemed J E Health* 2014;20:769–800.

5. Bashshur RL, Shannon GW, Bashshur N, et al. The empirical evidence for telemedicine interventions in mental disorders. *Telemed J E Health* 2016;22:87–113.

6. de la Torre-Diez I, Lopez-Coronado M, Vaca C, et al. Cost-utility and cost-effectiveness studies of telemedicine, electronic, and mobile health systems in the literature: a systematic review. *Telemed J E Health* 2015;21:81–85.

7. Ward MM, Jaana M, Natafgi N. Systematic review of telemedicine applications in emergency rooms. *Intl J Med Inform* 2015;84:601–616.

8. Gooden AM. Telemedicine: a guide to online resources. *Coll Res Lib News* 2016;77:135–139.

9. Arizona Telemedicine Program Service Provider Directory. http://telemedicine.arizona.edu/servicedirectory. Accessed October 1, 2016.

10. Schmidt S. 10 companies to watch in the field of telemedicine. http://blog.marketresearch.com/10-companies-to-watch-in-the-field-of-telemedicine. Accessed September 15, 2016.

11. American Telemedicine Association's Accreditation Program for Online Patient Consultations. http://www.americantelemed.org/ata-accreditation. Accessed September 17, 2016.

12. Bryan S, Weatherburn GC, Watkins JR, et al. The benefits of hospital-wide picture archiving and communication systems: a survey of clinical users of radiology services. *Br J Radiol* 1999;72:469–478.

13. Reiner BI, Siegel EL, Hooper F, et al. Impact of filmless imaging on the frequency of clinician review of radiology images. *J Digit Imag* 1998;11:149–150.

14. Roehrig H, Frost M, Baker R, et al. High-resolution low-light-level video systems for diagnostic radiology. *Proc SPIE Low Light Level Dev Science Tech* 1976; 0078:102–107.

15. Kruger RA, Mistretta CA, Crummy AB, et al. Digital K-edge subtraction radiography. *Radiol* 1977;125:243–245.

16. Frost MM, Fisher HD, Nudelman S, et al. A digital video acquisition system for extraction of subvisual information in diagnostic medical imaging. *Proc SPIE Appl Opt Instrum Med VI* 1977;0127:208.

17. Nudelman S, Fisher HD, Frost MM, et al. A study of photoelectric-digital radiology – Part I: the photoelectric-digital radiology department. *Proc IEEE* 1982;70:700–707.

18. Crummy AB, Strother CM, Sackett JF, et al. Computerized fluoroscopy: digital subtraction for intravenous angiocardiography and arteriography. *Am J Roentgenol* 1980;135:1131–1140.

19. Thrall JH. Teleradiology. Part I. History and clinical applications. *Radiol* 2007;243:613–617.

20. Li Q, Nishikawa RM. *Computer-aided Detection and Diagnosis in Medical Imaging*. New York, NY, CRC Press; 2015.

21. Arenson RL, Chakraborty DP, Seshardi SB, et al. The digital imaging workstation. *Radiol* 1990;176:303–315.

22. Krupinski EA, Johnson J, Roehrig H, et al. Use of a human visual system model to predict observer performance with CRT vs LCD display of images. *J Digit Imag* 2004;17:258–263.

23. Krupinski EA, Roehrig H. Pulmonary nodule detection and visual search: P45 and P104 monochrome versus color monitor displays. *Acad Radiol* 2002;9:638–645.

24. Kagadis G, Walz-Flannigan A, Krupinski EA, et al. Medical imaging displays and their use in image interpretation. *RadioGraphics* 2013;33:275–290.

25. Krupinski EA, Kallergi M. Choosing a radiology workstation: technical and clinical considerations. *Radiol* 2007;242:671–682.

26. Krupinski EA, McNeill K, Haber K, et al. High-volume teleradiology service: focus on radiologist satisfaction. *J Digit Imag* 2003;16:203–209.

27. Krupinski EA, McNeill K, Ovitt T, et al. Patterns of use and satisfaction with a university-based teleradiology system. *J Digit Imag* 1999;12:166–167.

28. Krupinski EA. Medical image perception issues for PACS deployment. *Semin Roentgenol* 2003;38:231–243.

29. Samei E, Siebert JA, Andriole K. et al. AAPM/RSNA tutorial on equipment selection: PACS equipment overview: general guidelines for purchasing and acceptance testing of PACS equipment. *RadioGraphics* 2004;24:313–334.

30. Krupinski E, Roehrig H, Furukawa T. Influence of film and monitor display luminance on observer performance and visual search. *Acad Radiol* 1999;6:411–418.

31. Fifadara DH, Averbukh A, Channin DS, et al. Effect of viewing angle on luminance and contrast for a five-million-pixel monochrome display and a nine-million-pixel color liquid crystal display. *J Digit Imag* 2004;17:264–270.

32. Krupinski EA, Johnson J, Roehrig H. et al. On-axis and off-axis viewing of images on CRT displays and LCDs: observer performance and vision model predictions. *Acad Radiol* 2005;12:957–964.

33. Badano A. AAPM/RSNA tutorial on equipment selection: PACS equipment overview: display systems. *Radiographics* 2004;24:879–889.

34. Krupinski EA, Roehrig H. The influence of a perceptually linearized display on observer performance and visual search. *Acad Radiol* 2000;7:8–13.

35. Krupinski EA. Medical grade vs. off-the-shelf color displays: influence on observer performance and visual search. *J Digit Imag* 2009;22:363–368.

36. McIlgorm DJ, Lawinski C, Ng S, et al. Could standardizing "commercial off-the-shelf" (COTS) monitors to the DICOM part 14: GSDF improve the performance of dental images? A visual grading characteristic analysis. *Dentimaxilo Radiol* 2013;42:2013–2021.

37. Hirschorn DS, Krupinski E, Flynn MJ. PACS displays: how to select the right display technology. *J Am Coll Radiol* 2013;11:1270–1276.

38. Norweck JT, Seibert JA, Andriole K, et al. ACR-AAPM-SIIM technical standard for electronic practice of medical imaging. *J Digit Imag* 2013;26:38–52.

39. Kanal KM, Krupinski E, Berns EA, et al. ACR-AAPM-SIIM practice guidelines for determinants of image quality in digital mammography. *J Digit Imag* 2013;26:10–25.

40. Andriole KP, Ruckdescel TG, Flynn MJ, et al. ACR-AAPM-SIIM practice guideline for digital radiography. *J Digit Imag* 2013;26:26–37.

41. Faggioni L, Nrei E, Bargellini I, et al. iPad-based primary 2D reading of CT angiography examinations of patients with suspected acute gastrointestinal bleeding: preliminary experience. *Br J Radiol* 2015;88:20140477.

42. O'Connell TW, Patlas MN. Mobile devices and their prospective future role in emergency radiology. *Br J Radiol* 2015;89:20150820.

43. Schlechtweg PM, Kammerer FJ, Seuss H, et al. Mobile image interpretation: diagnostic performance of CT exams displayed on a tablet computer in detecting abdominopelvic hemorrhage. *J Digit Imag* 2016;29:183–188.

44. Kim C, Kang B, Choi HJ, et al. A feasibility study of real-time remote CT reading for suspected acute appendicitis using an iPhone. *J Digit Imag.* 2015;28:399–406.

45. Krupinski E, Gonzales M, Gonzales C, et al. Evaluation of a digital camera for acquiring radiographic images for telemedicine applications. *Telemed J E Health.* 2000;6:297–302.

46. Licurse MY, Kim SH, Kim W, et al. Comparison of diagnostic accuracy of plain film radiographs between original film and smartphone capture: a pilot study. *J Digit Imag* 2015;28:646–653.

47. Khodaie M, Askari A, Bahaadinbeigy K. Evaluation of a very low-cost and simple teleradiology technique. *J Digit Imag* 2015;28:295–301.

48. Digital Imaging and Communications in Medicine (DICOM). *Part 14: Grayscale Standard Display Function.* Rosslyn, VA: National Electrical Manufacturers Association; 2004.

49. Pianykh O. *Digital Imaging and Communications in Medicine (DICOM): A Practical Introduction and Survival Guide.* New York, NY: Springer; 2012.

50. Badano A, Revie C, Casertano A, et al. Consistency and standardization of color in medical images: a consensus report. *J Digit Imag* 2015;28:41–52.

51. Roth CJ, Lannum LM, Dennison DK, et al. The current state and path for enterprise image viewing: HIMSS-SIIM collaborative white paper. *J Digit Imag* 2016;29:567–573.

52. Thrall JH. Teleradiology. Part II. Limitations, risks, and opportunities. *Radiol* 2007;244:325–328.

53. Thrall JH. Teleradiology: two-edged sword or friend of radiology practice? *J Am Coll Radiol* 2009;6:73–75.

54. Bradley WG. Special focus—outsourcing after hours radiology—another point of view: use of a nighthawk service in an academic radiology department. *J Am Coll Radiol* 2007;4:675–677.

55. Bradley WG. Off-site teleradiology: the pros. *Radiol* 2008;248:337–341.

56. Boland GW. Teleradiology coming of age: winners and losers. *Am J Roentgenol* 2008;190:1161–1162.

57. Brant-Zawadzki M. The goose and the nighthawk: a bedtime fable for young radiologists (with apologies to the Brothers Grimm). *J Am Coll Radiol* 2006;3:231–232.

58. Levin DC, Rao VM. Outsourcing to teleradiology companies: bad for radiology, bad for radiologists. *J Am Coll Radiol* 2011;8:104–108.

59. Kaye AH, Forman HP, Kapoor R, et al. A survey of radiology practices' use of after-hours radiology services. *J Am Coll Radiol* 2008;5:748–758.

60. Sherry CS. Outsourcing off-hour imaging services. *J Am Coll Radiol* 2010;7:222–223.

61. Lewis RS, Sunshine JH, Bhargavan M. Radiology practices' use of external off-hours teleradiology services in 2007 and changes since 2003. *Am J Roentgenol* 2009;19:1333–1339.

62. Gunderman R, Dodson S. Is it time for radiology to embrace commoditization? *J Am Coll Radiol* 2016;13:754–755.

63. Hunter TB, Krupinski EA, Weinstein RS. Factors in the selection of a teleradiology provider in the United States. *J Telemed Telecare* 2013;19:354–359.

64. European Society of Radiology. ESR white paper on teleradiology: an update from the teleradiology subgroup. *Insights Imaging* 2014;5:1–8.

65. Silva E, Breslau J, Barr RM, et al. ACR white paper on teleradiology practice: a report from the Task Force on Teleradiology Practice. *J Am Coll Radiol* 2013;10:575–585.

66. Raenschaert ER, Boland G, Duerinckx AJ. Comparison of European (ESR) and American (ACR) white papers on teleradiology: patient primacy is paramount. *J Am Coll Radiol* 2015;12:174–182.

67. American Colege of Radiology: Teleradiology (Federal Level). http://www.acr.org/Advocacy/Legislative-Issues/Teleradiology. Accessed October 4, 2016.

68. American Colege of Radiology: Report of the ACR Task Force on International Teleradiology. http://www.acr.org/Membership/Legal-Business-Practices/Telemedicine-Teleradiology/Report-of-the-ACR-Task-Force-on-International-Teleradiology. Accessed October 4, 2016.

69. Major J. Telemedicine room design. *J Telemed Telecare* 2005;11:10–14.

70. Thompson AC, Kremer MJ, Biswal S, et al. Factors associated with repetitive strain, and strategies to reduce injury among breast-imaging radiologists. *J Am Coll Radiol* 2014;11:1074–1079.

71. Rodrigues JCL, Morgan S, Augustine K, et al. Musculoskeletal symptoms amongst clinical radiologists and the implications of reporting environment ergonomics – a multicenter questionnaire study. *J Digit Imag* 2014;27;255–261.

72. Krupinski EA, Berbaum KS. Measurement of visual strain in radiologists. *Acad Radiol* 2009;16:947–950.

73. Krupinski EA, Berbaum KS, Caldwell RT, et al. Long radiology workdays reduce detection and accommodation accuracy. *J Am Coll Radiol* 2010;7:698–704.

74. Krupinski EA, MacKinnon L, Reiner BI. Feasibility of using a biowatch to monitor GSR as a measure of radiologists' stress and fatigue. *Proc SPIE Med Imag* 2015;9416:941613.

75. Krupinski EA, Berbaum KS, Caldwell RT, et al. Do long radiology workdays affect nodule detection in dynamic CT interpretation? *J Am Coll Radiol* 2012;9:191–198.

76. Taylor-Phillips S, Elze MC, Krupinski EA, et al. Retrospective review of the drop in observer detection performance over time in lesion-enriched experimental studies. *J Digital Imag* 2015;28:32–40.

77. Occupational and Safety Health Administration Computer Workstations eTool. https://www.osha.gov/SLTC/etools/computerworkstations/. Accessed September 15, 2016.

78. Hoffmann JC, Mittal S, Hoffmann CH, et al. Combating the health risks of sedentary behavior in the contemporary radiology reading room. *Am J Roentgen* 2016;206:1135–1140.

Clinical Services— Adult

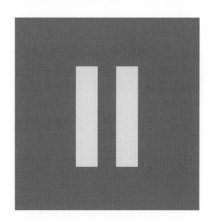

Telestroke

Andrew M. Southerland, MD, MSc, Nina J. Solenski, MD
and Lee H. Schwamm, MD

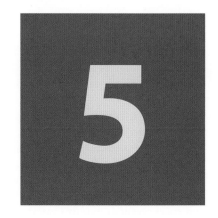

CASE STUDY

Mr. Taylor is a 45-year-old man enjoying a summer vacation camping in rural southwest Virginia. He has been enjoying hiking and swimming with his wife and two young daughters for the last two days. Today at 5:25 P.M., his wife finds him in their tent "slumped over" with incomprehensible speech. She had just talked to him no more than 10 minutes prior and he seemed fine. She sees that his right side is paralyzed and immediately knows he needs emergency help. Emergency medical services (EMS) are summoned by the clerk at the park entrance. Mr. Taylor is lifted into the ambulance to be transported to the nearest hospital, which is a small 16-bed critical access hospital serving the surrounding rural area. During ambulance transport, the EMS provider identifies the patient as having a potential "stroke" using a validated prehospital stroke scale. Under a new protocol, the EMS provider connects with a telestroke neurologist at a regional academic medical center using a mounted tablet with 4G LTE connectivity. The neurologist reviews the history, medications, and vital signs with EMS and performs the NIH Stroke Scale (NIHSS). The neurologist's assessment suggests a severe stroke that may be eligible for thrombolytic treatment and perhaps a large vessel occlusion that may warrant endovascular therapy with clot retrieval. This information is relayed to the local emergency department physicians.

Upon arrival to the hospital, Mr. Taylor is rapidly taken to the computed tomography (CT) scanner, and the images are digitally transferred to the hub hospital's radiology server. A videoconference telemedicine cart is placed at the foot of the bed, and the telestroke consulting neurologist rapidly repeats the NIHSS to confirm the deficits. She discusses her findings with the patient's wife, explaining that he is a good candidate for the clot-busting drug, intravenous tissue plasminogen activator (tPA), and recommends immediate treatment. The tPA is administered at 6:35 P.M., 80 minutes since Mr. Taylor was last seen normal. The neurologist has notified the on-call interventional neuroradiologist at the hub hospital. Using multipoint videoconferencing, they discuss the patient's neurovascular imaging, including a CT angiogram that demonstrates an abrupt "cut-off" sign indicating an embolus in the left middle cerebral artery. The emergency department (ED) physician, the neurologist, and the interventionalist discuss with the patient's family by live videoconferencing and recommend that Mr. Taylor be air-lifted to the hub stroke center for immediate clot retrieval. Mr. Taylor successfully undergoes the procedure and is able to discharge to home with minimal neurological deficits several days later. He is independent and back to work at 3 months.

INTRODUCTION

The paradigm of acute stroke care shifted in the 1990s with the approval of intravenous (IV) tPA, rendering stroke a time-sensitive condition requiring rapid availability of neurological expertise.[1] For many hospitals and communities unable to provide continual stroke expertise, particularly in rural and underserved areas,[2,3] the emerging practice of telemedicine offered a virtual bridge to support rapid tPA decision making between centrally based consultants and remote-access patients and emergency providers. This concept was crystalized with the term *telestroke* in 1999 by Levine and Gorman.[4,5]

Over the past two decades, telestroke systems of care have expanded to take a prominent role in the practice of stroke medicine in the United States, Europe, and around the world. According to a 2009 nationwide survey, there were over 50 active telestroke programs in the United States, predominantly serving small and rural hospitals, but this number has undoubtedly grown over the past 5 years (Figure 5-1).[6] Additionally, numerous for-profit telestroke companies have cropped up in recent years, producing a nationwide network of independent teleconsultants and blurring the traditional geographic demarcations of regional stroke care. Moreover, advances in acute stroke treatment, including the recently established prominence of endovascular therapy (EVT) for severely affected patients with large vessel occlusions (LVO),[7] have

placed a renewed premium on the role of telemedicine to help restructure our stroke systems of care. In this way, telestroke models are being explored to facilitate better interfacility access to endovascular services, and in the prehospital setting, to guide earlier diagnosis and triage decisions.

In this chapter, we highlight both the established aspects of telestroke care and burgeoning concepts in its ongoing evolution. We will explore various telestroke models and modalities, traditional and emerging technology, the underlying evidence base, financial and regulatory considerations, quality of care and limitations, and relevant guidelines and statements on the practice of telestroke. Of note, we will not cover applications of telestroke in subacute or chronic care, including stroke telerehabilitation and preventive telestroke services in the ambulatory setting, both of which could be expounded upon in their own form.

From this chapter, we hope that readers will not only learn the practical tenets of stroke telemedicine, but also appreciate the unique and pivotal role of telestroke in the wider world of telehealth.

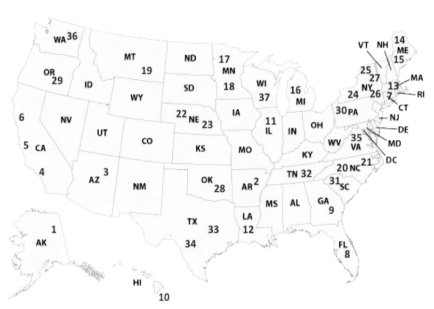

▲ **Figure 5-1.** 2009 nationwide survey of U.S. telestroke programs, with 38 of 56 active telestroke programs participating. (Published with permission from Silva GS, Farrell S, Shandra E, et al. The status of telestroke in the United States: a survey of currently active stroke telemedicine programs. *Stroke* 2012;43(8):2078–2085.)

THE TELESTROKE CONSULTATION

Performing a high-quality telestroke consultation requires a real-time virtual partnership between the consultant neurologist at the hub and the emergency room staff at the spoke facility. Although the technology to support this interaction must be reliable and secure, it is the personal connection between the tele-provider, telepresenter, and the patient that serves as the foundation for a successful telestroke encounter. The Star Telehealth Alliance offers certification training for bedside telepresenters assisting during acute telestroke encounters and can be accessed at the following link: http://www.startelehealth.org/.

The principal features of the acute telestroke consultation include:

– Establish a remote audiovisual (AV) link

– Obtain a brief history, including key elements such as "time of last known well"

– Perform the NIHSS with the assistance of a local telepresenter (Figure 5-2)

– Review initial brain imaging, typically a noncontrast head CT via teleradiology

– Determine eligibility for IV tPA or other acute stroke treatments

– Offer guidance for further management or transfer to a higher level of care (eg, *drip and ship*)

– Provide feedback to the spoke facility and emergency medical team

Although the telestroke evaluation has proven reliable for performing the standardized NIHSS, it is not validated in nonstroke diagnoses or as a substitute for the full neurological exam. For instance, in the absence of a neurologically trained telepresenter, visual observation alone is not reliable for complex visual field testing, manual assessment of tone and motor strength, obtaining reflexes, distinguishing fine sensory modalities, and additional bedside maneuvers (eg, vestibular testing, discerning organic from nonorganic findings).

In some large series, up to 20% of patients treated with IV tPA receive a nonstroke discharge diagnosis.[8] However, the challenge of treating stroke mimics was no different between telestroke and face-to-face encounters.[9] More common stroke mimics include migraine headaches with neurological accompaniments, seizures, metabolic/toxic/infectious encephalopathies, mass effect, reactivation of old stroke symptoms/signs, and psychogenic etiologies. In an attempt to minimize treating mimics during complex, time-critical telestroke evaluations, the TeleStroke Mimic Score (TM-Score) was devised.[10] The score is based on factors independently associated with stroke mimic status, including age, medical history (eg, atrial fibrillation, hypertension, seizures), facial weakness, and NIHSS >14. The TM-Score performed well on receiver operator curve (ROC) analysis (internal validation area under curve = 0.71, external validation area under curve = 0.77) and perhaps should be utilized more often in acute telestroke evaluations.

MODALITIES/MODELS

There are a variety of telestroke clinical care models, including hospital-based hub and spoke, for-profit telemedicine company based, hub and spoke, hubless private practice physicians, and multipoint telestroke consults (Figure 5-3).[6]

The "hub and spoke" model is the traditional telemedicine model, with the hub consisting of the providing consulting hospital, and the "spoke" the network of hospitals that the providers service. The hub is either a Joint Commission–certified Primary Stroke Center or a certified larger Comprehensive Stroke Center tertiary care medical center. This model is well suited for either nonprofit or for-profit medical systems of care.

The for-profit telemedicine company-based model is in essence a spoke and hub model, with the hub being the company but the provider pool decentralized and consisting of physicians across the United States with service also rendered from homes, offices, or other site. Another model, the "hubless private practice physicians," has been gaining in popularity, particularly with physicians who are contracted by a hospital system or are practicing in an urban setting. Leaving a busy office practice in the middle of the day to cover an emergency stroke care call is not practical for patient care. Instead, in this model the practice uses an office-based telestroke program to efficiently see stroke consultations in the ED. These four models can be used for either acute or nonacute consultation, in a variety of settings, from the ED, to neurological intensive care units (ICUs), to inpatient wards, or community health centers.

N I H
STROKE
SCALE

Patient Identification. ___ ___-___ ___ ___-___ ___ ___

Pt. Date of Birth ___ ___/___ ___/___ ___

Hospital _____(___ ___-___ ___)

Date of Exam ___ ___/___ ___/___ ___

Interval: [ ] Baseline   [ ] 2 hours post treatment   [ ] 24 hours post onset of symptoms ±20 minutes   [ ] 7-10 days
         [ ] 3 months   [ ] Other _____(___ ___)

Time: ___ ___:___ ___   [ ]am [ ]pm

Person Administering Scale _____

Administer stroke scale items in the order listed. Record performance in each category after each subscale exam. Do not go back and change scores. Follow directions provided for each exam technique. Scores should reflect what the patient does, not what the clinician thinks the patient can do. The clinician should record answers while administering the exam and work quickly. Except where indicated, the patient should not be coached (i.e., repeated requests to patient to make a special effort).

Instructions	Scale Definition	Score
1a. Level of Consciousness: The investigator must choose a response if a full evaluation is prevented by such obstacles as an endotracheal tube, language barrier, orotracheal trauma/bandages. A 3 is scored only if the patient makes no movement (other than reflexive posturing) in response to noxious stimulation.	0 = **Alert;** keenly responsive. 1 = **Not alert**; but arousable by minor stimulation to obey, answer, or respond. 2 = **Not alert**; requires repeated stimulation to attend, or is obtunded and requires strong or painful stimulation to make movements (not stereotyped). 3 = Responds only with reflex motor or autonomic effects or totally unresponsive, flaccid, and areflexic.	_____
1b. LOC Questions: The patient is asked the month and his/her age. The answer must be correct - there is no partial credit for being close. Aphasic and stuporous patients who do not comprehend the questions will score 2. Patients unable to speak because of endotracheal intubation, orotracheal trauma, severe dysarthria from any cause, language barrier, or any other problem not secondary to aphasia are given a 1. It is important that only the initial answer be graded and that the examiner not "help" the patient with verbal or non-verbal cues.	0 = **Answers** both questions correctly. 1 = **Answers** one question correctly. 2 = **Answers** neither question correctly.	_____
1c. LOC Commands: The patient is asked to open and close the eyes and then to grip and release the non-paretic hand. Substitute another one step command if the hands cannot be used. Credit is given if an unequivocal attempt is made but not completed due to weakness. If the patient does not respond to command, the task should be demonstrated to him or her (pantomime), and the result scored (i.e., follows none, one or two commands). Patients with trauma, amputation, or other physical impediments should be given suitable one-step commands. Only the first attempt is scored.	0 = **Performs** both tasks correctly. 1 = **Performs** one task correctly. 2 = **Performs** neither task correctly.	_____
2. Best Gaze: Only horizontal eye movements will be tested. Voluntary or reflexive (oculocephalic) eye movements will be scored, but caloric testing is not done. If the patient has a conjugate deviation of the eyes that can be overcome by voluntary or reflexive activity, the score will be 1. If a patient has an isolated peripheral nerve paresis (CN III, IV or VI), score a 1. Gaze is testable in all aphasic patients. Patients with ocular trauma, bandages, pre-existing blindness, or other disorder of visual acuity or fields should be tested with reflexive movements, and a choice made by the investigator. Establishing eye contact and then moving about the patient from side to side will occasionally clarify the presence of a partial gaze palsy.	0 = **Normal.** 1 = **Partial gaze palsy;** gaze is abnormal in one or both eyes, but forced deviation or total gaze paresis is not present. 2 = **Forced deviation,** or total gaze paresis not overcome by the oculocephalic maneuver.	_____

Rev 10/1/2003

▲ **Figure 5-2.** The National Institutes of Health Stroke Scale.

N I H
STROKE
SCALE

Patient Identification. ___ ___-___ ___ ___-___ ___ ___

Pt. Date of Birth ___ ___/___ ___/___ ___

Hospital _____(___ ___-___ ___)

Date of Exam ___ ___/___ ___/___ ___

Interval: [ ] Baseline   [ ] 2 hours post treatment   [ ] 24 hours post onset of symptoms ±20 minutes   [ ] 7-10 days
[ ] 3 months   [ ] Other _____(___ ___)

3. Visual: Visual fields (upper and lower quadrants) are tested by confrontation, using finger counting or visual threat, as appropriate. Patients may be encouraged, but if they look at the side of the moving fingers appropriately, this can be scored as normal. If there is unilateral blindness or enucleation, visual fields in the remaining eye are scored. Score 1 only if a clear-cut asymmetry, including quadrantanopia, is found. If patient is blind from any cause, score 3. Double simultaneous stimulation is performed at this point. If there is extinction, patient receives a 1, and the results are used to respond to item 11.	0 = **No visual loss.** 1 = **Partial hemianopia.** 2 = **Complete hemianopia.** 3 = **Bilateral hemianopia** (blind including cortical blindness).	_____
4. Facial Palsy: Ask – or use pantomime to encourage – the patient to show teeth or raise eyebrows and close eyes. Score symmetry of grimace in response to noxious stimuli in the poorly responsive or non-comprehending patient. If facial trauma/bandages, orotracheal tube, tape or other physical barriers obscure the face, these should be removed to the extent possible.	0 = **Normal** symmetrical movements. 1 = **Minor paralysis** (flattened nasolabial fold, asymmetry on smiling). 2 = **Partial paralysis** (total or near-total paralysis of lower face). 3 = **Complete paralysis** of one or both sides (absence of facial movement in the upper and lower face).	_____
5. Motor Arm: The limb is placed in the appropriate position: extend the arms (palms down) 90 degrees (if sitting) or 45 degrees (if supine). Drift is scored if the arm falls before 10 seconds. The aphasic patient is encouraged using urgency in the voice and pantomime, but not noxious stimulation. Each limb is tested in turn, beginning with the non-paretic arm. Only in the case of amputation or joint fusion at the shoulder, the examiner should record the score as untestable (UN), and clearly write the explanation for this choice.	0 = **No drift;** limb holds 90 (or 45) degrees for full 10 seconds. 1 = **Drift;** limb holds 90 (or 45) degrees, but drifts down before full 10 seconds; does not hit bed or other support. 2 = **Some effort against gravity;** limb cannot get to or maintain (if cued) 90 (or 45) degrees, drifts down to bed, but has some effort against gravity. 3 = **No effort against gravity;** limb falls. 4 = **No movement.** UN = **Amputation** or joint fusion, explain: _____ **5a. Left Arm** **5b. Right Arm**	 _____ _____
6. Motor Leg: The limb is placed in the appropriate position: hold the leg at 30 degrees (always tested supine). Drift is scored if the leg falls before 5 seconds. The aphasic patient is encouraged using urgency in the voice and pantomime, but not noxious stimulation. Each limb is tested in turn, beginning with the non-paretic leg. Only in the case of amputation or joint fusion at the hip, the examiner should record the score as untestable (UN), and clearly write the explanation for this choice.	0 = **No drift;** leg holds 30-degree position for full 5 seconds. 1 = **Drift;** leg falls by the end of the 5-second period but does not hit bed. 2 = **Some effort against gravity;** leg falls to bed by 5 seconds, but has some effort against gravity. 3 = **No effort against gravity;** leg falls to bed immediately. 4 = **No movement.** UN = **Amputation** or joint fusion, explain: _____ **6a. Left Leg** **6b. Right Leg**	 _____

Rev 10/1/2003

▲ **Figure 5-2.** (*Continued*)

N I H
STROKE
SCALE

Patient Identification. ___ ___-___ ___ ___-___ ___ ___

Pt. Date of Birth ___ ___/___ ___/___ ___

Hospital _____(___ ___-___ ___)

Date of Exam ___ ___/___ ___/___ ___

Interval: [ ] Baseline   [ ] 2 hours post treatment   [ ] 24 hours post onset of symptoms ±20 minutes   [ ] 7-10 days
        [ ] 3 months   [ ] Other _____(___ ___)

7. Limb Ataxia: This item is aimed at finding evidence of a unilateral cerebellar lesion. Test with eyes open. In case of visual defect, ensure testing is done in intact visual field. The finger-nose-finger and heel-shin tests are performed on both sides, and ataxia is scored only if present out of proportion to weakness. Ataxia is absent in the patient who cannot understand or is paralyzed. Only in the case of amputation or joint fusion, the examiner should record the score as untestable (UN), and clearly write the explanation for this choice. In case of blindness, test by having the patient touch nose from extended arm position.	0 = **Absent.** 1 = **Present in one limb.** 2 = **Present in two limbs.** UN = **Amputation** or joint fusion, explain: _____	_____
8. Sensory: Sensation or grimace to pinprick when tested, or withdrawal from noxious stimulus in the obtunded or aphasic patient. Only sensory loss attributed to stroke is scored as abnormal and the examiner should test as many body areas (arms [not hands], legs, trunk, face) as needed to accurately check for hemisensory loss. A score of 2, "severe or total sensory loss," should only be given when a severe or total loss of sensation can be clearly demonstrated. Stuporous and aphasic patients will, therefore, probably score 1 or 0. The patient with brainstem stroke who has bilateral loss of sensation is scored 2. If the patient does not respond and is quadriplegic, score 2. Patients in a coma (item 1a=3) are automatically given a 2 on this item.	0 = **Normal;** no sensory loss. 1 = **Mild-to-moderate sensory loss;** patient feels pinprick is less sharp or is dull on the affected side; or there is a loss of superficial pain with pinprick, but patient is aware of being touched. 2 = **Severe to total sensory loss;** patient is not aware of being touched in the face, arm, and leg.	_____
9. Best Language: A great deal of information about comprehension will be obtained during the preceding sections of the examination. For this scale item, the patient is asked to describe what is happening in the attached picture, to name the items on the attached naming sheet and to read from the attached list of sentences. Comprehension is judged from responses here, as well as to all of the commands in the preceding general neurological exam. If visual loss interferes with the tests, ask the patient to identify objects placed in the hand, repeat, and produce speech. The intubated patient should be asked to write. The patient in a coma (item 1a=3) will automatically score 3 on this item. The examiner must choose a score for the patient with stupor or limited cooperation, but a score of 3 should be used only if the patient is mute and follows no one-step commands.	0 = **No aphasia;** normal. 1 = **Mild-to-moderate aphasia;** some obvious loss of fluency or facility of comprehension, without significant limitation on ideas expressed or form of expression. Reduction of speech and/or comprehension, however, makes conversation about provided materials difficult or impossible. For example, in conversation about provided materials, examiner can identify picture or naming card content from patient's response. 2 = **Severe aphasia;** all communication is through fragmentary expression; great need for inference, questioning, and guessing by the listener. Range of information that can be exchanged is limited; listener carries burden of communication. Examiner cannot identify materials provided from patient response. 3 = **Mute, global aphasia;** no usable speech or auditory comprehension.	_____
10. Dysarthria: If patient is thought to be normal, an adequate sample of speech must be obtained by asking patient to read or repeat words from the attached list. If the patient has severe aphasia, the clarity of articulation of spontaneous speech can be rated. Only if the patient is intubated or has other physical barriers to producing speech, the examiner should record the score as untestable (UN), and clearly write an explanation for this choice. Do not tell the patient why he or she is being tested.	0 = **Normal.** 1 = **Mild-to-moderate dysarthria;** patient slurs at least some words and, at worst, can be understood with some difficulty. 2 = **Severe dysarthria;** patient's speech is so slurred as to be unintelligible in the absence of or out of proportion to any dysphasia, or is mute/anarthric. UN = **Intubated** or other physical barrier, explain:_____	_____

Rev 10/1/2003

▲ **Figure 5-2.** (*Continued*)

N I H
STROKE
SCALE

Patient Identification. ___ ___-___ ___ ___-___ ___

Pt. Date of Birth ___ ___/___ ___/___ ___

Hospital _____(___ ___-___ ___)

Date of Exam ___ ___/___ ___/___ ___

Interval: [ ] Baseline   [ ] 2 hours post treatment   [ ] 24 hours post onset of symptoms ±20 minutes   [ ] 7-10 days
         [ ] 3 months   [ ] Other _____(___ ___)

11. Extinction and Inattention (formerly Neglect): Sufficient information to identify neglect may be obtained during the prior testing. If the patient has a severe visual loss preventing visual double simultaneous stimulation, and the cutaneous stimuli are normal, the score is normal. If the patient has aphasia but does appear to attend to both sides, the score is normal. The presence of visual spatial neglect or anosagnosia may also be taken as evidence of abnormality. Since the abnormality is scored only if present, the item is never untestable.	0 = **No abnormality.** 1 = **Visual, tactile, auditory, spatial, or personal inattention** or extinction to bilateral simultaneous stimulation in one of the sensory modalities. 2 = **Profound hemi-inattention or extinction to more than one modality;** does not recognize own hand or orients to only one side of space.	_____

Rev 10/1/2003

▲ **Figure 5-2.** (*Continued*)

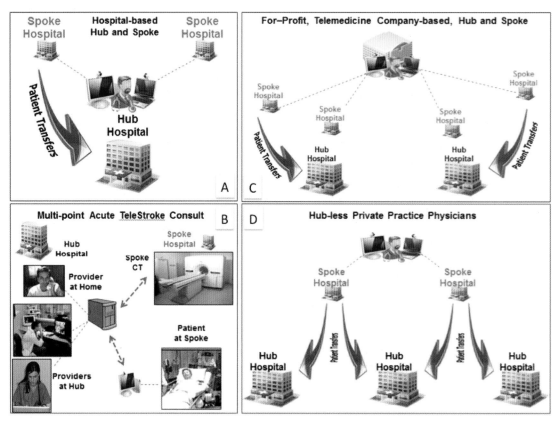

▲ Figure 5-3. Various models of telestroke systems. **A.** Traditional hub and spoke. **B.** Multipoint consultation. **C.** For-profit company consultant based. **D.** Hubless private practice consultant based. (Published with permission from Silva GS, Farrell S, Shandra E, et al. The status of telestroke in the United States: a survey of currently active stroke telemedicine programs. *Stroke* 2012;43(8):2078–2085.)

Focusing on acute telestroke consultation in the hub and spoke model, the primary goal is to provide neurological support for the local ED physicians in determining eligibility for IV thrombolysis or IV tPA. In this scenario, acute stroke patients are often treated locally and then transferred to the hub or another primary stroke center for further inpatient or ICU management. This model has been dubbed "drip and ship," and observational studies suggest improved outcomes for patients transferred to a higher level of care at certified stroke centers compared to those who remain at the initiating facility.[11–13]

▶ Emerging Models

A burgeoning model of telestroke advances care to the prehospital setting, facilitating remote neurological consultation with EMS providers prior to hospital arrival. The 2009 AHA/ASA *Review of the Evidence for the Use of Telemedicine Within Stroke Systems of Care* addressed the possibility of ambulance-based telestroke by stating, "It is clear that existing technology can provide some degree of interactive video and audio communication with preshoptial units in transport, although current published applications have unacceptably low frame rates, and broad application of this technology to large fleets of EMS vehicles is not yet practical … The usefulness of this intervention in real practice is uncertain, and further research is required."[14]

Although the concept of mobile or ambulance-based telestroke dates to the late 1990s with the TeleBAT pilot studies,[15–17] feasibility has improved in the last several years with the rapid evolution in mobile, or m-health, technologies and high-fidelity 4G cellular connectivity to support real-time AV streaming,[18-22] Efforts to make prehospital telestroke more practical using tablet-based endpoints and low-cost, off-the-shelf components have been demonstrated in both rural and urban EMS networks, including the *Improving Treatment with Rapid Evaluation of Acute Stroke Using Mobile Telemedicine (iTREAT) Study*.[23-26] Pilot trials of ambulance-based telestroke suggest the possibility of faster stroke treatment times,[27] and future trials will seek to translate technical feasibility into improved clinical outcomes.

The prehospital telestroke model has been taken a step further with the development of so-called "mobile stroke units," customized ambulances equipped with a portable CT scanner and other advanced diagnostics, with the capability of administering IV thrombolysis in the field.[28-31] Although effective in significantly reducing stroke onset to treatment times, these units have primarily been deployed in urban or suburban EMS networks with limited coverage areas, and cost utility remains a barrier to widespread adoption and generalizability across health systems.[32] Nonetheless, telemedicine and teleradiology may help streamline efficient mobile stroke unit deployment.[33-35] Mobile stroke units could also enhance prehospital diagnosis and select triage for patients with LVO to facilities capable of providing EVT,[36,37] but further research and systems-of-care considerations are needed.

TECHNOLOGIES

At its inception in the 1990s, a telestroke consult required that the physician use a fixed workstation and in some cases a second computer for documentation of the encounter or reviewing films. However, because the "time is brain" concept mandates instant access to the patient for a rapid evaluation for potential therapy, this was not an ideal 24/7 telestroke model.

Telemedicine workstations continue to exist in the hospital or physician's office, but are complemented by more mobile technology options such as laptops, tablets, and smart phones. Cloud-based technology (circa 2006) facilitated doing telestroke consultations using these mobile technologies. Consultations can be provided wherever there is a secure Internet connection and via "hot spot"–generating cellular connections. These advances allow the provider significant access to web-based tools for documentation, imaging, and electronic medical records review.

Furthermore, telestroke-tailored, software-bundled applications allow for live video consultation (VC) encounters, with the consultation documentation and the HCT imaging for review, all into one convenient screen. The development of "multipoint" capacity, having more than two terminals connected by a single communications channel, allows for two or more physicians to join the VC encounter and confer on the clinical case. For example, the neurointerventionalist can enter the call to discuss the candidacy of a patient with the stroke neurologist "live" and directly with the ED physician, the patient, and/or their family.

▶ Brain/Vascular Imaging Transfer (Teleradiology)

First conceived in 1982, Picture Archiving and Communication Systems (PACS) is a medical imaging-based technology that provides convenient access to images from multiple modalities. PACS allows electronic images and reports to be rapidly transmitted digitally via a PACS link. In the United States, the University of Kansas developed one of the first PACS, and the University of California Los Angeles deployed pilot PACS in their pediatric radiology department. The first filmless fully digital radiology department using PACS was in the Danube Hospital in Vienna in 1991. The current PACS is critical for fast interpretation of head CT scans in the evaluation of the stroke patient who may qualify for the time-sensitive thrombolytic TPA. Today, most PACS can be accessed securely using cellular or Internet connections.

Telestroke patient imaging includes an emergency noncontrast CT brain scan to identify any intracranial hemorrhage (which is a contraindication for thrombolytic treatment). In selected cases, CT angiography of the head and neck, brain magnetic resonance imaging (MRI), and/or magnetic resonance (MR) angiography are obtained. A newer modality, a multiphase CT, has been used to assist in the selection of patients who may benefit from thrombectomy. This technique generates time-resolved cerebral angiograms of brain vasculature from the skull base to the vertex in three phases after contrast material injection. By evaluating the potential for collateral vessels at the later phases, the teleprovider can better predict outcome.

VC equipment has advanced tremendously since the first "peer to peer" VC device proposed by AT&T at the New York's World's Fair in the 1960s. The technology improved with the introduction of the Network Video Protocol, and in the 1980s, the availability of digital transmission of voice and video by electrical pulses, through the Integrated Services Digital Network. In 1991, IBM introduced the first personal computer VC product, followed by Multipoint VC by Apple Macintosh. In 1995 the first VC occurred internationally between North America and Africa. During this time frame, high-capacity broadband services and more powerful computing processors followed high-definition systems, "icloud" applications, and lower-cost video-capturing technologies, leading to today's highly sophisticated VC equipment and systems. A critical shift occurred from company-based proprietary equipment and software to standards based technology. The Unified Communications Interoperability Forum (UCIF), a nonprofit alliance between communications vendors, was launched in May 2010. The UCIF created VC standards and protocols to ensure interoperability regardless of the platform.

Telestroke VC equipment requires the ability to perform an observational bedside assessment that includes components of alertness and cognition, vision, speech, motor, sensory, and coordination (ie, NIHSS). Optimally the system has a high-definition, remote-controlled video camera with a "pan-tilt" and zoom capability, or "PTZ," camera. In addition, omnidirectional microphones are essential for quality sound transmission.

Current Internet speeds can easily handle transmission of most radiological images required to evaluate the patient. Cellular 4G (50 Mbps download/350 Mps upload), broadband wireless (600 Mbps – 2007), and LAN/fiber-optics (10 Gbs – 2010) will undoubtedly continue to advance in the future. Initiatives to expand the footprint for telemedicine include federal programs, such as the FCC's *Connect America Fund* (https://www.fcc.gov/encyclopedia/connecting-america) and HRSA's regional funding of Telehealth Resource Centers (http://www.telehealthresourcecenter.org).

The evolution of mobile media, or m-health, will also shape the future application of mobile technologies in telestroke.[38] Telestroke assessments have been validated across a range of mobile endpoints, including smart phones and tablet-based devices.[39–41] Advances in mobile imaging may lead to the ability to evaluate brain hemorrhage using handheld devices in the future.[42]

Regarding security, telestroke providers must ensure that telemedicine networks are secure and encrypted. Although this is crucial, doing so without compromising the real-time flow of voice and video is challenging. The American Telemedicine Association has issued guidelines for a variety of subspecialties, and currently, FIPS 140-2, known as the Federal Information Processing Standard, is the U.S. government security standard used to accredit software encryption standards and lists encryption techniques such as AES (Advanced Encryption Standard) as providing acceptable levels of security.[43] All providers must use extreme caution and restraint in using personal devices to provide clinical care.

SUMMARY EVIDENCE/LITERATURE

To date, only a few prospective randomized and comparative trials have assessed the clinical efficacy of telestroke intervention. The Stroke Team Remote Evaluation Using a Digital Observation Camera (STRokE DOC) trial randomized acute stroke patients at four remote spoke sites (n = 222) to AV telestroke (intervention) versus telephone-only consultation (control), with the primary outcome of accuracy for thrombolysis treatment decision as assessed by masked central adjudication. The trial was stopped early for superiority of video-based telestroke with an absolute difference in correct decision making of 16% favoring the intervention (98% versus 82% correct; odds ratio [OR], 10.9; 95% confidence interval [CI], 2.7–44.69; p = 0.0009).[44] Although the trial failed to show any difference in clinical outcomes between the two groups, the study was not powered for these secondary measures.

The STRokE DOC AZ TIME trial was a follow-up study conducted in a single-hub, two-spoke system in rural Arizona. Using similar methods and patient selection (n = 54), there were no differences between AV telestroke and telephone-only consultation regarding thrombolysis decision making; however, the intervention was limited by technical issues (74%).[45] A pooled analysis from the STRokE DOC trials further supported the efficacy of AV telestroke versus telephone-only consultation to enhance decision making for thrombolysis eligibility (96% versus 83% correct; OR, 4.2; 95% CI, 1.7–10.5; p = 0.002), but results were driven largely by data from the original trial.[46]

From the Telemedic Project for Integrative Stroke Care (TEMPiS) network in Bavaria, Germany, a non-randomized, open-label study found that patients treated in network hospitals were less likely to have a poor outcome (moderate to severe disability) at 90 days compared to out-of-network community hospitals (OR 0.62, 95% CI 0.52–0.74; p < 0.0001).[47] Review of the longitudinal experience in this network demonstrated sustained benefit in increased proportion of acute stroke patients receiving IV thrombolysis, reduction in median treatment times, and improved clinical outcomes.[48,49] Similar observational results have been reported from numerous retrospective cohorts and case series.[50]

Supplementing the limited number of comparative telestroke trials is a robust body of literature supporting the feasibility and generalizability of telestroke in practice. Fundamentally, numerous studies have confirmed the interrater reliability of performing the NIHSS via remote, real-time AV consultation, although some components are less reliable than others.[51–53] NIHSS reliability has further been confirmed across multiple telemedicine endpoints, including smart phone and tablet devices as previously mentioned.[39,40,41,54,]

Several studies have assessed the level of agreement for head CT interpretation in the telestroke encounter, essential to acute management and determination for thrombolysis eligibility.[55,56] A pooled analysis of data from the STRokE DOC trials (n = 261) found excellent agreement in head CT interpretation between spoke radiologists and hub neurologists (95.4%, kappa = 0.74, 95% CI 0.59–0.88).[57] Additionally, at least one other observational study found no difference in final diagnosis of stroke, confirmed by brain imaging, in thrombolysis-treated patients at the telestroke hub versus spoke hospitals.[58]

In addition to studies supporting the practice of telestroke in a hub and spoke model, emphasis has focused on telestroke systems of care to improve access to treatment and neurological expertise in rural and underserved areas.[59–62] In 2014, the Health Resources and Services Administration (HRSA) announced grants worth more than $22 million to support health care in rural areas, including funds to improve emergency services. The HRSA "Evidence-Based Tele-Emergency Network Program" was created to determine the effectiveness of tele-emergency care for rural patients and providers, including telestroke care.

In the Rural "EQUITe" Project, designed to evaluate the effectiveness of telestroke to improve access and timeliness of treatment for rural patients in Virginia, data were pooled from 46 rural hospitals encompassing 3,257 emergency telestroke consults.[63] Nineteen percent of patients were treated with tPA, and the majority (73%) were treated within 3 hours from the time of last known normal. In the majority of cases, the median "door-to-needle" time was 83 minutes, and about a fourth of the patients received tPA in less than or equal to 60 minutes from their arrival to the ED. Although this was in many cases an improvement from pre-telestroke benchmarks, it revealed that systems improvements were needed to augment the efficiency of the telestroke encounter at many of these rural hospitals.

As the treatment of acute ischemic stroke has evolved with evidence supporting EVT for select patients, there is a dire need to improve stroke systems of care capable of rapid identification and triage between first-arrival spoke hospitals and endovascular-capable facilities.[64] Although observational experience suggests these processes may be enhanced by telestroke systems,[65] further research is needed to examine the impact of telestroke in the endovascular era.

REIMBURSEMENT/LEGAL/REGULATORY/ LICENSING-RELATED ISSUES

Telestroke shares the same barriers in reimbursement, regulation, and licensing as with other telemedicine subspecialties.[66–68]

At the time of this writing (2017) not all 50 U.S. states have parity insurance reimbursement with the same "in-person" insurance reimbursement schedule for the same service. Strides are being made in rural telestroke reimbursement from the Centers for Medicare & Medicaid Services (CMS), but many needful urban-based encounters remain unreimbursable, which is a disincentive for hospitals to develop the service. For Medicaid, the majority of states cover telemedicine services statewide without distance restrictions or geographic designations.[69]

For Medicare, the originating site—where the patient is located—must be a facility located within a primary care health professional shortage area (HPSA) and/or outside of a metropolitan statistical area (MSA). By definition, these are sites with fewer than one primary care physician per 3,500 people and cities with no more than 50,000 residents.[70,71] Twenty-two states and Washington, DC, have private insurance telemedicine parity laws providing statewide coverage, with no provider, technology, or patient setting restrictions.[69]

Federal legislation has been introduced in the United States to increase access and reimbursement for telemedicine services. Specific to telestroke, the bipartisan bill "Furthering Access to Stroke Telemedicine," or the FAST Act (H.R. 2799 and S.1465), was introduced in 2015 to broaden the definition of the originating site to include both rural and urban spoke facilities for CMS reimbursement. At the time of this writing, the FAST Act legislation, widely supported by professional bodies, including the American Telemedicine Association, American Heart Association/American Stroke Association (AHA/ASA), and American Academy of Neurology, has subsequently been referred

for committee review in the House and the Senate and awaits final determination.

Beyond coverage reimbursement, the economic sustainability of telestroke networks requires buy-in and ongoing support by key stakeholders ranging from hospital leadership to nurses and first responders at the point of care. Additional financial considerations include contract negotiations between hub and spoke sites, adequate salary support or incentives for telestroke providers, capital budgeting for technology startup and maintenance, return on investment, and marketing strategies to promote the telestroke program in the surrounding community.[66]

Numerous studies have also assessed the cost effectiveness and cost utility of telestroke programs in both

Table 5-1. Evidence-Based Recommendations for Telestroke Systems of Care

Class I recommendations
1. High-quality videoconferencing systems are recommended for performing an NIHSS-telestroke examination in nonacute stroke patients, and this is comparable to an NIHSS-bedside assessment. Similar recommendations apply for the European and Scandinavian Stroke scales (Class I, Level of Evidence A).
2. The NIHSS-telestroke examination, when administered by a stroke specialist using high-quality videoconferencing, is recommended when an NIHSS-bedside assessment by a stroke specialist is not immediately available for patients in the acute stroke setting, and this assessment is comparable to an NIHSS-bedside assessment (Class I, Level of Evidence A).
3. Teleradiology systems approved by the FDA (or equivalent organization) are recommended for timely review of brain CT scans in patients with suspected acute stroke (Class I, Level of Evidence A).
4. Review of brain CT scans by stroke specialists or radiologists using teleradiology systems approved by the FDA (or equivalent organization) is useful for identifying exclusions for thrombolytic therapy in acute stroke patients (Class I, Level of Evidence A).
5. When implemented within a telestroke network, teleradiology systems approved by the FDA (or equivalent organization) are useful in supporting rapid imaging interpretation in time for thrombolysis decision making (Class I, Level of Evidence B).
6. It is recommended that a stroke specialist using high-quality videoconferencing provide a medical opinion in favor of or against the use of intravenous tPA in patients with suspected acute ischemic stroke when onsite stroke expertise is not immediately available (Class I, Level of Evidence B).
7. When the lack of local physician stroke expertise is the only barrier to the implementation of inpatient stroke units, telestroke consultation via high-quality videoconferencing is recommended (Class I, Level of Evidence B).
8. Assessment of occupational, physical, or speech disability in stroke patients by allied health professionals via high-quality videoconferencing systems using specific standardized assessments is recommended when in-person assessment is impractical, the standardized rating instruments have been validated for high-quality videoconferencing use, and administration is by trained personnel using a structured interview (Class I, Level of Evidence B).
9. Telephonic assessment for measuring functional disability after stroke is recommended when in-person assessment is impractical, the standardized rating instruments have been validated for telephonic use, and administration is by trained personnel using a structured interview (Class I, Level of Evidence B).

Class II recommendations
1. High-quality videoconferencing is reasonable for performing a general neurological examination by a remote examiner with interrater agreement comparable to that between different face-to-face examiners (Class IIa, Level of Evidence B).
2. Implementation of telestroke consultation in conjunction with stroke education and training for healthcare providers can be useful for increasing the use of intravenous tPA at community hospitals without access to adequate onsite stroke expertise (Class IIa, Level of Evidence B).
3. Compared with traditional bedside evaluation and use of intravenous tPA, the safety and efficacy of intravenous tPA administration based solely on telephone consultation without CT interpretation via teleradiology are not well established (Class IIb, Level of Evidence C).
4. Prehospital telephone-based contact between emergency medical personnel and stroke specialists for screening and consent can be effective in facilitating enrollment into hyperacute neuroprotective trials (Class IIa, Level of Evidence B).
5. Delivery of occupational or physical therapy to stroke patients by allied health professionals via high-quality videoconferencing systems is reasonable when in-person assessment is impractical (Class IIa, Level of Evidence B).

(Used with permission from Schwamm LH, Holloway RG, Amarenco P, et al. A review of the evidence for the use of telemedicine within stroke systems of care: a scientific statement from the American Heart Association/American Stroke Association. *Stroke* 2009;40(7): 2616–2634.)

centralized and decentralized health care systems. Most analyses have concluded a favorable incremental cost-effectiveness ratio (ICER) well below societal thresholds for reimbursement, particularly when considering outcomes across the lifespan.[72–78] Whereas most of the attendant costs in a telestroke system are in startup, societal return on investment is substantial when considering long-term savings in reduced lifelong disability for stroke patients.

From a business model perspective, hospitals can realize a return on investment incurred by an increased number of patients treated with tPA (ie, higher diagnosis-related group billing) at the spoke, transfers to the hub for EVT, and patients discharged from both hub and spoke.[79]

QUALITY IMPROVEMENT, STANDARDS, AND GUIDELINES

Since the inception of telestroke systems in the early 2000s, there have been several evidence-based guidelines and policy statements guiding practice and implementation for acute stroke care. Given limited data from prospective randomized trials, the literature supporting the implementation of telestroke primarily reflects analyses of practical feasibility, observational experience, and recommendations from a systems-of-care perspective (Table 5-1).[80,81]

A recent scientific statement from the AHA/ASA suggested new recommendations for monitoring quality and outcomes in telestroke programs.[82] Specifically, these recommendations include measuring processes such as time to treatment and hospital transfers, documenting patient outcomes and safety events, and technical quality metrics of the telestroke system. Many of these recommendations overlap with previous stroke guidelines and hospital-reporting requirements for certified stroke centers; however, a number of additional metrics may serve as new quality standards and benchmarks for telestroke practice going forward (Table 5-2 and 5-3).

In 2017, the American Telemedicine Association drafted *Practice Guidelines for Telestroke* "to assist practitioners in providing assessment, diagnosis,

Table 5-2. Telestroke Quality Measures Overlapping with Existing Acute Stroke Quality Standards

Telestroke Quality Measure	AHA/GWTG	BAC Articles	Hospital Accrediting Bodies[*]
Patient characteristics on arrival after transfer	Yes	Yes	Yes
CT scan completion time	Yes	Yes	Yes
tPA treatment (eligibility, door-to-needle time, protocol adherence)	Yes	Yes	Yes
The percent of tPA in patients seen in the ED with the initial diagnosis of stroke, arriving in the ED within the 3- and 4.5-h time windows, and eligible for tPA	Yes	No	Yes
Patient disposition after telestroke consultation	Yes	Yes	Yes
Short-term patient outcomes (length of stay, symptomatic and asymptomatic ICH, in-hospital or 7-d mortality)	Yes	Yes	Yes
Functional outcome at discharge	Yes	No	No
Longer-term outcomes (90-d mRS score) for patients treated with thrombolysis	Yes	No	Yes
Quality performance should be collected in a standardized fashion and shared across the network	Yes	Yes	Yes
Certification should be conducted by an independent, external organization	Yes	Yes	Yes

AHA, American Heart Association; BAC, Brain Attack Coalition; CT, computed tomography; ED, emergency department; GWTG, Get With The Guidelines; ICH, intracranial hemorrhage; mRS, modified Rankin Scale; tPA, tissue-type plasminogen activator.
[*]The Joint Commission, DNV Healthcare, Healthcare Facilities Accreditation Program, and Center for Improvement in Healthcare Quality.
(Used with permission from Wechsler LR, Demaerschalk BM, Schwamm LH, et al. Telemedicine quality and outcomes in stroke: a scientific statement for healthcare professionals from the American Heart Association/American Stroke Association. *Stroke* 2017;48(1):e3–e25.)

Table 5-3. Unique Telestroke Quality Measures

Telestroke Quality Measure	Comments
Telestroke workflow times (consult notification, phone response, video-consult initiation, consult completion)	BAC suggests telemedicine link be established within 20 min of consult request
Quality metrics on phone and audiovisual consults	
Tracking transfers between facilities (time of arrival and departure at originating site and arrival at receiving facility)	AHA/ASA policy and HFAP recommend only tracking the median facility-to-facility transfer times
Telestroke consultant preliminary diagnosis and final discharge diagnosis	GWTG only tracks patients with discharge diagnosis of stroke; this recommendation extends the collection of diagnosis to all patients seen as a telestroke consult, whether stroke or not
Patient satisfaction with the telestroke consult	
Provider feedback on network operation	
Monitoring of technical failures/limitations during consults, including the frequency that technical issues affect patient care (for both ED-based and EMS-based systems)	Although this is new, as it applies solely to telestroke systems, it is in the spirit of general hospital quality monitoring
Investigation of any telestroke security breaches	Although this is new, as it applies solely to telestroke systems, it is in the spirit of general hospital quality monitoring
Quality monitoring of CT image quality, technical failures, operational failures, or workflow issues should be recorded and regularly reviewed, along with other technology quality measures	Although this is new, as it applies solely to telestroke systems, it is in the spirit of general hospital quality monitoring
The responsibility for collecting quality data should be a component of the agreement between telestroke sites and either a coordinating stroke center or distributed partner	Although this is new, as it applies solely to telestroke systems, it is in the spirit of general hospital quality monitoring

AHA, American Heart Association; *ASA*, American Stroke Association; *BAC*, Brain Attack Coalition; *CT*, computed tomography; *ED*, emergency department; *EMS*, emergency medical services; *GWTG*, Get With The Guidelines; *HFAP*, Healthcare Facilities Accreditation Program.
(Used with permission from Wechsler LR, Demaerschalk BM, Schwamm LH, et al. Telemedicine quality and outcomes in stroke: a scientific statement for healthcare professionals from the American Heart Association/American Stroke Association. *Stroke* 2017;48(1):e3–e25.)

management, and/or remote consultative support to patients exhibiting symptoms and signs consistent with an acute stroke syndrome, using telemedicine communication technologies." This comprehensive document covers a broad scope, including clinical, administrative, and technical guidelines, and seeks to highlight "the unique aspects of delivering collaborative bedside and remote care through the telestroke model." Although these guidelines are currently under review at the time of this writing, they represent another important step in the effort to standardize high-quality telestroke care for patients and communities (http://hub.americantelemed.org/resources/telemedicine-practice-guidelines).

CONCLUSIONS

By any account, the establishment of telestroke is a true success story in the annals of telehealth. Throughout much of the world, telestroke partnerships are now an integral component of emergency care and have helped ameliorate geographic disparities in access to acute stroke treatment. Despite widespread acceptance of telestroke in clinical practice, much work remains to broaden the evidence base and integrate quality improvement metrics across telestroke systems of care. As many hospitals explore telestroke programs for the first time, efforts are underway to utilize telestroke for novel means, particularly with innovations in mobile technology for prehospital stroke care and as a tool to facilitate enhanced regionalization of care in the endovascular era. Financial and regulatory considerations will continue to shape the expansion of telestroke, as proponents await the outcome of important legislation such as the FAST Act to guide reimbursement in years to come.

Despite much progress, stroke persists as one of the most disabling and devastating medical conditions, with stroke incidence estimated to more than double by 2050 as the population ages.[83] Thus, great opportunity remains to further utilize telemedicine to improve the outcomes for stroke patients and lessen the burden of stroke on society.

REFERENCES

1. The National Institute of Neurological Disorders and Stroke rt-PA Stroke Study Group. Tissue plasminogen activator for acute ischemic stroke. *N Engl J Med* 1995;333(24):1581–1587.

2. Kleindorfer D, Xu Y, Moomaw CJ, et al. US geographic distribution of rt-PA utilization by hospital for acute ischemic stroke. *Stroke* 2009;40(11):3580–3584.

3. Mullen MT, Judd S, Howard VJ, et al. Disparities in evaluation at certified primary stroke centers: reasons for geographic and racial differences in stroke. *Stroke* 2013;44(7):1930–1935.

4. Hess DC, Audebert HJ. The history and future of telestroke. *Nat Rev Neurol* 2013;9(6):340–350.

5. Levine SR, Gorman M. "Telestroke": the application of telemedicine for stroke. *Stroke* 1999;30(2):464–469.

6. Silva GS, Farrell S, Shandra E, et al. The status of telestroke in the United States: a survey of currently active stroke telemedicine programs. *Stroke* 2012;43(8):2078–2085.

7. Powers WJ, Derdeyn CP, Biller J, et al. 2015 American Heart Association/American Stroke Association focused update of the 2013 guidelines for the early management of patients with acute ischemic stroke regarding endovascular treatment: a guideline for healthcare professionals from the American Heart Association/American Stroke Association. *Stroke* 2015;46(10):3020–3035.

8. Chernyshev OY, Martin-Schild S, Albright KC, et al. Safety of tPA in stroke mimics and neuroimaging-negative cerebral ischemia. *Neurology* 2010;74(17):1340–1345.

9. Yaghi S, Rayaz S, Bianchi N, et al. Thrombolysis to stroke mimics in telestroke. *J Telemed Telecare* 2012 Oct 3. [Epub ahead of print]

10. Ali SF, Viswanathan A, Singhal AB, et al. The TeleStroke mimic (TM)-score: a prediction rule for identifying stroke mimics evaluated in a telestroke network. *J Am Heart Assoc* 2014;3(3):e000838.

11. Pervez MA, Silva G, Masrur S, et al. Remote supervision of IV-tPA for acute ischemic stroke by telemedicine or telephone before transfer to a regional stroke center is feasible and safe. *Stroke* 2010;41(1):e18–e24.

12. Heffner DL, Thirumala PD, Pokharna P, et al. Outcomes of spoke-retained telestroke patients versus hub-treated patients after intravenous thrombolysis: telestroke patient outcomes after thrombolysis. *Stroke* 2015;46(11):3161–3167.

13. Yaghi S, Harik SI, Hinduja A, et al. Post t-PA transfer to hub improves outcome of moderate to severe ischemic stroke patients. *J Telemed Telecare* 2015;21(7):396–399.

14. Saver JL, Gornbein J, Grotta J, et al. Number needed to treat to benefit and to harm for intravenous tissue plasminogen activator therapy in the 3- to 4.5-hour window: joint outcome table analysis of the ECASS 3 trial. *Stroke* 2009;40(7):2433–2437.

15. Gagliano D. Wireless ambulance telemedicine may lessen stroke morbidity. *Telemed Today* 1998;6(1):22.

16. LaMonte MP, Cullen J, Gagliano DM, et al. TeleBAT: mobile telemedicine for the Brain Attack Team. *J Stroke Cerebrovasc Dis* 2000;9(3):128–135.

17. LaMonte MP, Xiao Y, Hu PF, et al. Shortening time to stroke treatment using ambulance telemedicine: TeleBAT. *J Stroke Cerebrovasc Dis* 2004;13(4):148–154.

18. Ziegler V, Rashid A, Müller-Gorchs M, et al. Mobile computing systems in preclinical care of stroke. Results of the Stroke Angel initiative within the BMBF project PerCoMed. *Anaesthesist* 2008;57(7):677–685.

19. Audebert HJ, Boy S, Jankovits R, et al. Is mobile teleconsulting equivalent to hospital-based telestroke services? *Stroke* 2008;39(12):3427–3430.

20. Bergrath S, Reich A, Rossaint R, et al. Feasibility of prehospital teleconsultation in acute stroke—a pilot study in clinical routine. *PLoS One* 2012;7(5):e36796.

21. Liman TG, Winter B, Waldschmidt C, et al. Telestroke ambulances in prehospital stroke management: concept and pilot feasibility study. *Stroke* 2012;43(8):2086–2090.

22. Van Hooff RJ, Cambron M, Van Dyck R, et al. Prehospital unassisted assessment of stroke severity using telemedicine: a feasibility study. *Stroke* 2013;44(10):2907–2909.

23. Levine SR, Switzer JA. Acute stroke in the field: iTREAT, you treat, we all one day will treat … better. *Neurology* 2016;87(1):13–14.

24. Lippman JM, Smith SN, McMurry TL, et al. Mobile telestroke during ambulance transport is feasible in a

rural EMS setting: the iTREAT Study. *Telemed J E Health* 2016;22(6):507–513.

25. Chapman Smith SN, Govindarajan P, Padrick MM, et al. A low-cost, tablet-based option for prehospital neurologic assessment: the iTREAT Study. *Neurology* 2016;87(1):19–26.

26. Barrett KM, Pizzi MA, Kesari V, et al. Ambulance-based assessment of NIH Stroke Scale with telemedicine: a feasibility pilot study. *J Telemed Telecare* 2017 May; 23(4):476-483.

27. Belt GH, Felberg RA, Rubin J, Halperin JJ. In-transit telemedicine speeds ischemic stroke treatment: preliminary results. *Stroke* 2016;47(9):2413–2415.

28. Fassbender K, Walter S, Liu Y, et al. "Mobile stroke unit" for hyperacute stroke treatment. *Stroke* 2003;34(6):e44.

29. Parker SA, Bowry R, Wu TC, et al. Establishing the first mobile stroke unit in the United States. *Stroke* 2015;46(5):1384–1391.

30. Walter S, Kostopoulos P, Haass A, et al. Diagnosis and treatment of patients with stroke in a mobile stroke unit versus in hospital: a randomised controlled trial. *Lancet Neurol* 2012;11(5):397–404.

31. Ebinger M, Winter B, Wendt M, et al. Effect of the use of ambulance-based thrombolysis on time to thrombolysis in acute ischemic stroke: a randomized clinical trial. *JAMA* 2014;311(16):1622–1631.

32. Rajan SS, Baraniuk S, Parker S, et al. Implementing a mobile stroke unit program in the United States: why, how, and how much? *JAMA Neurol* 2015;72(2): 229–234.

33. Wu TC, Nguyen C, Ankrom C, et al. Prehospital utility of rapid stroke evaluation using in-ambulance telemedicine: a pilot feasibility study. *Stroke* 2014;45(8):2342–2347.

34. Wu TC, Parker SA, Jagolino A, et al. Telemedicine can replace the neurologist on a mobile stroke unit. *Stroke* 2017;48(2):493–496.

35. Itrat A, Taqui A, Cerejo R, et al. Telemedicine in prehospital stroke evaluation and thrombolysis: taking stroke treatment to the doorstep. *JAMA Neurol* 2016;73(2):162–168.

36. Weber J, Ebinger M, Audebert HJ. Prehospital stroke care: telemedicine, thrombolysis and neuroprotection. *Expert Rev Neurother* 2015;15(7):753–761.

37. Southerland AM, Johnston KC, Molina CA, et al. Suspected large vessel occlusion: should emergency medical services transport to the nearest primary stroke center or bypass to a comprehensive stroke center with endovascular capabilities? *Stroke* 2016;47(7):1965–1967.

38. Blodget H, Danova T. *The Future of Mobile*. Business Insider [Online]. March 21, 2014 [cited August 19, 2015]; United States:[Slide deck]. http://www.busines sinsider.com/future-of-mobile-slides-2014-3.

39. Binz S, Carroll J, Prusakov P, Chang F. *The Feasibility of iPad Technology for Remote Acute Ischemic Stroke Assessment (P05.203)*. Neurology 2013; 80. Meeting Abstracts 1. 2013. San Diego, CA.

40. Anderson ER, Smith B, Ido M, Frankel M. Remote assessment of stroke using the iPhone 4. *J Stroke Cerebrovasc Dis* 2013;22(4):340–344.

41. Gonzalez MA, Hanna N, Rodrigo ME, et al. Reliability of prehospital real-time cellular video phone in assessing the simplified National Institutes of Health Stroke Scale in patients with acute stroke: a novel telemedicine technology. *Stroke* 2011;42(6):1522–1527.

42. Leon-Carrion J, Dominguez-Roldan JM, Leon-Dominguez U, Murillo-Cabezas F. The Infrascanner, a handheld device for screening in situ for the presence of brain haematomas. *Brain Inj* 2010;24(10):1193–1201.

43. Turvey C, Coleman M, Dennison O, et al. ATA practice guidelines for video-based online mental health services. *Telemed J E Health* 2013;19(9):722–730.

44. Meyer BC, Raman R, Hemmen T, et al. Efficacy of site-independent telemedicine in the STRokE DOC trial: a randomised, blinded, prospective study. *Lancet Neurol* 2008;7(9):787–795.

45. Demaerschalk BM, Bobrow BJ, Raman R, et al. Stroke team remote evaluation using a digital observation camera in Arizona: the initial Mayo Clinic experience trial. *Stroke* 2010;41(6):1251–1258.

46. Demaerschalk BM, Raman R, Ernstrom K, Meyer BC. Efficacy of telemedicine for stroke: pooled analysis of the Stroke Team Remote Evaluation Using a Digital Observation Camera (STRokE DOC) and STRokE DOC Arizona telestroke trials. *Telemed J E Health* 2012;18(3):230–237.

47. Audebert HJ, Schenkel J, Heuschmann PU, et al. Effects of the implementation of a telemedical stroke network: the Telemedic Pilot Project for Integrative Stroke Care (TEMPiS) in Bavaria, Germany. *Lancet Neurol* 2006;5(9):742–748.

48. Muller-Barna P, Hubert GJ, Boy S, et al. TeleStroke units serving as a model of care in rural areas: 10-year experience of the TeleMedical project for integrative stroke care. *Stroke* 2014;45(9):2739–2744.

49. Audebert HJ, Schultes K, Tietz V, et al. Long-term effects of specialized stroke care with telemedicine support in community hospitals on behalf of the Telemedical Project for Integrative Stroke Care (TEMPiS). *Stroke* 2009;40(3):902–908.

50. Jhaveri D, Larkins S, Sabesan S. Telestroke, tele-oncology and teledialysis: a systematic review to analyse the outcomes of active therapies delivered with telemedicine support. *J Telemed Telecare* 2015;21(4):181–188.

51. Handschu R, Littmann R, Reulbach U, et al. Telemedicine in emergency evaluation of acute stroke: interrater agreement in remote video examination with a novel multimedia system. *Stroke* 2003;34(12):2842–2846.

52. Shafqat S, Kvedar JC, Guanci MM, et al. Role for telemedicine in acute stroke. Feasibility and reliability of remote administration of the NIH Stroke Scale. *Stroke* 1999;30(10):2141–2145.

53. Wang S, Lee SB, Pardue C, et al. Remote evaluation of acute ischemic stroke: reliability of National Institutes of Health Stroke Scale via telestroke. *Stroke* 2003;34(10):e188–e191.

54. Demaerschalk BM, Vegunta S, Vargas BB, et al. Reliability of real-time video smartphone for assessing National Institutes of Health Stroke Scale scores in acute stroke patients. *Stroke* 2012;43(12):3271–3277.

55. Demaerschalk BM, Bobrow BJ, Raman R, et al. CT interpretation in a telestroke network: agreement among a spoke radiologist, hub vascular neurologist, and hub neuroradiologist. *Stroke* 2012;43(11):3095–3097.

56. Johnston KC, Worrall BB. Teleradiology Assessment of Computerized Tomographs Online Reliability Study (TRACTORS) for acute stroke evaluation. *Telemed J E Health* 2003;9(3):227–233.

57. Spokoyny I, Raman R, Ernstrom K, et al. Pooled assessment of computed tomography interpretation by vascular neurologists in the STRokE DOC telestroke network. *J Stroke Cerebrovasc Dis* 2014;23(3):511–515.

58. Agrawal K, Raman R, Ernstrom K, et al. Accuracy of stroke diagnosis in telestroke-guided tissue plasminogen activator patients. *J Stroke Cerebrovasc Dis* 2016;25(12):2942–2946.

59. Hess DC, Wang S, Gross H, et al. Telestroke: extending stroke expertise into underserved areas. *Lancet Neurol* 2006;5(3):275–278.

60. Hess DC, Wang S, Hamilton W, et al. REACH: clinical feasibility of a rural telestroke network. *Stroke* 2005;36(9):2018–2020.

61. Ickenstein GW, Horn M, Schenkel J, et al. The use of telemedicine in combination with a new stroke-code-box significantly increases t-PA use in rural communities. *Neurocrit Care* 2005;3(1):27–32.

62. Switzer JA, Hall C, Gross H, et al. A web-based telestroke system facilitates rapid treatment of acute ischemic stroke patients in rural emergency departments. *J Emerg Med* 2009;36(1):12–18.

63. Solenski N, Southerland A, Shephard T, et al. Improving telestroke performance in rural systems of care – The EQUITe Initiative (P6.084). *Neurology* 2016;86(16 Supplement).

64. Smith EE, Schwamm LH. Endovascular clot retrieval therapy: implications for the organization of stroke systems of care in North America. *Stroke* 2015;46(6):1462–1467.

65. Pedragosa A, Alvarez-Sabín J, Rubiera M, et al. Impact of telemedicine on acute management of stroke patients undergoing endovascular procedures. *Cerebrovasc Dis* 2012;34(5-6):436–442.

66. Switzer JA, Demaerschalk BM. Overcoming challenges to sustain a telestroke network. *J Stroke Cerebrovasc Dis* 2012;21(7):535–540.

67. de Bustos EM, Moulin T, Audebert HJ. Barriers, legal issues, limitations and ongoing questions in telemedicine applied to stroke. *Cerebrovasc Dis* 2009;27(Suppl 4):36–39.

68. Fanale CV, Demaerschalk BM. Telestroke network business model strategies. *J Stroke Cerebrovasc Dis* 2012;21(7):530–534.

69. Neufeld JD, Doarn CR, Aly R. State policies influence Medicare telemedicine utilization. *Telemed J E Health* 2016;22(1):70–74.

70. Shuaib FM, Durant RW, Parmar G, et al. Awareness, treatment and control of hypertension, diabetes and hyperlipidemia and area-level mortality regions in the Reasons for Geographic and Racial Differences in Stroke (REGARDS) study. *J Health Care Poor Underserved* 2012;23(2):903–921.

71. Hassol A, Gaumer G, Grigsby J, et al. Rural telemedicine: a national snapshot. *Telemed J* 1996;2(1):43–48.

72. Demaerschalk BM, Hwang HM, Leung G. Cost analysis review of stroke centers, telestroke, and rt-PA. *Am J Manag Care* 2010;16(7):537–544.

73. Nelson RE, Saltzman GM, Skalabrin EJ, et al. The cost-effectiveness of telestroke in the treatment of acute ischemic stroke. *Neurology* 2011;77(17):1590–1598.

74. Rudolph SH, Levine SR. Telestroke, QALYs, and current health care policy: the Heisenberg uncertainty principle. *Neurology* 2011;77(17):1584–1585.

75. Demaerschalk BM, Switzer JA, Xie J, et al. Cost utility of hub-and-spoke telestroke networks from societal perspective. *Am J Manag Care* 2013;19(12):976–985.

76. Fearon P, Quinn TJ. Making the call: is telestroke cost effective? *Expert Rev Pharmacoecon Outcomes Res* 2012;12(1):15–18.

77. Nelson RE, Okon N, Lesko AC, et al. The cost-effectiveness of telestroke in the Pacific Northwest region of the USA. *J Telemed Telecare* 2016;22(7):413–421.

78. Handschu R, Scibor M, Nückel M, et al. Teleneurology in stroke management: costs of service in different organizational models. *J Neurol* 2014;261(10):2003–2008.

79. Switzer JA, Demaerschalk BM, Xie J, et al. Cost-effectiveness of hub-and-spoke telestroke networks for the management of acute ischemic stroke from the hospitals' perspectives. *Circ Cardiovasc Qual Outcomes* 2013;6(1):18–26.

80. Schwamm LH, Chumbler N, Brown E, et al. Recommendations for the implementation of telehealth in cardiovascular and stroke care: a policy statement from the American Heart Association. *Circulation* 2017;135(7):e24–e44.

81. Schwamm LH, Holloway RG, Amarenco P, et al. A review of the evidence for the use of telemedicine within stroke systems of care: a scientific statement from the American Heart Association/American Stroke Association. *Stroke* 2009;40(7):2616–2634.

82. Wechsler LR, Demaerschalk BM, Schwamm LH, et al. Telemedicine quality and outcomes in stroke: a scientific statement for healthcare professionals from the American Heart Association/American Stroke Association. *Stroke* 2017;48(1):e3–e25.

83. Howard G, Goff DC. Population shifts and the future of stroke: forecasts of the future burden of stroke. *Ann N Y Acad Sci.* 2012;1268:14–20.

High-Risk Obstetrics and Telehealth

Curtis Lowery, MD

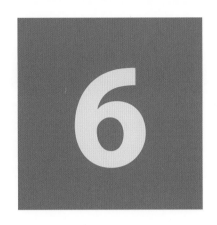

High-risk pregnancies "threaten the health or life of the mother or her fetus" and are often prompted by certain risk factors like "existing health conditions, such as high blood pressure, diabetes, or being HIV-positive; overweight and obesity; multiple births, and young or old maternal age."[1] The National Institutes of Health recommend that high-risk pregnancies receive the care of a "special team of health care providers" to ensure healthy outcomes for both mothers and their infants.[1] However, such a "special team" represents a professional resource that is swiftly dwindling. The American Congress of Obstetricians and Gynecologists project that the United States will lack 6,000 to 8,000 obstetricians by the year 2020, with a potential shortage of 22,000 by 2050.[2] Even scarcer are obstetricians, like maternal-fetal medicine specialists, prepared to handle high-risk pregnancies. Considering this need and shortage, telemedicine becomes a natural means of distributing specialty high-risk obstetrical expertise in an efficient manner.

MODALITIES

High-risk obstetrical telehealth has been used to provide a number of support, diagnostic, and ancillary services, including nonstress testing, fetal echocardiograms, hypertension and diabetes counseling, and monitoring. Nonstress testing, meaning no stress placed on the fetus, is done by placing a belt with a sensor on the abdomen of the mother to monitor fetal heart rate in response to fetal movement.[3] Fetal echocardiograms use ultrasound to evaluate the heart of

the fetus and assess for cardiac abnormalities prior to birth. These tests are performed most often in the second trimester and provide a more detailed image than a regular ultrasound, showing blood flow, structure, and heart rhythm.[4] Each of these test results can be read in the office or remotely via real-time teleultrasounds and video technology. Common medical complications in high-risk pregnancies, such as hypertension and diabetes, can also be remotely monitored through the use of a handheld or wearable device and can be used as an educational/counseling tool. Increasingly, high-risk obstetrical telehealth is making its way into the home, providing patients the opportunity to increase time between required clinic visits, replace visits, or offer physicians rich data on patients in between appointments. This amazing evolution of high-risk obstetrical care is currently underway and is expected to change drastically in the future, with the anticipation that obstetrical societies and authorities will endorse certain practices for clinical reliability.

There are a number of different ways to incorporate telehealth in high-risk obstetrics. Each of these modalities can be used to consult, diagnose, treat, and educate. First and foremost, these modalities all have a common theme in consulting and treating high-risk obstetrical patients: each provides gateways for expectant mothers to receive specialized care needed to achieve optimal maternal and antenatal health.

Live, two-way synchronous audio and video allows specialists, local providers, and obstetrical patients to see and hear each other in real time to discuss high-risk obstetrical conditions (see Figure 6-1). This modality

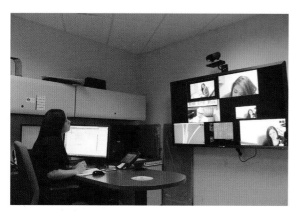

▲ **Figure 6-1.** A high-risk obstetrical specialty team consults with patient and local health care provider through live two-way synchronous audio and video.

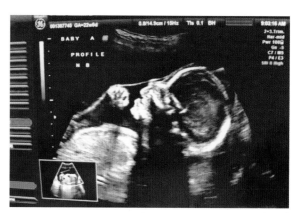

▲ **Figure 6-2.** High-definition ultrasound image.

places the specialist virtually into the remote patient consultation, allowing him or her to play an active role in the patient's diagnosis and care. Combined with teleultrasound technology, as discussed in the following section, it affords the care team the capacity to detect fetal anomalies, discuss treatment plans and options, and provide genetic counseling as needed.

The model for high-risk obstetrical synchronous telehealth has evolved over time. Initially, this real-time care was primarily found in hospitals and clinics where secure live audio and video connections were in place between partnering specialists, tertiary hospitals or other specialty facilities.[5] Although this has been the standard of high-risk obstetrical telehealth for a number of years, accessibility to live audio and video has been greatly increased through computers, smart phones, tablets, and handheld devices that have the capacity to connect to remote parties through wireless and broadband technologies. Hence, the model for high-risk obstetrical telehealth has expanded to include home-based support, with patients even directing and recording fetal heart rate at home when given the proper tools and training.[5] Therefore, specialty advice, genetic counseling, and other potentially valuable high-risk obstetrical services are beginning to make a presence in home-based synchronous telehealth interventions.

However, for this discussion about high-risk obstetrical care as delivered by synchronous telehealth, further testing, training, and tweaking of these new technologies will be needed to ensure that home-based synchronous telehealth yields accurate results. With the complexity of high-risk pregnancies, for the time being, it is advised that this model stays within the walls of hospitals, clinics, and other places in which patients are treated, which have the medical personnel, Health Insurance Portability and Accountability Act (HIPAA) security, technology infrastructure, and the medical diagnostic and analytical equipment needed to provide sound high-risk obstetrical advice to patients in need. In sum total, synchronous telemedicine delivered in the clinical care setting is the gold standard for all high-risk obstetrical telehealth modalities, yet home-based synchronous telehealth may be possible to support high-risk patients in between appointments or as needed when obstetrical problems occur.

Store-and-forward, also referred to as asynchronous telemedicine, sends medical images (eg, X-rays, photos, ultrasound recordings, or other static and video medical imaging) to remote specialists for analysis and future consultation (see Figure 6-2).

The use of store-and-forward is growing at a rapid pace worldwide to reach populations where the likelihood of receiving adequate medical care is severely low, with obstetrics seeing the same growth. For example, a cervical cancer prevention program was successfully implemented in Zambia, one of the poorest countries in the world. The "screen and treat" approach used a telecommunications matrix to capture digital images (cervigrams) and then provide access to offsite experts for consultation. The program was used as a model to train other providers and public health experts in other disparate settings.[6] Other uses in obstetrics include ultrasound images that are saved, stored on a computer, and reviewed by a physician at a later time. Video images and clips from a fetal echocardiograph might also be transmitted and stored using this modality.

Remote patient monitoring collects personal health and medical data from an individual in one location and electronically, and oftentimes wirelessly, transmits that data to a provider in a different location for use in care and related support. Remote patient monitoring may use medically designated handheld or wearable devices to collect health data remotely or may use smart phones with applications ("apps") that leverage wireless or Bluetooth technologies to track patients while away from the clinic setting. The use of smart phones and related devices is often referred to as mobile health ("m-health"). Health data collected can include weight, heart rate, blood pressure, and other vitals specific to the health condition being treated. Remote patient monitoring is used in a wide variety of medical disciplines, especially to monitor patients with chronic diseases such as diabetes and hypertension to not only help with symptoms and treatment, but for ease of the patient with regard to time and expense.[7]

Hypertensive disorders in pregnancy are common and require constant monitoring and in many cases will lead to preeclampsia and infant complications such as low birth weight.[8] Without remote monitoring, it is left up to the mother to assess her own symptoms and report them to her physician at her regular follow-up visits, which may be infrequent, especially at the beginning of the pregnancy. Early intervention is important, and monitoring of the high-risk mother can decrease complications and increase health of the infant. In a study done by Barton, et al., remote monitoring included patient education combined with daily measurement of blood pressure, weight, pulse using a physiologic data recorder, proteinuria assessment, and fetal movement using an automated monitor.[8] In addition, nursing assessment was provided on a scheduled and as-needed basis. Remote patient monitoring may provide better support for high-risk pregnant women in between pregnancies, while giving the monitoring physician or nurse the opportunity to catch obstetrical issues as they occur and before they worsen.

M-health, although similar to remote patient monitoring, is self-managed patient care and does not necessarily involve monitoring by a provider. It is most commonly used to deliver or reinforce patient education about preventive care and provide medication reminders, appointment reminders, and other essential self-care steps that patients should undertake to maintain optimal obstetrical health.[9] Text4baby, which was launched in 2010, was the first national text messaging service in the United States and was designed to provide health information related to a woman's pregnancy as well as her baby's developmental stage. The strengths of this program, along with lessons learned, have led to further evolution and design of additional remote monitoring tools for obstetrics.[10]

These telehealth modalities should be utilized in delivery models that not only provide access to specialty care for remote patients or providers, but also access to resources necessary to make them run smoothly for all users. Because technical troubleshooting is a necessity for any type of telehealth effort, this discussion will not focus on the need for such services beyond stating that such services are essential to make telehealth endeavors work for all users. For high-risk obstetrics, call centers also offer patients and providers an easy-to-access, familiar modality to seek help and care that can support and reinforce the use of high-risk obstetrical telehealth modalities. Like many other medical specialties, it is common for the telephone to be used as a method of communication, not only for appointments, but also for patients to ask questions, get advice, and many times, for reassurance alone. Communication is even more pertinent in obstetrics where the contact should occur on a 24/7 basis when timeliness is of the essence.

High-risk pregnant women may experience immediate health conditions that warrant emergent triage of the situation, either by connecting with a specialist or arranging transport to a clinical facility.[11] Call centers can be an effective and efficient tool to provide immediate access to medical assistance before and after normal clinic hours. A number of triage systems specific to obstetrics have been implemented, and some have been in existence for many years, such as midwifery triage.[11] Other systems utilize nurses experienced in obstetrics or physicians

Table 6-1. High-Risk Obstetrical Telemedicine Modalities

Live two-way synchronous audio and video	Places specialist virtually in consultation with patient	• Detect fetal anomalies • Discuss treatment plans • Provide genetic counseling
Store-and-forward	Sends medical images to specialist for further analysis	• Digital images • Video images or clips
Remote patient monitoring	Collects individual patient data in one location and transmits to a provider at a different location	• Vitals such as weight, heart rate, blood pressure • Fetal movement
M-health	Used to deliver patient education on preventative care and usually not monitored by a provider	• Patient reminders such as medication and appointments • Self-care steps • Baby's development tracking

themselves to triage and assess patients according to clinical standards or algorithms.[11] Call centers may also assist the patient in other areas such as making referrals, scheduling appointments, or arranging for emergency transfers if needed. According to Lowery et al., some call centers, such as the ANGELS Call Center, have also structured their support services with the ability to connect providers to specialists through video teleconferencing to discuss complex patient cases or seek advice on best practices, making the call center all the more pertinent to high-risk obstetrical telehealth programs.[12]

A summary of the list of high-risk obstetrical telemedicine modalities is included in Table 6-1.

TECHNOLOGIES

From high-definition video to mobile health applications, high-risk obstetrical telehealth employs technologies similar to any clinical telehealth endeavor; however, some technologies are unique to this clinical field and deserve special attention.

▶ The Basics

First, it is essential to identify the technological building blocks of a high-quality, secure, high-risk obstetrical telehealth practice (see Figure 6-3). At a minimum these include,

- High-definition video cameras – Cameras are required at both the remote and local sites that can achieve at least 720p (1280 × 720 px or HD Ready) to ensure high-quality images.
- Video screens – A screen size of no less than 20 inches diagonal is recommended with at least 1280 × 720 pixel resolution.
- Software – Must have the ability to dial H.323 via Internet Protocol (IP) or E.164 and be connected to transverse firewalls of participating sites.
- Broadband – At least 1.5 Mbps download, with 6 Mbps download and 1 Mbps upload speeds recommended to ensure real-time, live video transmission without significant delays.
- Security – HIPAA-compliant firewalls and encryption are required.

▶ High-Definition Video

The use of high-definition video in obstetrics is implemented in a variety of ways. Primary care physicians may use it to consult with maternal-fetal medicine specialists or other specialists who may not be available locally or in remote locations where access is not feasible. Specialists can also remotely examine patients, giving them the ability to directly observe and assess the patient. It can also be used as a tool to provide continuing education to health care professionals or to disseminate information through teleconferences or discuss

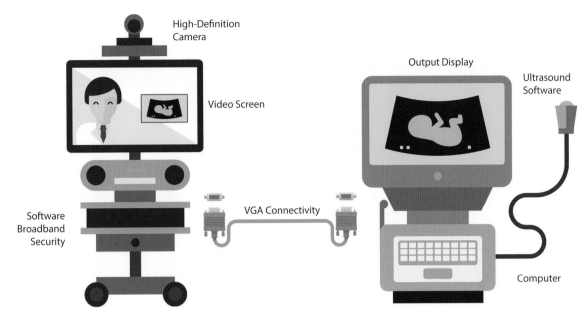

▲ **Figure 6-3.** Essential technology used in high-risk obstetrical telemedicine.

high-risk obstetric cases in the form of grand rounds. High-definition video can educate patients on topics such as birth, breastfeeding, or nutrition. The use of high-definition video in high-risk obstetrics provides a conduit for a multidisciplinary approach and comanagement to coordinate and provide treatment options for women with heightened medical needs and/or a diagnosis of a fetal anomaly or genetic or chromosomal abnormality.

▶ Teleultrasound

Currently, live, real-time video level 2 ("targeted") ultrasounds ("teleultrasounds") represent the gold standard of high-risk obstetrical telemedicine delivered in the clinic. Traditionally conducted face to face in a hospital or clinic, a targeted ultrasound provides women in their second trimester of pregnancy levels of scanning detail not possible through a level 1 ultrasound, making it possible for physicians to determine the sex of the fetus along with a range of other valuable pieces of information for expectant families. However, this type of ultrasound can also detect potential fetal anomalies and complications that may prompt the involvement

of maternal-fetal medicine specialists, geneticists, and other specialists to determine how to ensure the best obstetrical outcome for high-risk pregnancies. Should an obstetrician, family medicine provider, or other medical provider detect a potential problem with a pregnancy—whether based on patient history or the imagery derived from an ultrasound—a targeted teleultrasound can enable distant specialists to view the ultrasound imaging in real time through high-definition video, while also conversing with the patient and her provider in real time over secure video and audio. This clinical exchange, in effect, provides all parties the opportunity to explore the pregnancy and its potential benefits and complications and to collectively formulate a plan of care based on best practices.

Specialists may also analyze teleultrasounds through store-and-forward technologies through the collection and transmission of still images and/or video for later analysis.[13] Store-and-forward teleultrasounds are typically less costly and more feasible in low resource settings, which include countries and regions that have underserved populations and difficulties accessing specialty care. Store-and-forward teleultrasound also allows less need to coordinate schedules of patients and specialists, which can be a great benefit in such low-resource settings. Whereas synchronous teleultrasound allows for immediate consultation between specialist and patient, asynchronous teleultrasound has been cited as a useful tool in low-resource settings and has demonstrated its clinical usefulness, sustainability, and cost effectiveness.[14]

One might wonder why targeted teleultrasound is so important in the care of high-risk pregnancies. Complicated pregnancies occur everywhere, rural and urban, yet access to specialty care does not occur everywhere. Most importantly, rural areas without the means to employ maternal-fetal medicine specialists, geneticists, or even obstetricians within their community hospitals or clinics do not have equal access to high-risk obstetrical care. Therefore, even if a community provider can perform a targeted ultrasound in his or her clinic, the means to accurately interpret such images with specialty obstetrical knowledge may not be readily available to that provider, nor may the knowledge of best practices be as readily available as at academic medical centers.

This is how telemedicine revolutionizes high-risk obstetrical care—using teleultrasound technology, HIPAA-compliant broadband connections, and high-definition video, a patient need not leave her hometown hospital or clinic to receive the expert advice and care offered by obstetrical subspecialists. Before teleultrasound technology, such pregnant patients had no choice: travel to town for subspecialty care. The alternative was to receive no subspecialty care at all, which only further endangers a complicated pregnancy. With the stress of traveling to receive care, the costs of hiring babysitters or missing work, the psychological toll of a problematic pregnancy, and the countless other barriers to making such a journey, high-risk pregnant women too often may elect to receive no subspecialty care at all, with potentially disastrous outcomes on the lives of the family and the health care system. Telemedical comanagement of patients also provides a protective legal barrier for rural providers by giving the best possible collaborative care to complicated pregnancies.

The anatomy of a teleultrasound setup is made possible through the following technologies and partnerships:

To forge a *high-risk obstetrical telemedicine partnership* that utilizes teleultrasound or any other in-clinic services, a specialist should ideally unite forces with a community provider. This may be more difficult than it sounds. As with any clinical application of telemedicine, a partnership must be built on the idea that such specialist support will not steal patients from community providers, but instead support them so they may reinforce their available care with supplemental specialty support. In effect, instead of losing a patient, the community provider is actually gaining a clinical ally with whom she or he can comanage complicated pregnancies leading up to delivery. Because evidence shows pregnancy outcomes fare better at tertiary hospitals,[15] this comanagement must agree that in the interests of the patient and her baby, complicated deliveries should be transported and/or arranged at the nearest tertiary centers, otherwise known as perinatal regionalization. Emphasizing that this partnership balances on the contribution of both the specialist and the community provider to provide the best possible care will better ensure that the telehealth partnership lays the ground rules for collaboration.

Next, an *ultrasound unit* with an output display, ultrasound software, and computer is needed at the patient site to make real-time teleultrasound possible. For real-time encounters the ultrasound device can be integrated with a telemedicine cart that manages the transmission and other aspects required for real-time interaction. For store-and-forward of an ultrasound, the equipment should include an ultrasound unit and Picture Archiving Communications System (PACS) or other dedicated storage and transmission software. Alternatively, the operator may use the ultrasound unit and a CD or other storage device to copy and send the images to the consulting site. These computers and/or telemedicine carts must be connected to secure broadband, as noted earlier. With the necessary broadband and technology in place, next comes technology training.

Teleultrasound training is key to success of any new high-risk obstetrical telemedicine program, and retraining is necessary whenever new personnel join an existing program or the skills of existing personnel need updating and further refinement. The sonographer controlling the teleultrasound equipment and performing the actual ultrasound on the patient should receive orientation to introduce him or her to the new roles of teleultrasound. Training should be conducted sonographer to sonographer, including an introduction to the equipment, shadowing during a normal ultrasound and teleultrasound, and the reinforcement of best practices in ultrasound and how they apply in full to teleultrasound. A technologist can aid the process by explaining and troubleshooting telemedicine technology to new users.

Home Monitoring

The increase in remote monitoring in obstetrics has led to the development of a number of systems and devices to enable the patient to be monitored from the convenience of her own home. The Sense4Baby system was developed specifically to remotely monitor high-risk pregnancies for real-time fetal heart rate and allows the provider to access data directly on their smart phone or tablet.[16]

High-risk obstetrical fetal heart remote monitoring devices have flooded the "at home" market, with some devices being dedicated solely to the collection of specific obstetrical readings or advice and others being used on smart phones through apps. Although these at-home Dopplers may provide the patient with a new tool, they may not be accurate when it comes to fetal heartbeat detection, thus creating unwarranted patient anxiety, worry, or even false reassurance.[17] Such a case in Great Britain occurred in 2009 when a woman 38 weeks pregnant used a home monitor to listen for the baby's heartbeat when she no longer felt movement. Having thought she heard a heartbeat, she delayed medical help, unfortunately losing the baby.[18] Currently, this is a rapidly evolving telemedicine technology, and further testing for safety and clinical reliability is needed before such monitoring can replace clinical monitoring.

M-health has also assisted pregnant women in tracking their personal health at home, empowering patients with advice and data never as easily accessible to any patient prior to the advent of such technology. This technology is constantly evolving as developers are continually devising apps that address obstetrical issues ranging from fertility advice based on individualized menstrual cycles, to patient-directed abdominal scanning to detect fetal heart rate. This technology is as exciting as it is concerning due to its need to be thoroughly validated to ensure the data generated are reliable and valid before patients can rely on the technology's ability to accurately address complicated monitoring, such as fetal heart rate. M-health will undoubtedly provide patients unique tools never before available in their home. It will take time and scientifically based testing to ensure these tools provide accurate and trustworthy advice to expectant families. Patient education and training on how to use this technology are advised for any complex collection of patient data to help prevent false-positives through inaccurate reading techniques.

Mobile Health Applications

Because over half of American adults own a smart phone, mobile health applications are increasing in popularity. In fact, one in five smart phone users have at least one health-related app on their phone,[19] and the Apple App Store has at least 1,800 obstetrics and gynecology apps currently available for download.[20] Moreover, industry estimates predict that by 2018 half or more of 3.4 billion smart phone and tablet users worldwide will be using a health care application.[21] The money spent by digital health companies specifically for women's health has been rapidly increasing, with an estimated $2 million spent in 2011 to $111 million spent in 2015 before year end, a development that has resulted in an influx of women's health apps.[22] Women are more invested than ever in taking charge of their health and need ready access to trustworthy educational resources. M-health apps that provide educational, reliable, and trustworthy information are in high demand among pregnant women.[22] Although many apps are available, their reliability and trustworthiness must be further scrutinized before clinical endorsement is possible. Some apps transcend patient education to provide actual one-on-one clinical consultation. Some apps host virtual clinics specifically designed for women that provide visits with doctors including pediatricians and OB/GYNs, lactation consultants, nurse practitioners, doulas, and nutritionists. Apps such as these are predicted "to make a visit to a women's health professional affordable and easy" considering such resources are available on any smart phone.[23] The U.S. Food and Drug Administration (FDA) has taken a lead in reviewing and regulating certain moderate-risk and high-risk mobile medical apps, which include "apps that are intended to be used as an accessory to a regulated medical device or transform a mobile platform into a regulated mobile device."[21] This regulation helps identify FDA-approved apps, which are accessible through an online searchable database.[24]

SUMMARY OF EVIDENCE/LITERATURE

Although telehealth is still new to many people and has become quite the buzzword in the last few years, telecommunication technologies have been used for more than 30 years. Moreover, some of the greatest opportunities telehealth has offered are in women's health, specifically pregnancy and prenatal care.[25] The earliest application of telemedicine in obstetrics was in 1979 for fetal evaluation, when Boehm and Haire transmitted fetal monitoring data through a Xerox telecopier to tertiary care centers.[26] Obstetrical telehealth has expanded over the past 30 years to integrate ultrasound, fetal echocardiogram, fetal surgery, diabetes management, obstetrical counseling and consultation, and cardiotocography.

▶ Fetal Ultrasound

Throughout the years, studies have focused on the feasibility and accuracy of diagnosis by teleultrasound. For instance, an Australian study published in 2000 tested ultrasound practices at general clinics followed by teleultrasound overseen by tertiary centers on the same pool of patients. Physicians from the general clinics established an initial diagnosis; then a secondary diagnosis was established upon collaboration with the tertiary center specialist through teleultrasound. Overall, the clinical diagnosis changed in 45.8% of the cases and minor changes to the management plan in 33.3% of the cases when comparing the findings of the generalist versus the comanagement team of specialist and generalist. Because all pregnancies were completed at the time of publishing, all diagnoses were confirmed to be accurate postnatally. Furthermore, 95% of the pregnant women were pleased with the protection of their privacy and would highly recommend videoconferencing to others.[27] Fisk, et al. completed a 6-month study in 1995 that administered teleultrasound to women who were at risk of a fetal abnormality. Through the provision of teleultrasound, significantly fewer specialist referrals resulted, with only four women requiring referral to a specialist as compared to 13 referrals that would have been recommended had the women not received teleultrasound.[28]

▶ Live Two-Way Synchronous Audio and Video

Through live two-way video, telemedicine can be used to offer consultations to high-risk obstetrical patients for a number of various subspecialties. For instance, a retrospective study by Rabie, et al. analyzed live teleconsultations given to women who had been diagnosed with fetal urologic disorders. Because the teleconsultation could combine maternal-fetal medicine and urologic consultations, patients benefited from the coordination of clinical resources through time savings and reassurance of further coordination of local delivery and follow-up.[29]

▶ Fetal Echocardiography

Congenital heart defects, the most common type of birth defect, affect about 40,000 births each year in the United States.[30] Telemedicine has been at the forefront in fetal echocardiography to improve neonatal outcomes. Therefore, research involving feasibility and accuracy in diagnosis is ongoing. One prospective study performed over 20 months with fetal cardiologists providing live guidance of telemedicine-enabled fetal echocardiograms found fetal diagnosis of congenital heart disease by telemedicine accurate in 97% of the cases.[31]

▶ Remote Patient Monitoring

Fetal monitoring is currently being used to monitor fetal movement in high-risk pregnancies at home. A limited number of studies have explored remote patient fetal monitoring. A Chinese study published in 2002 analyzed remote fetal monitoring in a total of 116 high-risk pregnant women. The results found remote fetal monitoring to be not only reliable, but also found a decrease in the rate of neonatal asphyxia and preterm delivery.[32] A 5-year study by Quemere, et al. concluded in 1997 also explored at-home fetal monitoring in high-risk pregnancies. This study found this technology to be safe and technically reliable, and participants experienced a decrease in their number of hospital stays.[33]

▶ Indications for Future Research

Although the first use of telemedicine dates back to 1950,[34] obstetrical telemedicine did not emerge until the late 1970s. Initial concerns included efficacy, poor technology, high cost, and patient–physician satisfaction. Perinatal telemedicine has improved over time with developing technologies and more accessible, affordable high-speed Internet. Evidence suggests telehealth provides comparable health outcomes when compared with traditional methods of health care delivery without compromising the patient–doctor relationship. Barriers to access of care and the cost and emotional burden of neonatal and maternal morbidity and mortality are significant in obstetrics, and there is no doubt that telehealth has played a role in alleviating some of this burden. Significant future high-quality studies should be focused on validating efficacy and evidence of improved maternal and neonatal outcomes. Based on the review of the literature, telehealth has demonstrated its usefulness as a new form of health care delivery in areas with limited access to care, making it an effective adjunct to traditional methods.[35] A 2013 study specifically evaluated expectant mothers' experiences when learning poor pregnancy prognoses through live telemedicine. The results showed women positively viewed telemedicine in general under these stressful circumstances, yet their experience was markedly improved by tailoring the personal encounter and emotional response of the physician, preparing patients regarding the telemedicine visit, and considering the potential for technical issues.[36]

Therefore, future studies should continue to test all telemedicine high-risk obstetrical technologies to determine whether these technologies are comparable to traditional care delivery and affect patient outcomes and to identify limitations among certain patients or conditions. Studies should specifically test the accuracy, reliability, and trustworthiness of emerging high-risk obstetrical m-health apps and remote monitoring devices. Studies should also evaluate patient understanding of prenatal care guidelines and improvement in perinatal outcomes with the use of pregnancy-specific apps and to determine patient acceptability of and reception to pregnancy-specific smart phone applications as a means of patient education. Ultimately, development of a comprehensive, more medically tailored app that conveys more prenatal care guidelines and functions as a supplement to prenatal care is needed to deliver more complete health-related messages and patient education during pregnancy.[37]

In 2016, the Agency for Healthcare Research and Quality (AHRQ) published *Telehealth: Mapping the Evidence for Patient Outcomes from Systematic Reviews* that assessed the applications and implications of telehealth interventions and what further research is needed. Overall, research on telemedicine/telehealth is vast but clinically generic. There is evidence to support telehealth can be effective, but future systematic reviews are needed, specifically in maternal health, that look at barriers and how to implement on a larger scale and to adapt easily for policy development.[38]

REIMBURSEMENT/LEGAL/REGULATORY/ LICENSING ISSUES

Current issues affecting the expansion of telemedicine include licensing and credentialing rules, reimbursement policies, data security and confidentiality of patient information, legal issues, and malpractice liability. These issues affect every clinical application of telemedicine, not only obstetrics. Single-state licensure systems are cumbersome, expensive, and act as a deterrent to the practice of telemedicine across state lines. Moreover, telemedicine parity laws and regulations vary from state to state, making the full adoption of obstetrical telemedicine—or that of any clinical application—a practice that must take close consideration of state laws. In 2015, 48 Medicaid programs had some type of coverage for telemedicine and 24 states had enacted telemedicine parity laws,[39] numbers that are rapidly changing each year. In Arkansas, for example, the state's Medicaid agency funded a high-risk obstetrical telemedicine program long before telemedicine parity laws were in place in the state. Collaborative measures between physician groups and insurance companies are necessary in states where parity does not exist, where telemedical interventions can be targeted to beneficiaries that, given proper management, may make better use of available resources and experience healthier births.

Despite parity laws and licensure limitations, there are "telemedicine" companies in the market that deliver one-on-one clinical consultations with distant patients. These fee-for-service clinical services oftentimes practice without proper state licensure and seek consumer-direct payment, thus negating the need for telemedicine parity. Again, oftentimes, these telemedicine services do not require or seek to establish a physician–patient relationship, making such consultations a true isolated encounter. Such practices in any clinical discipline are discouraged, especially in high-risk clinical encounters such as high-risk obstetrics, where uninformed decisions can result in myriad legal and physical problems. Patients asking about these services should be directed to telemedicine services provided by in-state, licensed specialists who can practice legally for the safety of physician and patient alike, while also potentially developing a physician–patient relationship and relating teleconsultation encounters back to the patient's primary care physician.

M-health also has exploded onto the market with a range of informed and uninformed high-risk obstetrical applications. In light of the rapid expansion of mobile applications, the FDA issued a guidance document in February 2015 that explains how the agency intends to regulate the use of medical mobile applications, specifically focusing on those that meet the guidelines and are classified as a medical device and could potentially be a safety risk. The guidance also provides examples of mobile devices classified as medical devices and those that are not medical devices, along with regulatory requirements.[40]

Credentialing and licensure present a tangled web for telemedical physicians, yet are essential to consider before delivering high-risk obstetrical care or other clinical services through telemedicine. In a nutshell, physician credentialing in telemedicine depends on the facility requirements of the patient's physical location and the source of service payment or reimbursement. Further, The Joint Commission also has requirements for physician credentialing in accredited facilities, and the Center for Medicaid and Medicare Services also has credentialing requirements that determine whether such services are Medicare eligible. In effect, credentialing should be determined on a site-by-site basis to ensure telemedical care is, indeed, cognizant of myriad organizations' many rules and regulations; however, as a general rule of thumb, telemedicine physicians very

likely should be credentialed at the facility where the patient is located, and physicians, nurses, and other providers should be licensed in the state in which the patient receiving telemedicine care is located.[41] Credentialing and licensure rules are subject to all clinical areas of telemedical care in which a remote physician provides individualized care to a distant patient.

QUALITY IMPROVEMENT/CARE IMPROVEMENT/ETHICS/PITFALLS

One of the most controversial topics in telemedicine falls within the realm of high-risk obstetrics. Teleabortion is the practice of using real-time teleconsultation to administer a two-step medication regimen using mifepristone and misoprostol to women in distant clinics as a means of aborting unwanted pregnancies. The teleconsultation offers the woman clinical insight on the pregnancy and abortion in collaboration with a consulting specialist and a local physician or nurse. Following the consultation, should the woman wish to proceed with the abortion, the medication is administered in a two-step process: one pill of mifepristone is administered to the woman while in the office and under the care of a physician, and a dose of misoprostol is self-administered by the woman when she is at home some 24 to 48 hours later. This is a telemedical procedure that is currently performed by Planned Parenthood.[42]

Teleabortion is controversial for myriad reasons, and the laws and regulations on it vary from state to state. Some states enforce a "demand-side" law that requires women to receive detailed information and consultation about the health risks of abortion 24 to 48 hours prior to the procedure. Other states enforce a "supply-side" law that requires women at or beyond 16 weeks' gestation to receive the procedure in an ambulatory surgical center by means of surgical abortion, a practice that teleabortion has not currently breeched. Of special note, the "supply-side" laws saw the most dramatic impact on abortions. For example, Texas employs such a supply-side law, and the state's post–16-week abortion rate "dropped 88 percent after the law went into effect, and the number of residents who left the state for abortion quadrupled."[43] Further, 19 states have enacted laws that require the physical presence of an abortionist when administering a medical abortion.[44] Although relevant studies are limited, Grindlay and Grossman in 2011 determined teleabortion to be "highly acceptable and effective."[45]

Whatever the law may be in a given state, teleabortion has made abortion easier to access for those who live distant from an abortion clinic. For example, at the time of this publication, Mississippi, Missouri, South Dakota, and North Dakota each only have a single abortion clinic to serve their entire state and Wyoming has none. It is estimated that roughly a quarter of all abortions could be done nonsurgically and, therefore, through teleabortion. However, state lawmakers will weigh ethical and moral concerns before accepting the practice in their state, and it can be assumed that adoption of teleabortion will be slow in coming for many states. Many decisions requiring in-person exams and visits are "influenced by political factors and not explicitly made based on medical evidence."[42]

The patient–physician relationship has been an ongoing ethical concern in telemedicine care, especially for those cases in which an actual face-to-face relationship may never be established between remote physicians and their telemedicine patients. The patient–physician relationship is important in the delivery of health care in all areas, but the relationship can become even more apparent when a mother entrusts the care of her unborn baby to her physician. There is still much debate on whether that relationship is cultivated in telemedicine, where there is an absence of the face-to-face encounter, and some state telemedicine parity laws may define and address this topic specifically as a means to provide the basis for insurer reimbursement qualification. Therefore, as technology increases and enhances access to care, it is imperative to ensure the patient–physician relationship is upheld and valued in the treatment plan,[46] and telemedical physicians should closely examine their respective state parity law and state medical board definitions to ensure their practices are in compliance.

High-risk obstetrics also must be focused on quality improvement and navigating pitfalls in rapidly developing technologies that serve patients directly, like m-health applications. A recent study done on the characteristics of pregnant women using m-health found women frequently use smart phones as sources of information.[22] As such, physicians must look toward identifying and developing high-quality m-health apps and tools accompanied by patient and physician guidance on how such technologies can be used to improve health and health care. Physicians and national obstetric organizations have ethical and quality improvement responsibilities to

assess this new technology for patient risk and clinical integration. With a field as young as m-health, established protocols and advisories from national organizations are currently not available, but are being drafted to assist in guiding physicians attempting to understand how new technologies affect their patients and how such technologies may enhance patient management and practice. Moreover, some guidance will be needed on how patient self-collected data can be integrated within the medical record and be considered for future clinical decision making. Even with guidelines in place, staying abreast of an ever-evolving field will remain a challenge to health care providers.[47]

STANDARDS/GUIDELINES

The standards and guidelines that govern high-risk obstetrical telemedicine are true of all clinical disciplines delivered through telemedical technologies. As a rule, high-risk obstetrical telemedicine should equal the quality of care received in person within a clinic or hospital. Furthermore, the guidelines and standards of care should not differ within telemedical care and traditional care.[48] Some authoritative telemedicine organizations have outlined standards and guidelines for the practice of telemedicine across general clinical applications. These standards and guidelines, too, are entirely applicable to the practice of high-risk obstetrical telemedicine.

Practice guidelines for telemedicine are imperative to ensure safety in health care delivery. Although a number of governing bodies are actively developing standards and guidelines for telemedicine, the American Telemedicine Association (ATA) is the organization with the broadest focus and covers a variety of clinical specialties that can be adapted and used in high-risk obstetrical telemedicine, which oftentimes covers multiple disciplines due to the nature of women's health. Although the ATA does not currently have guidelines specific to high-risk obstetrics, several ATA-published guidelines are highly applicable to high-risk obstetrical telemedicine and worth special note. The following guidelines are available to download from the website (www.americantelemed.org)[49]:

- *Practice Guidelines for Live, On Demand Primary and Urgent Care*: These guidelines cover the provision of patient-initiated primary and urgent care services by licensed health care providers using real-time, interactive technologies, including mobile devices.

- *Core Operational Guidelines for Telehealth Services Involving Provider–Patient Interactions:* These guidelines are general requirements to be followed when utilizing any form of telecommunication technology.

Additionally, in 2014, as part of their State Best Practice Series, ATA analyzed state telehealth policies and highlighted components of best policy models for telehealth services in *State Medicaid Best Practices Telehealth for High-Risk Pregnancy.* These represent the benchmarks for best practices in obstetrical telemedical reimbursement policies and/or state parity laws.[50]

- "Inclusive definitions of technology with little to no restrictions on the types of technology approved for use in a clinical service;
- Unrestricted geographic coverage areas or patient settings;
- Applicable health services related to obstetrical or natal care, and conditions such as high blood pressure, gestational diabetes, chronic illness, or history of preterm labor or genetic disorder;
- Eligible telehealth providers such as physicians, maternal-fetal specialists, neonatal specialists, certified midwives, clinical nurse specialists, and nutrition and diabetes educators;
- Allowances for innovative payment models other than fee-for-service;
- Reimbursement considerations should be made for managed care, medical homes, accountable care organizations, and other service and payment innovations; and
- Parity coverage for services that are also provided in-person as well as coverage under Medicaid expansion plans created under the Affordable Care Act (ACA)."

At the time of the report in 2014, only three states were highlighted for their notable policies, including Arkansas, Pennsylvania, and Virginia.

In 2016 at its annual meeting, the American Medical Association (AMA) adopted ethical guidelines for the use of telemedicine and included the following recommendations[51]:

"Managing Conflicts of Interest
- Physicians should disclose any financial or other interests in the telehealth/telemedicine application

or service used by the physician and should manage or reduce potential conflicts of interest.
- Physicians should provide objective and accurate information when producing content for mobile health applications or services.

Privacy and Security
- The telehealth application or services must have appropriate protocols to protect the security of patient information and prevent unauthorized access to such information both throughout the electronic encounter and during any subsequent provision of care.

Patient Information
- Physicians should inform users about any limitations resulting from care being provided via telemedicine, advise patients on how to arrange for follow-up care when medically indicated, and encourage users to inform their primary care physicians about the telemedicine consultation.

Standards of Care
- Physicians should uphold the standards of professionalism expected for in-person interactions and adhere to applicable law governing the practice of telemedicine.
- Physicians should be proficient in the use of relevant technologies.
- Given the inability to conduct a physical examination, physicians should ensure that they have sufficient information to make well-informed clinical recommendations.
- Physicians should be "prudent" in carrying out evaluation or prescribing medications by confirming the patient's identity, confirming that telemedicine services are appropriate given the patient's circumstances and medical needs, evaluating the appropriateness and safety of any prescription, and documenting the diagnostic evaluation and prescription.
- When physicians would otherwise be expected to obtain informed consent, physicians should tailor the informed consent process to provide information about telemedicine features.
- Physicians should promote continuity of care and information sharing with the patient's primary provider or other specialists.

Professional Organizations/Health Care Institutions

- Through their professional organizations and health care institutions, physicians should support refinement to telemedicine technologies, advocate for policies to improve access to telemedicine services, and monitor the telemedicine landscape."

The American Congress of Obstetricians and Gynecologists (ACOG) is the leading professional membership organization dedicated to the advancement of women's health through continuing medical education, practice, research, and advocacy.[52] ACOG has not developed a set of guidelines specific to telemedicine, but routinely develops and publishes updates, reports, and guidelines regarding telemedicine in clinical practice.

Telehealth has reenergized and rethought the delivery of care in every possible clinical area, with high-risk obstetrics being no exception. With constantly evolving technologies, it is certain that the observations and recommendations contained herein will evolve at the same pace to adapt to emerging trends and technological advances. However, the same principles will remain true in high-risk obstetrical telehealth: patient safety and clinical integrity will be held foremost, and technology will be used to make specialty obstetrical care more accessible, with the anticipation that telemedicine care will equal the quality of traditional, face-to-face care without compromising any aspect of the patient experience.

REFERENCES

1. NIH Eunice Kennedy Shriver National Institute of Child Health and Human Development. *What Is High-Risk Pregnancy?* 2013. https://www.nichd.nih.gov/health/topics/pregnancy/conditioninfo/pages/high-risk.aspx.

2. Advisory Board. *There's a Shortage of OB-GYNs and Midwives. Here's What's Being Done About It.* 2016. https://www.advisory.com/daily-briefing/2016/09/01/ob-gyn-shortage. 2016.

3. The American Congress of Obstetricians and Gynecologists. *Special Tests for Monitoring Fetal Health.* http://www.acog.org/Patients/FAQs/Special-Tests-for-Monitoring-Fetal-Health#test. 2016.

4. NIH U.S. National Library of Medicine. *Medline Plus: Fetal Echocardiography.* https://www.nlm.nih.gov/medlineplus/ency/article/007340.htm.

5. Magann EF, McKelvey SS, Hitt WC, et al. The use of telemedicine in obstetrics: a review of the literature. *Obstet Gynecol Surv* 2011;66(3):170–178.

6. Parham GP, Mwanahamuntu MH, Pfaendler KS, et al. eC3—a modern telecommunications matrix for cervical cancer prevention in Zambia. *J Low Gen Tract Dis* 2010;14(3):167–173.

7. Meystre S. The current state of telemonitoring: a comment on the literature. *Telemed J E Health* 2005;11(1):63–69.

8. Barton JR, O'Brien JM, Bergauer NK, et al. Mild gestational hypertension remote from term: progression and outcome. *Am J Obstet Gynecol* 2001;184(5):979–983.

9. Search Health IT. *mHealth.* 2011. http://searchhealthit.techtarget.com/definition/mHealth.

10. Whittaker R, Matoff-Stepp S, Meehan J, et al. Text4baby: development and implementation of a national text messaging health information service. *Am J Public Health* 2012;102(12):2207–2213.

11. Manning NA, Magann EF, Rhoads SJ, et al. Role of telephone triage in obstetrics. *Obstet Ggynecol Surv* 2012;67(12):810–816.

12. Lowery C, Bronstein J, McGhee J, et al. ANGELS and University of Arkansas for Medical Sciences paradigm for distant obstetrical care delivery. *Am J Obstet Gynecol* 2007;196(6):534e1–e9.

13. U.S. Department of Veteran Affairs. VA Telehealth Services. 2015. http://www.telehealth.va.gov/sft/.

14. Wooton R, Bonnardot L. Telemedicine in low-resource settings. *Front Public Health* 2015;3:5–7.

15. Chien LY, Whyte R, Aziz K, et al. Improved outcome of preterm infants when delivered in tertiary care centers. *Obstet Gynecol* 2001;98(2):247–252.

16. Airstrip. *Wireless Maternal-Fetal Monitoring.* 2016. http://www.airstrip.com/fetal-monitoring.

17. What to Expect. *At-Home Fetal Heart Monitors.* 2016. http://www.whattoexpect.com/pregnancy/ask-heidi/fetal-heart-monitors.aspx.

18. Well. *The Risk of Home Fetal Heart Monitors.* 2009. http://well.blogs.nytimes.com/2009/11/06/the-risk-of-home-fetal-heart-monitors/?_r=0.

19. Pew Research Center. *Mobile Health 2012.* 2012. http://www.pewinternet.org/2012/11/08/mobile-health-2012/.

20. Farag S, Chyjek K, Chen KT. Identification of iPhone and iPad applications for obstetrics and gynecology providers. *Obstet Gynecol* 2014;124(5):941–945.

21. U.S. Food & Drug Administration. *Mobile Medical Applications.* 2015. http://www.fda.gov/MedicalDevices/DigitalHealth/MobileMedicalApplications/default.htm.

22. Rock Health. *Entrepreneurs Have Many Reasons to Tackle Women's Health.* 2015. https://rockhealth.com/

entrepreneurs-have-many-reasons-to-tackle-womens-health/.

23. Contemporary OB/GYN. *Can Telemedicine Boost Our Ailing Healthcare System*. 2015. http://contemporaryobgyn.modernmedicine.com/contemporary-obgyn/news/can-telemedicine-boost-our-ailing-healthcare-system-1?page=full.

24. U.S. Food & Drug Administration. *510(k) Premarket Notification*. 2016. http://www.accessdata.fda.gov/scripts/cdrh/cfdocs/cfPMN/pmn.cfm.

25. ObGyn.net. *Telemedicine in Women's Health Care*. 2011. http://www.obgyn.net/infertility/telemedicine-women%E2%80%99s-health-care.

26. Boehm FH, Haire MF. Xerox telecopier transmission of fetal monitor tracings: a 4-year experience. *Obstet Gynecol* 1979;53(4): 520–523.

27. Chan FY, Soong B, Lessing K, et al. Clinical value of real-time tertiary fetal ultrasound consultation by telemedicine: preliminary evaluation. *Telemed J* 2000;6(2):237–242.

28. Fisk NM, Sepulveda W, Drysdale K, et al. Fetal telemedicine: Six month pilot of real-time ultrasound and video consultation between the Isle of Wight and London. *Brit J Obstet Gynaec* 1996;103(11):1092–1095.

29. Rabie NZ, Canon S, Patel A, et al. Prenatal diagnosis and telemedicine consultation of fetal urologic disorders. *J Telemed Telecare* 2016;22(4):234–237.

30. Hoffman JL, Kaplan S. The incidence of congenital heart disease. *J Am Coll Cardiol* 2002;39(12):1890–1900.

31. McCrossan BA, Sands AJ, Kileen T, et al. Fetal diagnosis of congenital heart disease by telemedicine. *Arch Dis Child-Fetal* 2011;96:(6), F394–F397.

32. Qi H, Sun J, Liu J, He X, et al. Clinical value of remote fetal monitoring network in high-risk pregnancy. *Chinese J Obstet Gynecol* 2002;37(8):455–458.

33. Quemere MP, Boutroy JL, Fresson J, et al. Fetal home telemonitoring: the Nancy experience from 1992-1997. Analysis of 12,649 recordings. *J Gynecol Obstet Biol Reprod* 2000;29(6):571–578.

34. Institute of Medicine (US) Committee on Evaluating Clinical Applications of Telemedicine; Field MJ (Ed.). *Telemedicine: A Guide to Assessing Telecommunications in Health Care*. Washington, DC: National Academies Press; 1996:34.

35. Odibo IN, Wendel PJ, Magann EF. Telemedicine in obstetrics. *Clin Obstet Gynecol* 2013;56(3):422–433.

36. Wyatt SN, Rhoads SJ, Green AL, et al. Maternal response to high-risk obstetric telemedicine consults when perinatal prognosis is poor. *Aust N Z J Obstet Gynecol* 2013;53(5):494–497.

37. O'Donnell BE, Lewkowitz AK, Vargas JE, et al. Examining pregnancy-specific smartphone applications: what are patients being told? *J Perinatol* 2016;36(10):802–807.

38. Agency for Healthcare Research and Quality. *Effective Health Care Program*. 2016. https://effectivehealthcare.ahrq.gov/ehc/products/624/2254/telehealth-report-160630.pdf.

39. Thomas L., Capistrano G. *State Telemedicine Gaps Analysis*. January 2016.

40. U.S. Food & Drug Administration. *Medical Devices*. 2015. http://www.fda.gov/MedicalDevices/DigitalHealth/MobileMedicalApplications/default.htm.

41. Telehealth Resource Centers. *Credentialing and Licensing*. 2016. http://www.telehealthresourcecenter.org/toolbox-module/credentialing-and-licensing.

42. Health News. *Telemedicine Could Expand Access to Medical Abortions*. 2016. http://www.reuters.com/article/us-health-abortions-telemedicine-idUSKCN0WU1N4.

43. Joyce T. The supply-side economics of abortion. *N Engl J Med* 2011;365(16):1466–1469.

44. National Right to Life. *State Legislative Center*. http://www.nrlc.org/uploads/stateleg/StateLawsWebCamBan.pdf.

45. Grossman D, Grindlay K, Buchacker T, et al. Effectiveness and acceptability of medical abortion provided through telemedicine. *Obstet Gynecol* 2011;118(2 Pt 1): 296–303.

46. Mehta SJ. Telemedicine's potential ethical pitfalls. *Virtual Mentor* 2014;16(12):1014–1017.

47. Ganju N, DeNicola NG. *Mobile and Digital Technologies in Obstetrics and Gynecology*. Unpublished.

48. Krupinski EA, Bernard J. Standards and guidelines in telemedicine and telehealth. *Healthcare* 2014;2(1): 74–93.

49. American Telemedicine Association. *Telemedicine Practice Guidelines*. 2012. http://www.americantelemed.org/resources/telemedicine-practice-guidelines/telemedicine-practice-guidelines#.V-BRi_krJpg.

50. American Telemedicine Association. *State Policy Resource Center*. 2012. http://www.americantelemed.org/docs/default-source/policy/state-medicaid-best-practices-telehealth-for-high-risk-pregnancy.pdf?sfvrsn=4.

51. Health Care Law Today. *AMA Adopts Ethical Guidelines for Telemedicine Providers*. 2016. https://www.healthcarelawtoday.com/2016/07/28/ama-adopts-ethical-guidelines-for-telemedicine-providers/.

52. American Congress of Obstetricians and Gynecologists. *About ACOG*. 2016. http://www.acog.org/About-ACOG.

Teleophthalmology

Alice Yang Zhang, MD, Christine Y. Yoon and
Ingrid E. Zimmer-Galler, MD

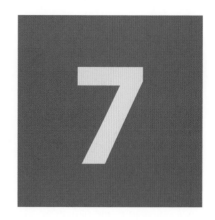

PG is a 56-year-old male with a 17-year history of suboptimally controlled type 2 diabetes mellitus. He has always had good vision and requires only over-the-counter reading glasses. Because of the inconvenience of having his pupils dilated and because he has no vision symptoms, he has not had an eye examination for diabetic retinopathy in more than 7 years. Recently his primary care physician began offering screening evaluations for diabetic retinopathy. At a regularly scheduled primary care follow-up visit, PG elected to have nonmydriatic (with undilated pupils) retinal photographs taken. The images were sent to a remote reading center for evaluation by an ophthalmologist. A report was returned to the primary care physician the next day with a diagnosis of high-risk proliferative diabetic retinopathy in the right eye and severe nonproliferative diabetic retinopathy in the left eye (Figure 7-1). He was immediately referred to a retina specialist and underwent panretinal laser photocoagulation in the right eye within the following 2 weeks. He now understands the severity of his eye disease and regularly returns to his retina specialist for follow-up and management of his diabetic retinopathy.

Without treatment, half of patients with proliferative diabetic retinopathy will lose their vision within 2 years. Individuals treated with panretinal photocoagulation reduce the risk of severe vision loss by 50% compared with untreated patients with the same severity of disease. Clearly having access to telemedicine diabetic retinopathy screening had a significant impact on the likelihood of preserving vision in this patient.

Teleophthalmology allows for the delivery of eye care at a distance using telecommunications technology to transmit information to a remote eye care provider. Teleophthalmology is an excellent example of the alignment of telemedicine with the Triple Aim health policy, a benchmark for health care reform in the United States.[1] The Triple Aim objectives are to 1) *improve the health of populations*, 2) *improve the patient experience of their care*, and 3) *reduce per capita cost of health care*. Although teleophthalmology is still in the relatively early stages of adoption, there is clear evidence that it is a useful adjunct to traditional face-to-face eye care in achieving the Triple Aim goals. This chapter outlines the current status of teleophthalmology and ocular telehealth, including the common modalities and technologies being used. Validation, quality assurance,

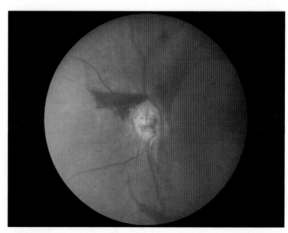

▲ **Figure 7-1.** Neovascularization of the disc in proliferative diabetic retinopathy with pre-retinal and vitreous hemorrhage.

reimbursement and practice recommendations, and guidelines for the most common teleophthalmology applications will be discussed.

MODALITIES

Telemedicine is mature, technology is no longer a barrier, connectivity is a reality in most geographies, and the benefits are proven and real. Telemedicine can be performed in a synchronous or real-time face-to-face interaction with video technology or more simply with asynchronous store-and-forward technology, which does not require the patient and provider to be present simultaneously. Ophthalmology is a highly visual specialty, and digital imaging devices are used with many eye diseases for diagnosis and intervention. Ophthalmology is therefore ideally suited to take advantage of telemedicine, especially with store-and-forward platforms. With asynchronous modalities of teleophthalmology, images are obtained and transmitted to a reading site either with or without compression. This utilizes much lower bandwidth than synchronous video visits and allows high-resolution images to be delivered to a reading center for evaluation and interpretation, often with the use of image enhancement tools.

Imaging systems are only one of multiple critical components for the efficient operation of a teleophthalmology program.

Ophthalmic imaging encompasses a wide variety of modalities ranging from digital photography to optical coherence tomography (OCT), all of which can be captured and easily transmitted for remote interpretation. Most of the imaging performed for ocular care is noninvasive. The external eye, eyelids, and ocular adnexa can be easily documented with external ocular photography. Off-the-shelf digital cameras now largely have at least 10 to 14 megapixel resolution and provide appropriate color reproduction and resolution for medical imaging of the external eye.

A fundus camera is the optical instrument used to visually document the retina. Excellent automated nonmydriatic fundus cameras, which do not require pupil dilation, are now readily available necessitating only limited training to obtain excellent retinal images. The information derived from retinal images depends on the field of view, which determines the extent of the retina imaged, stereoscopic versus monoscopic views, and color versus monochromatic images. Special-use fundus cameras are also available to provide wide-angle imaging, stereo imaging, and handheld imaging options. Although legacy 30-degree color images of the retina are still widely used in ophthalmology, wide field photography using low-power coherence laser beams to scan the retina enables photographs covering up to 80% or more of the retina in a single high-resolution, 120- to 200-degree image. This becomes a consideration for diseases that include significant peripheral retinal pathology and is even essential for conditions such as retinopathy of prematurity (ROP). Although such improvements in digital imaging systems further enhance the delivery of care by decreasing the unreadable image rate and allowing more efficient access to a larger at-risk population, their cost and size limit the use for telemedicine applications.[2,3]

Imaging the anterior segment of the eye is more complex and requires a slit lamp with a built-in digital camera or an adapter to attach an off-the-shelf camera. Slit lamps offer a variety of illuminating and observing methods and require a skilled operator. The slit lamp evaluation is a dynamic process involving changes in illumination and angle of view. Although significant information can be gleaned from single images, documentation of a complete slit lamp examination requires capturing a video or at least multiple images.

Additional specialty imaging modalities are being explored for use in telemedicine applications, including OCT. OCT uses light-scattering properties of tissue to provide cross-sectional images of the retina's distinctive layers with resolutions greater than 10 μm, allowing mapping and measuring of retinal layers and retinal thickness. These measurements provide diagnostic and treatment guidance for glaucoma and retinal diseases, including age-related macular degeneration and diabetic retinopathy. Although not yet widely used in teleophthalmology applications, partly due to its significant cost, OCT may be more useful for future telemedicine strategies than stereo fundus photographs in the detection of diabetic macular edema or swelling of the central retina, which is one of the two main causes for vision loss in diabetic retinopathy, and for assessing progression of glaucoma.

Numerous smart phone applications for telemedicine have been developed in recent years, including various adapters to allow capture of retinal images. For teleophthalmology screening applications, such as for diabetic retinopathy, to reach their full potential, imaging devices need to be deployed in all primary care settings, including remote and socioeconomically disadvantaged populations. Currently this is not feasible based on retinal imaging devices that cost $10,000 to $50,000 or more. Widely available smart phones with advanced imaging and integrated data transmission capability can be adapted for ophthalmoscopy and retinal photography.[4] Such devices are being explored as a low-cost portable solution and have shown clinical potential for screening applications. Early results are encouraging, at present, but validation of effectiveness compared to current established nonportable telemedicine systems is still lacking.[5] Additional concerns are that these new technologies are not standardized and have a short product life cycle. Teleophthalmology is an ideal platform to maximize the interaction of ongoing technological innovations with various digital ocular imaging modalities and pharmaceutical advances in response to the increasing demand for eye care and to more effectively prevent vision loss.

QUALITY AND SAFETY

Evaluation by remote telemedicine services must prove to be as safe as a traditional, in-person eye evaluation. Effectiveness refers to how well evidence-based practices are followed. The cornerstone of a safe and effective teleophthalmology program is clinical validation. The validation process, which should consider the entire program from image acquisition to data transmission, possible image compression, image review, and reporting, is a comprehensive assessment of the telemedicine system's safety and helps ensure that patients are not harmed by care that is intended to help them. Validation of ocular telehealth programs also provides a measure of the effectiveness of the system and is based on evidence and scientific knowledge.

The continuing relevance of a program's validation can only be ascertained with robust quality assurance. Given the increasing utilization of telemedicine as an alternative means of assessing patients with eye diseases and its realized benefits, efforts must now focus on ensuring that quality of care and long-term outcomes are not compromised with further implementation of large-scale ocular telehealth programs. Health care quality measures are mechanisms used to quantify the quality of a selected aspect of care by comparing it to an evidence-based criterion. Clinical performance measures, on the other hand, are mechanisms to assess the degree to which a provider competently and safely delivers appropriate clinical services to the patient in a timely manner. Together these domains of quality measures encompass the six aims outlined by the Institute of Medicine that a health care system must fulfill to provide quality health care: namely that health care should be safe, effective, patient centered, timely, efficient, and equitable.[6] The six aims are complementary, integrally connected with each other, and synergistic. Telemedicine health care delivery methods and ocular telehealth programs can be assessed in each of these dimensions through various performance indicators and quality measures, which must be specific, quantifiable, achievable, realistic, time bound, evidence based, and tailored to each program's objectives.

In ophthalmology, most telemedicine applications involve imaging in settings outside the traditional eye care arena, such as primary care venues for diabetic retinopathy screening and neonatal intensive care units for ROP screening. The majority of teleophthalmology services concentrate on screening and determining the need for referral for expert care. A literature review of over 2,000 publications on teleophthalmology or ocular telehealth revealed that more than one-third of the literature is on diabetic retinopathy screening.[7] Telemedicine for general ophthalmology, ROP, and glaucoma comprised the bulk of the remaining publications. Additionally, more than 80% of the teleophthalmology projects described utilized store-and-forward technology.

DIABETIC RETINOPATHY

It is estimated that by the year 2040, globally there will be 642 million persons with diabetes mellitus, and half of this population will develop diabetic retinopathy.[8] Despite recent advances in diagnostic capabilities and the availability of highly effective evidence-based treatment options, vision loss from complications of diabetic retinopathy remains the leading cause of legal blindness in working-age adults in most Western societies.[9] This is due to multiple factors, including that early stages of disease are asymptomatic and patients are unaware of the need for screening, poor access to care, and patient inconvenience.[10] As a result only about half of all patients with diabetes mellitus undergo annual retinal examinations as is recommended by widely accepted guidelines.[11] Appropriate screening and timely treatment of vision-threatening diabetic eye disease significantly affect vision outcomes in patients with diabetes, and most cases of severe vision loss are avoidable. Ocular telehealth technology is now well established as an effective adjunct method to increase adherence to guidelines for assessment of diabetic retinopathy and achieve all three Triple Aim goals.

Numerous programs have demonstrated that diabetic retinopathy telemedicine programs with acquisition of retinal images at the point of care in primary care locations can effectively increase rates of eye examinations among patients with diabetes and even reduce the rate of blindness and vision loss.[12,13] The benefits of ocular telehealth programs to remotely evaluate for diabetic retinopathy are perhaps best exemplified by the United Kingdom National Health Service (UK NHS), which reports that, for the first time in 5 decades, the leading cause of blindness in working-age adults in England and Wales is no longer diabetic retinopathy.[14] This outcome was largely achieved with the nationwide telemedicine diabetic retinopathy screening program, which is in place in England and Wales and has attained a very high uptake rate.

Both the American Academy of Ophthalmology (AAO) and the American Telemedicine Association (ATA) have stressed the need for validation of diabetic retinopathy screening programs.[15,16] The accepted gold standard for identifying diabetic retinopathy remains the Early Treatment Diabetic Retinopathy Study (ETDRS) 30-degree, stereoscopic, seven-standard field, color, 35-mm slides and, more recently digital images, evaluated by experienced readers.[17] Diagnostic accuracy is often measured with sensitivity (true positive rate) and specificity (true negative rate) with comparison to a gold standard reference. Additional standard statistical measures to assess reliability and reproducibility include kappa values for agreement of diagnosis, false-positive and false-negative readings, and positive predictive value and negative predictive value for identifying levels of retinopathy and macular edema.[16]

In the ATA Telehealth Practice Recommendations for Diabetic Retinopathy, four categories of validation are described for diabetic retinopathy telehealth programs using ETDRS seven-standard field photographs as the reference standard.[16] Category 1 validation indicates a system that can identify patients with no or minimal diabetic retinopathy from those who have more than minimal diabetic retinopathy. Category 2 validation indicates a system that can determine accurately if vision-threatening diabetic retinopathy (diabetic macular edema or severe nonproliferative or worse levels of diabetic retinopathy) is present or not. Ocular telehealth programs in the United States are most often Category 2 programs. Category 3 validation indicates a system that can identify ETDRS-defined levels of diabetic retinopathy and macular edema sufficiently accurately to allow patient management and treatment. A Category 4 validated system matches or exceeds ETDRS photographs in the ability to identify levels of diabetic retinopathy and diabetic macular edema. The category of validation required for an individual telemedicine diabetic retinopathy program depends on its specific goals and objectives.

In the UK NHS, a sensitivity of 80% and specificity of 95% has been suggested as a minimum performance threshold.[18] However, sensitivity and specificity measures will vary by the clinically relevant diagnostic target (ie, sensitivity and specificity for the presence of vision-threatening diabetic retinopathy versus presence of any diabetic retinopathy will be different). A meta-analysis of validated diabetic retinopathy telemedicine programs described in the literature revealed that the pooled sensitivity of telemedicine exceeded 80% in detecting the absence of diabetic retinopathy and low- or high-risk proliferative diabetic retinopathy.[19] It exceeded 70% in detecting mild or moderate nonproliferative diabetic retinopathy and clinically significant macular edema. The pooled sensitivity was 53% in detecting severe nonproliferative diabetic retinopathy. The pooled specificity of telemedicine was 89% or better. Diagnostic accuracy is generally higher with digital images obtained through dilated pupils and, in particular, with wide-angle imaging devices.[2,20] Although it is not the intended purpose of telemedicine diabetic retinopathy programs to evaluate for other ocular diseases, nondiabetic retinopathy ocular findings are relatively common.[21] Protocols must be in place to determine which findings would require referral and evaluation even in the absence of diabetic retinopathy.

Accuracy and reliability of ocular telehealth programs for diabetic retinopathy are also affected by the unreadable image rate. Published reports of unreadable image rates in various telehealth diabetic retinopathy programs range from 3% to 35%.[22] Image quality is affected by multiple factors, including age, media opacity such as cataract and vitreous hemorrhage, and small pupil size.[20,22] Telehealth diabetic retinopathy programs may utilize pupillary dilation, whereas others perform imaging with a nonmydriatic camera and undilated pupils. Some programs also utilize selective mydriasis based on age or image quality. Generally, a higher unreadable rate has been reported with undilated pupils, especially in older individuals who also have some degree of cataract formation.[16] In addition to patient inconvenience and time constraints, the potential risk of angle-closure glaucoma is sometimes cited as a reason for avoiding pupil dilation in the primary care setting. However, the risk of inducing angle-closure glaucoma with low-dose mydriatics is minimal with no reported cases in a large meta-analysis.[23] Nonetheless, offices with mydriatic systems should have a defined protocol to recognize and address this potentially serious complication.

State-of-the-art retinal imaging devices generally do not require a trained ophthalmic photographer to obtain quality retinal images. However, screening in the primary care setting with imaging obtained by office personnel rather than a dedicated imager may result in imagers who acquire only a small number of images at infrequent intervals, which may also affect the overall image quality. Personnel acquiring images should have demonstrated qualifications for obtaining images of adequate diagnostic quality and need to be monitored on an ongoing basis to ensure consistent image quality.

Another essential element of telehealth diabetic retinopathy programs is the remote reading center where images are evaluated. Image readers range from nonlicensed technical readers to ophthalmologists with specialty training in retina. In the United States, technical readers have been successfully used for many years at academic reading centers to support clinical trials. They are less often used for community-based telemedicine diabetic retinopathy programs. Technical readers may add business and operational efficiencies to a reading center but also require careful supervision by eye care providers, standardized procedures for training, and effective quality measures.[24] Image readers need to be qualified and, ideally, certified to grade and interpret retinal images, especially if nonlicensed nonophthalmic personnel are utilized. Protocols need to be in place to assess image reading capabilities of individual readers with intragrader and intergrader agreement, in an ongoing fashion with a sample size appropriate to the size of the screening program.

Quality assurance processes provide guidance on methods to ensure ongoing quality and performance improvement. They may be quite complex and difficult to execute for telemedicine diabetic retinopathy surveillance programs. Although no uniformly adopted quality assurance guidelines are in place in the United States, the UK NHS has developed comprehensive protocols for their national diabetic retinopathy screening program to assess performance and safety, including reading centers.[25] Quality assurance metrics and performance indicators will vary based on program goals and objectives. Certain clinical outcome measures, however, are important for all programs, such as the eye examination rate among patients with diabetes, the ungradable image rate, and image reviewer performance measures. Reasonable turnaround times for image evaluation and return of the report to the ordering physician need to be set and monitored. Additionally, recommendations need to be established for referral urgency and timing for varying levels of disease severity. More difficult to measure but equally important for an effective diabetic retinopathy program is the rate of compliance with referral recommendations, rate of intervention for advanced disease, and ultimately, the rate of vision loss in the population being screened. Only if such data are systematically collected and analyzed will we realize the full potential of telemedicine for diabetic retinopathy and how it aligns with the Triple Aim health care policy.

As one of the Triple Aim health policy objectives, comprehensive quality assurance programs will also assess patient satisfaction. Multiple studies show high levels of acceptance or preference for telemedicine as an alternative to conventional dilated retinal examination for diabetic retinopathy based on multiple factors, including patient convenience, cost, and perceived quality.[26]

The diagnostic accuracy of using digital imaging and the high sensitivity of telemedicine systems to detect clinical levels of diabetic retinopathy indicate that they may appropriately be widely utilized for diabetic retinopathy evaluation. A systematic review of the economic evidence for diabetic retinopathy screening reveals that all studies have demonstrated it is also a cost-effective modality.[27–29] Furthermore, cost avoidance for health systems may be appreciated if disease is detected early and prompt treatment is initiated. However, significant barriers to widescale implementation of telemedicine diabetic retinopathy screening remain in the United States. Economics are a substantial concern, with the high cost of acquiring and operating imaging equipment coupled with unreliable reimbursement for the diagnostic procedure. Although placing imaging equipment in all primary care settings would greatly benefit noncompliant patients and improve disease detection across the board, the expense of such an undertaking is not realistic in the current health care economies.

Reimbursement for telemedicine diabetic retinopathy screening remains unclear. Most commercial payors in the United States understand the benefits gained by timely evaluation for diabetic retinopathy and are covering telemedicine services for this purpose. The Centers for Medicare and Medicaid Services, however, do not have a uniform coverage policy. Most telemedicine diabetic retinopathy service providers are billing using the Current Procedural Terminology (CPT) code for fundus photography (92250) with varying reimbursement success. Retinal telescreening codes also exist, but are often not applicable or useful. CPT code 92227 describes "remote imaging for detection of retinal disease (e.g., retinopathy in a patient with diabetes) with analysis and report under physician supervision," whereas CPT code 92228 is designated for "remote imaging for monitoring and management of active retinal disease (e.g., diabetic retinopathy) with physician review, interpretation and report."[30] The descriptor for 92227 is not accurate for most telemedicine diabetic retinopathy screening programs, as the image interpretation is generally performed by a licensed eye care provider rather than by a nonlicensed technician under physician supervision. Because no physician work is involved, reimbursement for CPT 92227 is minimal and does not cover the actual costs of most programs. On the other hand, CPT code 92228 is assigned reasonable reimbursement but is only applicable if diabetic retinopathy (or other active eye disease) is present. As expected, most screening studies report a high percentage of patients have no appreciable diabetic retinopathy and therefore CPT code 92228 often does not come into play. Fortunately, as telemedicine diabetic retinopathy systems become more widely accepted and acknowledged as a useful adjunct to in-person examination, reimbursement is becoming more consistent. Additionally, pay-for-performance health care measures are aligned with the Triple Aim policies and provide incentives and/or penalties for achieving or missing target metrics for diabetic retinopathy screening rates among the population with diabetes mellitus.

Telemedicine diabetic retinopathy programs have matured rapidly in recent years and are being increasingly used worldwide to increase the rate of annual eye evaluations for patients with diabetes. Although a properly integrated telemedicine retinal imaging system does not replace a comprehensive eye examination, the resultant improved surveillance for diabetic retinopathy results in greater timely access to effective treatments and realization of improved clinical outcomes.

Due to the high current global prevalence of diabetes, it is estimated that seven retinal examinations must occur every second to fulfill guidelines of annual retinal screening for all diabetic patients.[8] Even though telemedicine has the potential of increasing efficiency of access for people, it can increase the burden of image interpretation by physicians and graders. Therefore, automated computer-based grading systems were developed to meet the increasing eye care demand. These systems are capable of distinguishing normal structures from diabetic lesions, such as hemorrhages or cotton wool spots.[28] Based on the type, severity, and extent, images are graded for the presence or absence of diabetic retinopathy. Furthermore, automated systems can be adjusted in order to improve the balance between sensitivity and specificity. To minimize false-negatives, a high sensitivity is a desirable characteristic of such a computerized system. The disadvantage would be a lower specificity, which requires more images to be regraded by physicians, reducing efficiency and increasing the cost of screening programs. However, such systems would serve a prescreening function and on a large scale, still decrease overall workload on the reading center staff.[31,32]

GLAUCOMA

Glaucoma is a progressive form of optic neuropathy associated with visual field defects and loss of retinal ganglion cells. High intraocular pressure (IOP) is a major modifiable risk factor for the development and progression of glaucoma but alone is not sufficient for a diagnosis of glaucoma. Glaucoma is a leading cause of irreversible visual impairment, affecting 60.5 million individuals worldwide in 2010.[33] This number is expected to increase to approximately 79.6 million by 2020.[34] Because there is no cure for glaucoma, this condition can progress to blindness if left untreated.[35] Moreover, older people are at a greater risk of developing glaucoma, and therefore, an aging population will require more frequent screening. The recommendation for screening exams for glaucoma is every 2 to 4 years for adults between the ages of 40 and 64 years and every 1 to 2 years at age 65 and older.[35,36]

The economic burden of the treatment of glaucoma is significant and increases with severity of disease.[34] Glaucoma typically progresses without symptoms and can present at advanced stages without the patient being aware of visual field loss. Therefore, similar to diabetic retinopathy, it is important to detect, diagnose, and treat patients at the earliest stages, both to prevent vision loss and improve quality of life and to decrease health care costs. Teleophthalmology in the field of glaucoma, or teleglaucoma, is a relatively new method of screening for and monitoring glaucoma and may improve access and early detection of disease.

Unlike diabetic retinopathy, which has very well-defined levels of severity that are uniformly accepted and detected with retinal imaging, glaucoma evaluation may involve a variety of diagnostic tools, including assessment of IOP or tonometry, corneal pachymetry or central corneal thickness measurements, visual field tests or perimetry, and imaging of the optic disc. The more tools that are used during the screening process, the greater the accuracy and effectiveness of the screening.[35] Stereoscopic fundus photographs, including images of the optic disc, may be evaluated for signs of glaucomatous damage, including an increased cup-to-disc ratio of the optic nerve and other characteristic features[37] (Figure 7-2). Glaucoma evaluation may involve more sophisticated diagnostic tools of optic nerve imaging such as OCT and confocal scanning laser ophthalmoscopy, which are instruments that provide more detailed topographic information about the three-dimensional structure of the cup and structural information about retinal nerve fiber layer thickness (Figure 7-3). However, the rapidity of evolving new structure analysis technology limits the number of longitudinal studies investigating progression with these techniques.

Standard in-person glaucoma screening typically includes history taking, slit lamp examination, visual field testing (Figure 7-4), and fundus photography performed by an eye care provider. Teleglaucoma screening platforms consist of various models, designed based on the resources of the program. Some programs consist of ophthalmologists evaluating images, and others involve a collaboration between ophthalmologists and optometrists.[38] Typically, patients undergo IOP and ultrasonic corneal thickness measurements by a specialized technician. These data, along with stereoscopic digital images of the optic disc, are then electronically transmitted to an ophthalmologist or glaucoma specialist for interpretation. Although remote grading services may be done after the patient visits, some sites offer real-time consultation.[38]

Goldmann applanation is considered the gold standard for IOP measurements. However, noncontact tonometers are more portable and require less skilled operators for effective use.[39] In the future, home monitoring may become possible using a contact lens

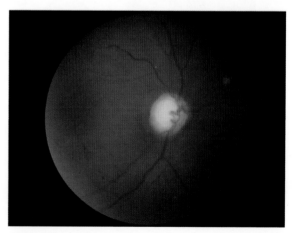

▲ **Figure 7-2.** Glaucomatous disc with increased vertical cup-to-disc ratio.

ONH and RNFL OU Analysis:Optic Disc Cube 200x200   OD ● | ● OS

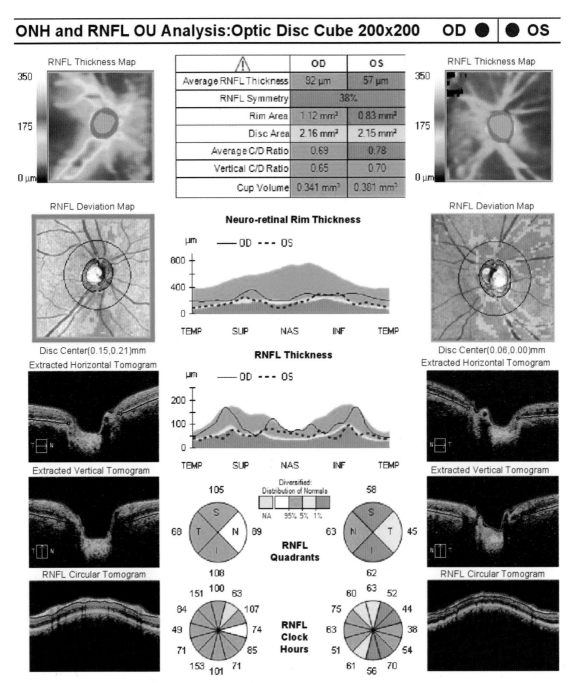

	⚠	OD	OS
Average RNFL Thickness		92 µm	57 µm
RNFL Symmetry		38%	
Rim Area		1.12 mm²	0.83 mm²
Disc Area		2.16 mm²	2.15 mm²
Average C/D Ratio		0.69	0.78
Vertical C/D Ratio		0.65	0.70
Cup Volume		0.341 mm³	0.381 mm³

RNFL Thickness Map

RNFL Deviation Map

Disc Center(0.15,0.21)mm

Extracted Horizontal Tomogram

Extracted Vertical Tomogram

RNFL Circular Tomogram

RNFL Thickness Map

RNFL Deviation Map

Disc Center(0.06,0.00)mm

Extracted Horizontal Tomogram

Extracted Vertical Tomogram

RNFL Circular Tomogram

Neuro-retinal Rim Thickness

RNFL Thickness

RNFL Quadrants

RNFL Clock Hours

▲ **Figure 7-3.** Optic nerve optical coherence tomography that illustrates a case of asymmetric glaucoma. The right eye has nerve fiber layer thickness within normal. The left eye has nerve fiber layer thinning, particularly superiorly and inferiorly, a larger cup-to-disc ratio, and decreased optic nerve rim area, suggestive of glaucomatous change.

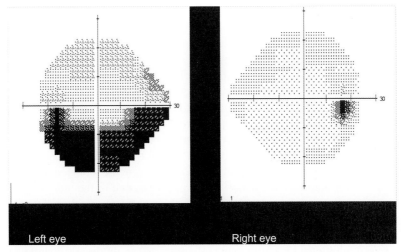

▲ Figure 7-4. The Humphrey visual field of the left eye shows a dense arcuate defect that spares central fixation. The visual field of the right eye is normal, showing only a scotoma at the physiologic location of the blind spot, which corresponds to the anatomic location of the optic nerve.

sensory device or other types of home tonometers, which allow more frequent monitoring of tonometry at various times of the day.[40–42] Such data can enable patients to become more actively involved in self-monitoring and in sharing data directly with screening centers and physicians.[43]

Because there is no single clear, gold-standard definition for glaucoma, validation studies for teleglaucoma programs remain challenging. The modalities that are used by different teleglaucoma programs can vary considerably, particularly the availability of the more expensive imaging devices such as OCT or confocal scanning laser ophthalmoscopy. Due to the differences between modalities and screening parameters used in various teleglaucoma programs, analyses comparing their findings are challenging. However, several studies have found that teleglaucoma has comparable diagnostic accuracy to in-person examination for the detection of glaucoma.

A review by Thomas et al. reported that teleglaucoma is less sensitive (83.2%) and more specific (79%) than face-to-face clinical examination in detecting glaucoma.[35] In comparison to an in-person slit lamp examination, the positive predictive value for a positive diagnosis was 77.5%, and the negative predictive value for a negative teleglaucoma diagnosis was 82.2%.[35]

Similar to diabetic retinopathy telemedicine programs, evaluation of photographs depends on the experience of the photographer as well as expertise of the grading physician. A study from Kenya found that 24% of teleglaucoma photographs were determined to be unreadable due to media opacities, patient cooperation, and poor photographic techniques.[44] Furthermore, if the image quality is low and the grading physician's expertise is variable, diagnostic accuracy can decrease. The sensitivity in this study was reported at 41.3% and specificity at 89.6%.[44]

Teleophthalmology can be used in the postsurgical management of glaucoma. Studies have evaluated images of postsurgical blebs (filtering site) acquired using a still slit lamp image as well as video images.[45] Remote assessment had high levels of agreement for the determination for vascularity, bleb leak, and anterior chamber depth.[46] However, agreement was variable for other assessments, including bleb height and bleb wall thickness. This model may be useful for postoperative care in remote regions. Long-term postoperative monitoring can be comanaged by local physicians and the surgeon via teleglaucoma in regions where surgical expertise is scarce.

Multiple studies agree that the majority of patients who undergo glaucoma screening do not require an in-person consultation with a glaucoma specialist. Therefore, glaucoma specialist expertise can be reallocated to patients with more advanced disease who require surgical management and closer monitoring or those who have a condition with greater diagnostic challenge. In a study conducted in the Netherlands, one-fourth of 1,729 subjects required additional examination, but only 11% consulted a specialist.[47] A teleglaucoma study in a remote region over 4 years demonstrated that most cases (three-fourths) did not require face-to-face consultation with a specialist and could be managed through remote collaboration.[48] The majority (69%) were managed by the referring local optometrist. Only 27% of patients were referred for in-person glaucoma evaluation and 48% of patients required repeat teleconsultation. There was additional benefit in being able to initiate treatment before the patient was seen for an in-person consultation. In the teleglaucoma program, 87% of patients with definite glaucoma and 28% of glaucoma suspects received earlier treatment.

The goal of teleglaucoma is to improve access to specialized care. Studies have shown that teleglaucoma improves access time, defined as time from patient referral to the date a visit is booked. In one study, this time was reduced from 88 days to 45 days.[49] Moreover, teleglaucoma reduced cycle time, which is the time spent from registration until departure from clinic, from 115 to 78 minutes.[35,49] In a meta-analysis, patient travel time was reduced and patient satisfaction with teleglaucoma was higher compared to in-person examination.[35]

As with other teleophthalmology programs, costs in teleglaucoma are associated largely with the type of diagnostic equipment. A meta-analysis of glaucoma cost analysis studies demonstrated that teleglaucoma costs varied by the capacity of service and type of equipment available.[35] The costs for sophisticated glaucoma equipment can be greater than $100,000. Cost effectiveness is difficult to compare across studies due to the variability in modalities used by different programs. Further analyses demonstrated that teleglaucoma saved $27,460 per quality adjusted life year per patient screened compared to in-person examination.[50] Reimbursement issues for teleglaucoma are similar to those for diabetic retinopathy telemedicine programs. There are no specific CPT codes for teleglaucoma. Glaucoma diagnostic procedures are generally covered by commercial and government payors in the United States. Teleconsults, however, are not typically billable for glaucoma screening.

Glaucoma can be classified as open angle or closed angle, based on the anatomical structure of the outflow channel or iridocorneal angle of the eye. This structure is evaluated by gonioscopy at the slit lamp, which requires a contact lens with mirrors enabling assessment of the iridocorneal angle. However, gonioscopy is a skill that is difficult to acquire and has only moderate agreement reported among observers.[51–53] The cases evaluated in the literature in teleglaucoma likely include glaucoma resulting from various mechanisms. Primary angle-closure glaucoma is more common in populations in East and Southeast Asia. Screening programs generally do not include gonioscopy and have the potential to underdiagnose angle-closure glaucoma, which can be treated very effectively and prevented with laser iridotomy.

Given the variability in teleglaucoma programs, quality assurance issues have not been addressed in any detail. However, similar to diabetic retinopathy telemedicine programs, performance metrics should include monitoring images from a technical standpoint as well as interpretation of images, reporting times, and referral/treatment times. In glaucoma management, the detection of false negatives can be a challenge, especially if cost limits use of diagnostic equipment. Therefore, in teleglaucoma, there is a risk of accepting an "unsafe" system.[39] However, repeated screening over time of a chronic condition should decrease the number of patients with true disease who are left undetected through telescreening. Further studies and outcomes data will be essential as teleglaucoma programs become incorporated into mainstream ophthalmology.

RETINOPATHY OF PREMATURITY

Worldwide ROP is a major potentially avoidable cause of childhood blindness. ROP is a vasoproliferative disease of the developing retina that can develop in low-birth-weight premature infants. The risk of severe irreversible vision loss is decreased significantly if the disease is detected and treated appropriately in a timely manner. To that end, ongoing screening examinations of these infants are required until the retinal vasculature has matured. The standard or reference examination technique is a bedside examination with binocular indirect ophthalmoscopy, which needs to be repeated at regular intervals until the infant is no longer at risk or the ROP has regressed. For a variety of reasons, including significant medicolegal liability concerns, an increasing rate of premature births and at-risk infants, the complexities of coordinating examinations, and the remote location of some neonatal intensive care units, there is an insufficient supply of qualified ophthalmologists willing to screen at-risk infants for ROP in the United States and elsewhere. Teleophthalmology services for ROP utilize wide-field imaging technology in a manner similar to imaging performed as part of diabetic retinopathy screening programs. Images are obtained from at-risk infants with a wide-angle retinal camera in the neonatal intensive care unit and are transmitted securely through the Internet to a viewing platform or reading center for review by an expert.

A number of studies provide level 1 evidence demonstrating that interpretation of wide-angle retinal photography by remote readers compared to the reference standard of bedside dilated ophthalmoscopic examination by an expert clinician has high accuracy for telemedicine detection of moderate and severe ROP disease.[54] As with diabetic retinopathy programs, there is significant variability among ROP telemedicine programs, including number of images taken per eye, background of personnel acquiring images, expertise of image readers, diagnostic outcome measures, and metrics of accuracy.[54] One of the largest studies, by Quinn and colleagues, reporting on a real-world operational telemedicine ROP screening program, revealed a sensitivity of 90% and a specificity of 87% of infants with referral-warranted ROP.[55] Although differences in methods preclude direct comparison, collectively, the level 1 studies reveal a sensitivity ranging between 57% and 100% and a specificity ranging from 37% to 98% for the detection of moderate to severe ROP by digital retinal photography.[54]

As previously mentioned, a major criterion for telemedicine programs in ophthalmology is rigorous performance validation relative to a reference or gold standard. The gold standard in diabetic retinopathy and other retinal diseases is based on retinal image evaluation and is well defined. For ROP, however, the gold standard is clinical examination with binocular indirect ophthalmoscopy. Interestingly, the availability of wide-field retinal imaging and telemedicine ROP programs raises questions about the appropriateness of the current gold standard.[56] In the e-ROP study (telemedicine approaches to evaluating acute-phase ROP), expert review of discrepant cases between readers reviewing images and the findings described by an examining ophthalmologist found that the consensus panel more often agreed with the image readers, suggesting that for certain findings, retinal imaging is better than clinical examination.[57] However, evaluation of the far peripheral retina, which cannot be reliably imaged even with existing wide-field technology, is still necessary in the staging of ROP. Even though the interpretation of digital retinal images, in some instances, may be more accurate than bedside examination and serves as a useful adjunct method to reduce the burden on examining ophthalmologists, it cannot be considered a replacement for binocular indirect ophthalmoscopy.

Reliably imaging the retinal periphery in infants is difficult, which sometimes results in poor image quality. Significant variability in image evaluation, even among experienced clinicians, presents another challenge.[58] On the other hand, documentation of findings with serial imaging may allow for better determination of disease progression compared with a traditional examination and documentation with retinal drawings and notes in the clinical record.

As with other teleophthalmology modalities, an inability to obtain interpretable images constitutes a screen-positive finding triggering a referral for an onsite examination. Once a diagnosis of referral-warranted ROP is made, resources and protocols for bedside examination and possible treatment, including transfer when necessary, must be in place.

The cost of implementing a telemedicine ROP screening service is largely driven by the cost of the retinal camera, but significant infrastructure needs must also be considered. A joint technical report by the AAO, American Academy of Pediatrics, and American Association of Certified Orthoptists provides useful recommendations and practical considerations for a telemedicine approach to ROP screening.[54] The guidelines discuss the importance of the health care team approach, including imaging protocols and standard image sets, infant monitoring, data transmission, return of interpretation report, and recommendations and termination criteria.

Quality assurance measures for telemedicine ROP programs are similar to those for diabetic retinopathy and, in addition to validation, include the ungradable image rate, image reviewer performance indicators, report return time, rate of intervention for advanced disease, and tracking of long-term visual and ocular structural outcomes.

Billing for telemedicine consults is generally not possible for ROP screening services, but reimbursement is often provided on a contractual basis between the neonatal intensive care unit and the eye care providers.

Although the implementation of telemedicine for ROP screening continues to increase, further studies on clinical and cost effectiveness, long-term outcomes, and validation of protocols are needed.

AGE-RELATED MACULAR DEGENERATION

In the past decade, public health attention has focused on age-related macular degeneration (AMD) as it remains a leading cause of vision loss in the United States and the world, and its prevalence is expected to increase with the rising elderly population.[9] If left untreated, exudative AMD leads to irreversible central vision loss. Recent availability of intravitreal anti–vascular endothelial growth factor (VEGF) therapy and other innovative treatments makes efficient screening for early detection crucial to identify patients at risk for vision loss. Despite recommendations for regular comprehensive eye examinations in older individuals, many elderly persons do not have access to specialist care for evaluation for AMD. Although telemedicine technology may be a valuable adjunctive tool to screen for AMD, there has been little utilization of this technology to date, possibly because effective treatments have only recently become available. Similar to telemedicine diabetic retinopathy programs, digital retinal images may be acquired and transferred to a remote reading center for detection of the characteristic clinical findings of AMD. Few studies have evaluated the feasibility, accuracy, and reliability of telemedicine AMD screening, and even fewer have discussed patient satisfaction and cost effectiveness.[26]

The use of OCT, which has transformed the management of AMD with its ability to identify exudation, will also need to be explored as telemedicine becomes more regularly incorporated into telemedical AMD care. A home telemedicine monitoring device to detect the progression of AMD is now also available and has shown early effectiveness.[59] However, questions about access, affordability, and cost effectiveness remain, and patients with the greatest chance at benefit need to be carefully selected.[60] Telemedicine approaches show promise for the evaluation of AMD, but additional studies and outcomes data are needed before widespread adoption is possible.

The role of teleophthalmology continues to expand rapidly, and its impact on providing adjunct methods of eye care delivery is being felt in all specialties of ophthalmology. Although most commonly used for diabetic retinopathy assessment and ROP screening, innovative technology solutions are allowing telemedicine systems to be utilized for screening, diagnosis, and management of an ever-growing number of ophthalmic diseases, including glaucoma, AMD, ocular trauma, anterior segment pathologies, and adnexal and orbital diseases. Early disease detection and improved access to specialty care are increasingly important as new treatment modalities become available, and teleophthalmology is assuming a vital role in filling the demand and helping to improve patient outcomes. Research to understand the progress that has been demonstrated to date and barriers to further implementation are important areas for future studies in teleophthalmology.

REFERENCES

1. Berwick DM, Nolan TW, Whittington J. The triple aim: care, health, and cost. *Health Aff (Millwood)* 2008;27(3):759–769.
2. Silva PS, Horton MB, Clary D, et al. Identification of diabetic retinopathy and ungradable image rate with ultrawide field imaging in a national teleophthalmology program. *Ophthalmology* 2016;123(6):1360–1367.
3. Silva PS, Cavallerano JD, Tolls D, et al. Potential efficiency benefits of nonmydriatic ultrawide field retinal imaging in an ocular telehealth diabetic retinopathy program. *Diabetes Care* 2014;37(1):50–55.
4. Micheletti JM, Hendrick AM, Khan FN, Ziemer DC, Pasquel FJ. Current and next generation portable screening devices for diabetic retinopathy. *J Diabetes Sci Technol* 2016;10(2):295–300.
5. Ryan ME, Rajalakshmi R, Prathiba V, et al. Comparison Among Methods of Retinopathy Assessment (CAMRA)

study: smartphone, nonmydriatic, and mydriatic photography. *Ophthalmology* 2015;122(10):2038–2043.

6. Institute of Medicine (U.S.). Committee on Quality of Health Care in America. *Crossing the quality chasm : a new health system for the 21st century.* Washington, DC: National Academy Press; 2001.

7. Bahaadinbeigy K, Yogesan K. A literature review of teleophthalmology projects from around the globe. In: Yogesan K, Goldschmidt L, Cuadros J, eds. *Digital Teleretinal Screening: Teleophthalmology in Practice.* Berlin: Springer; 2012:3–10.

8. Federation ID. *Diabetes Atlas.* http://www.idf.org/about-diabetes/facts-figures. Accessed January 22, 2017.

9. Congdon N, O'Colmain B, Klaver CC, et al. Causes and prevalence of visual impairment among adults in the United States. *Arch Ophthalmol* 2004;122(4):477–485.

10. Bressler NM, Varma R, Doan QV, et al. Underuse of the health care system by persons with diabetes mellitus and diabetic macular edema in the United States. *JAMA Ophthalmol* 2014;132(2):168–173.

11. *The State of Health Care Quality Report 2015.* Agency for Health Care Research and Quality; 2016.

12. Silva PS, Cavallerano JD, Aiello LM, Aiello LP. Telemedicine and diabetic retinopathy: moving beyond retinal screening. *Arch Ophthalmol* 2011;129(2):236–242.

13. Hautala N, Aikkila R, Korpelainen J, et al. Marked reductions in visual impairment due to diabetic retinopathy achieved by efficient screening and timely treatment. *Acta Ophthalmol* 2014;92(6):582–587.

14. Liew G, Michaelides M, Bunce C. A comparison of the causes of blindness certifications in England and Wales in working age adults (16-64 years), 1999-2000 with 2009-2010. *BMJ Open* 2014;4(2).

15. Williams GA, Scott IU, Haller JA, et al. Single-field fundus photography for diabetic retinopathy screening: a report by the American Academy of Ophthalmology. *Ophthalmology* 2004;111(5):1055–1062.

16. Li HK, Horton M, Bursell SE, et al. Telehealth practice recommendations for diabetic retinopathy. *Telemed J E Health* 2011;17(10):814–837.

17. Early Treatment Diabetic Retinopathy Study Research Group. Grading diabetic retinopathy from stereoscopic color fundus photographs–an extension of the modified Airlie House classification. ETDRS report number 10. *Ophthalmology* 1991;98(5 Suppl):786–806.

18. Scanlon PH. The English national screening programme for sight-threatening diabetic retinopathy. *J Med Screen* 2008;15(1):1–4.

19. Shi L, Wu H, Dong J, et al . Telemedicine for detecting diabetic retinopathy: a systematic review and meta-analysis. *Br J Ophthalmol* 2015;99(6):823–831.

20. Scanlon PH, Foy C, Malhotra R, Aldington SJ. The influence of age, duration of diabetes, cataract, and pupil size on image quality in digital photographic retinal screening. *Diabetes Care* 2005;28(10):2448–2453.

21. Silva PS, Cavallerano JD, Haddad NM, et al. Comparison of nondiabetic retinal findings identified with nonmydriatic fundus photography vs ultrawide field imaging in an ocular telehealth program. *JAMA Ophthalmol* 2016;134(3):330–334.

22. Murgatroyd H, Cox A, Ellingford A, et al . Can we predict which patients are at risk of having an ungradeable digital image for screening for diabetic retinopathy? *Eye (Lond)* 2008;22(3):344–348.

23. Pandit RJ, Taylor R. Mydriasis and glaucoma: exploding the myth. A systematic review. *Diabet Med* 2000;17(10):693–699.

24. Horton MB, Silva PS, Cavallerano JD, Aiello LP. Clinical components of telemedicine programs for diabetic retinopathy. *Curr Diab Rep* 2016;16(12):129.

25. Diabetic eye screening: programme overview. In: Public Health England ed. 2014.

26. Vaziri K, Moshfeghi DM, Moshfeghi AA. Feasibility of telemedicine in detecting diabetic retinopathy and age-related macular degeneration. *Semin Ophthalmol* 2015;30(2):81–95.

27. Jones S, Edwards RT. Diabetic retinopathy screening: a systematic review of the economic evidence. *Diabet Med* 2010;27(3):249–256.

28. Horton MB, Silva PS, Cavallerano JD, Aiello LP. Operational components of telemedicine programs for diabetic retinopathy. *Curr Diab Rep* 2016;16(12):128.

29. Mansberger SL, Sheppler C, Barker G, et al. Long-term comparative effectiveness of telemedicine in providing diabetic retinopathy screening examinations: a randomized clinical trial. *JAMA Ophthalmol* 2015;133(5):518–525.

30. *2017 CPT Professional Edition*, 4th ed. American Medical Association; 2016.

31. Sim DA, Keane PA, Tufail A, et al . Automated retinal image analysis for diabetic retinopathy in telemedicine. *Curr Diab Rep* 2015;15(3):14.

32. Abramoff MD, Folk JC, Han DP, et al. Automated analysis of retinal images for detection of referable diabetic retinopathy. *JAMA Ophthalmol* 2013;131(3):351–357.

33. Quigley HA, Broman AT. The number of people with glaucoma worldwide in 2010 and 2020. *Br J Ophthalmol* 2006;90(3):262–267.

34. Varma R, Lee PP, Goldberg I, Kotak S. An assessment of the health and economic burdens of glaucoma. *Am J Ophthalmol* 2011;152(4):515–522.

35. Thomas SM, Jeyaraman MM, Hodge WG, et al. The effectiveness of teleglaucoma versus in-patient examination for glaucoma screening: a systematic review and meta-analysis. *PLoS One* 2014;9(12).

36. Hatt S, Wormald R, Burr J. Screening for prevention of optic nerve damage due to chronic open angle glaucoma. *Cochrane Database Syst Rev* 2006;(4).

37. Li HK, Tang RA, Oschner K, et al . Telemedicine screening of glaucoma. *Telemed J* 1999;5(3):283–290.

38. Sreelatha OK, Ramesh SV. Teleophthalmology: improving patient outcomes? *Clin Ophthalmol* 2016;10:285–295.

39. Strouthidis NG, Chandrasekharan G, Diamond JP, Murdoch IE. Teleglaucoma: ready to go? *Br J Ophthalmol* 2014;98(12):1605–1611.

40. Gandhi NG, Prakalapakorn SG, El-Dairi MA, et al. Icare ONE rebound versus Goldmann applanation tonometry in children with known or suspected glaucoma. *Am J Ophthalmol* 2012;154(5):843–849, e841.

41. Mansouri K, Medeiros FA, Tafreshi A, Weinreb RN. Continuous 24-hour monitoring of intraocular pressure patterns with a contact lens sensor: safety, tolerability, and reproducibility in patients with glaucoma. *Arch Ophthalmol* 2012;130(12):1534–1539.

42. Flemmons MS, Hsiao YC, Dzau J, et al. Home tonometry for management of pediatric glaucoma. *Am J Ophthalmol* 2011;152(3):470–478, e472.

43. Dobkin BH, Dorsch A. The promise of mHealth: daily activity monitoring and outcome assessments by wearable sensors. *Neurorehabil Neural Repair* 2011;25(9):788–798.

44. Kiage D, Kherani IN, Gichuhi S, Damji KF, Nyenze M. The Muranga Teleophthalmology Study: comparison of virtual (teleglaucoma) with in-person clinical assessment to diagnose glaucoma. *Middle East Afr J Ophthalmol* 2013;20(2):150–157.

45. Kashiwagi K, Tanabe N, Go K, et al. Comparison of a remote operating slit-lamp microscope system with a conventional slit-lamp microscope system for examination of trabeculectomy eyes. *J Glaucoma* 2013;22(4):278–283.

46. Crowston JG, Kirwan JF, Wells A, Kennedy C, Murdoch IE. Evaluating clinical signs in trabeculectomized eyes. *Eye (Lond)* 2004;18(3):299–303.

47. de Mul M, de Bont AA, Reus NJ, Lemij HG, Berg M. Improving the quality of eye care with tele-ophthalmology: shared-care glaucoma screening. *J Telemed Telecare* 2004;10(6):331–336.

48. Verma S, Arora S, Kassam F, Edwards MC, Damji KF. Northern Alberta remote teleglaucoma program: clinical outcomes and patient disposition. *Can J Ophthalmol* 2014;49(2):135–140.

49. Arora S, Rudnisky CJ, Damji KF. Improved access and cycle time with an "in-house" patient-centered teleglaucoma program versus traditional in-person assessment. *Telemed J E Health* 2014;20(5):439–445.

50. Thomas S, Hodge W, Malvankar-Mehta M. The cost-effectiveness analysis of teleglaucoma screening device. *PLoS One* 2015;10(9).

51. Quek DT, Nongpiur ME, Perera SA, Aung T. Angle imaging: advances and challenges. *Indian J Ophthalmol* 2011;59(Suppl):S69–S75.

52. Foster PJ, Oen FT, Machin D, et al. The prevalence of glaucoma in Chinese residents of Singapore: a cross-sectional population survey of the Tanjong Pagar district. *Arch Ophthalmol* 2000;118(8):1105–1111.

53. Aung T, Lim MC, Chan YH, et al. Configuration of the drainage angle, intraocular pressure, and optic disc cupping in subjects with chronic angle-closure glaucoma. *Ophthalmology* 2005;112(1):28–32.

54. Fierson WM, Capone AJr, American Academy of Pediatrics Section on Ophthalmology, et al. Telemedicine for evaluation of retinopathy of prematurity. *Pediatrics* 2015;135(1):e238–e254.

55. Quinn GE, Ying GS, Daniel E, et al. Validity of a telemedicine system for the evaluation of acute-phase retinopathy of prematurity. *JAMA Ophthalmol* 2014;132(10):1178–1184.

56. Zimmer-Galler IE. Telemedicine for retinopathy of prematurity: an evolving paradigm. *JAMA Ophthalmol* 2016;134(11):1270–1271.

57. Quinn GE, Ells A, Capone AJr, et al. Analysis of discrepancy between diagnostic clinical examination findings and corresponding evaluation of digital images in the telemedicine approaches to evaluating acute-phase retinopathy of prematurity study. *JAMA Ophthalmol* 2016;134(11):1263–1270.

58. Wallace DK, Quinn GE, Freedman SF, Chiang MF. Agreement among pediatric ophthalmologists in diagnosing plus and pre-plus disease in retinopathy of prematurity. *J AAPOS* 2008;12(4):352–356.

59. Group AHSR, Chew EY, Clemons TE, et al. Randomized trial of a home monitoring system for early detection of choroidal neovascularization home monitoring of the Eye (HOME) study. *Ophthalmology* 2014;121(2):535–544.

60. Han DP. The ForeSeeHome device and the HOME study: a milestone in the self-detection of neovascular age-related macular degeneration. *JAMA Ophthalmol* 2014;132(10):1167–1168.

Adult Emergency and Critical Care Telehealth*

H. Neal Reynolds, MD, Marc T. Zubrow, MD,
Richard Alcorta, MD and Neal Sikka, MD

A picture is worth a thousand words (anonymous)
Every Second Counts
(< 3/100ᵗʰ of an R Adams Cowley's Golden Hour)

FUTURISTIC SCENARIO

Emergency medical services (EMS) is called to a road-side motor vehicle collision. EMS personnel are wearing helmet and body cameras, with head-mounted microphones and earphones. EMS notifies the regional telemedicine center EMS/MD that a single passenger in the driver position, belted with front air-bag deployment but no side-window airbags, was "T-boned" from the driver side with about 18 inches intrusion on the driver door. EMS connects the patient to a cellular-enabled vital signs monitor with connectivity to the telemedicine center. The driver is hypotensive, unconscious, and with obvious deformity to the left femur. The EMS doesn't hear breath sounds on the left chest, and neither does the telemedicine center EMS/MD. The telemedicine center EMS/MD recognizes the risk of tension pneumothorax, splenic rupture, lateral compression fracture of the pelvis, and possible traumatic brain injury. The EMS does a quick on-scene focused assessment with sonography for trauma (FAST) exam as the telemedicine center EMS/MD observes remotely but cannot see sliding pleural lines on the left. Additionally there is fluid in the left upper quadrant (LUQ). The remote physician confirms

no sliding pleura and authorizes needle decompression of the left hemithorax and advises 1 liter crystalloids immediately if blood pressure (BP) is no better after needle decompression. The telemedicine center EMS/MD recognizes this patient will need a tertiary trauma center and advises a bypass of local facilities. While the EMS decompresses the left chest and establishes an IV, the telemedicine center contacts aeromedical services to dispatch a medevac helicopter to global positioning system (GPS) coordinates transmitted from the EMS vehicle on scene. Airway patency is a concern in this unconscious critical patient. The paramedic begins a rapid sequence intubation with video laryngoscope and has difficulty. The telemedicine center EMS/MD views remotely and advises on an epiglottis lift with the blade of the scope. Immediately, both the paramedic and telemedicine EMS/MD can see the cords and endotracheal tube inserted. On scene the EMS places the patient in a pelvic binder on a back board after a cervical collar is placed. The medevac helicopter arrives 15 minutes later. The helicopter remains "hot" with rotors turning while the EMS and flight paramedic load the patient. Audio/video connection switches over to the flight paramedic during loading in addition to a portable screen in the aircraft. The patient becomes hypotensive again, and another liter of saline is authorized by the EMS/MD, who also recommends insertion of a left chest tube. The flight paramedic inserts a 32 F chest tube—there is a large gush of air. The helicopter lands on the roof of the trauma center 21 minutes after the crash. The telemedicine center physician follows the patient to the trauma bay with a portable audio–video

---

* Chapter author Dr. Marc T. Zubrow is currently the director of a tele-ICU program that deploys Philips technology.

screen and meets the trauma MD, hands off the patient, and advises of decompressed tension pneumothorax, risk of splenic rupture (which may account for the hypotension), and LUQ fluid on FAST exam. At the telemedicine center, the EMS/MD hands off to the intensivist/MD. Plain films confirm a pelvic fracture, and the rapid FAST is repeated by trauma staff and found to be positive for hemoperitoneum. The patient is taken as a "priority 1" to the operating room (OR) for splenectomy. A portable computed tomography (CT) of the head while in the OR reveals an expanding epidural hematoma. Images are transmitted immediately to radiology and neurosurgery. The neurosurgeon performs craniectomy while the general trauma team does the splenectomy and stabilizes the pelvic fractures. The telemedicine center intensivist/MD is intermittently observing the surgery from OR overhead cameras. After completion, trauma workup, and time-sensitive surgical interventions, the patient goes to the intensive care unit (ICU) with tele-ICU technology. The telemedicine center intensivist/MD appears on the video screen above the bed in the ICU and performs a hand-off to the bedside physician staff (intensivists, surgeon, anesthesiologists, etc.) to include OR blood products, estimated blood loss, difficulties seen with surgery, etc.

From the scene to the final destination in the ICU, the events are documented accurately and annotated with images by the EMS/MD in an electronic format. The electronic document is forwarded to the receiving physician in the ICU, leaving only the documentation of the physical exam for the ICU MD.

Technologies utilized

1. 700 megahertz public safety bandwidth
2. 700 megahertz deployable cellular systems
3. GPS transmitted to the telemedicine center from the EMS vehicle
4. Audio–video headsets and head/body cameras
5. Broadband cellular
6. Portable handheld ultrasonography visible to the telemedicine center
7. Electronic stethoscope audible to the telemedicine center
8. Portable vital signs monitor with broadband connectivity
9. Portable 12-inch screen for audio–video in the aircraft
10. Video laryngoscopy visible to the telemedicine center MD
11. Overhead audio–video technology in the operative suite
12. Teleradiology to radiologists
13. Radiology cellular technology link to the neurosurgeon
14. Tele-ICU technology

Although this scenario involved trauma, similar technology and process could apply to any nontraumatic unconscious patient, cardiac arrhythmias, etc.

This scenario provides the foundation for a proposed "Complete Emergency–Critical Care Telemedicine System." Generally, the concept is to have qualified, real-time, audio–video physician oversight from the first moment medical care begins to intervene on a critically ill patient at the scene, in route to a medical facility, through the emergency resuscitation, the operative suite, and on to the landing zone in the ICU. This proposed scenario (Figure 8-1) would take advantage of the changing demographics of the physician workforce to include more physicians with combined training in emergency medicine and critical care medicine (CCM). The rest of this chapter provides a summary of which pieces of this future model exist and where the challenges lie that require more effort to make it happen.

INTRODUCTION

There is an extremely close relationship between the prehospital realm, the emergency department (ED), and critical care services. In most cases, the largest percentage of hospital admissions come from the ED. Typically, 20% of acute hospital admissions are to an ICU, but up to 58% of ED admissions result in an ICU admission.[1] Often, critically ill patients are initially discovered "down"—unconscious—following cardiac arrest, blunt trauma, interpersonal violence, falls, entrapments, new intracerebral pathology, sepsis, respiratory failure, diabetic ketoacidosis, intoxication, or overdose. When a patient is discovered, he or she may not be breathing or protecting their airway,

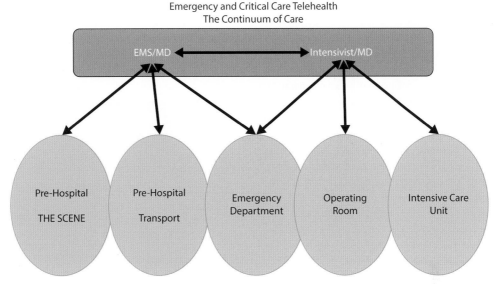

Emergency and Critical Care Telehealth
The Continuum of Care

EMS/MD   Intensivist/MD

Pre-Hospital

THE SCENE

Pre-Hospital

Transport

Emergency
Department

Operating
Room

Intensive Care
Unit

▲ **Figure 8-1.** Connecting critical care services from the scene, through prehospital transport, through the emergency department, to the OR if necessary and on to the ICU. All connected with currently available technology.

bleeding or hypotensive, and require immediate life-saving interventions. Critical care begins at the scene with initial stabilization; airway maintenance; oxygenation/ventilation; attempts to establish return of spontaneous circulation (ROSC); early resuscitation with fluids or vasoactive agents; decompression of tension pneumothorax; stabilization of cervical, thoracic, and lumbar spine, etc. The onsite EMTs and paramedics are expected to process huge amounts of information quickly, "stabilize the scene," make immediate lifesaving decisions and interventions, and participate in extraction efforts. Additionally, the on-scene care providers are gathering information as to mechanism of injury or illness and patient status in preparation for communication to the local medical facility.

The "information overload"[2] can be paralyzing, or at least overwhelming, partly due to normal human "limited attention capacity"[3] and difficulty assuring the information is the "right type."[4] Once moved from the scene, the patient spends time in transport. The mode of transport is essentially always compromised due to space constraints, noise, need to communicate with receiving facilities, limited personnel, and limited capabilities, with associated risk to the patient and

personnel.[5] Patient care must continue in route and response to therapy noted and shared with awaiting staff at the ED. With quick sharing of information, care shifts to the ED staff for ongoing stabilization, often with a visit to the OR, and subsequent transfer to the ICU for completion of resuscitation and management of life support equipment.

The concept of a second set of eyes has been well described in the tele-ICU[6] and in the corporate sphere.[7] A remote provider, away from the noise and chaos of the scene, protected from information overload could substantially add to decision making, data gathering, and information sharing as a patient moves from scene to ED to OR and on to the ICU. The purpose of this chapter is to expand upon this continuum of critical care and review applications of telehealth in all these arenas.

TELEHEALTH AT THE SCENE

There is increasing interest in the virtual presence of a high-level care provider "at the scene." In the trauma dogma, the six places patients lose blood are the pleural space, the retroperitoneal, the peritoneum, the pelvis, large extremities, and "the street". The trauma physician essentially never sees "the street" blood loss. Transmitting the images of a severe scalp wound with blood loss in situ could direct the trauma physician and avoid excessive searches for blood loss at the other sites. Injury prediction can be refined with direct visualization at the scene and patients directed to proper facilities initially. With recognition of injury risk, surgical interventions may be more rapid, leading to improved outcomes and a tightening of the "golden hour."

In 2012, the U.S. Congress enacted the Middle Class Tax Relief and Job Recovery Act of 2012, forming the First Responder Network Authority[8] within the U.S. Department of Commerce. FirstNet is charged with responsibility for deploying and operating the nationwide public safety broadband network and holds the license for the public safety broadband spectrum (763 to 769 MHz/793 to 799 MHz), commonly known as the *700 MHz public safety spectrum* (Figure 8-2).

The 700 MHz band is a 108 MHz-wide segment of the electromagnetic spectrum, from 698 to 806 MHz, available for both commercial wireless and public safety communications.

This segment of the spectrum became available with the transition away from analog television. Located just above the remaining TV broadcast channels, this 700 MHz signal will penetrate building walls and cover large geographic areas with relatively modest infrastructure required, providing ideal capability for EMS services. The National Institute on Standards and Technology[9] has promoted development of technology to accelerate the deployment of 700 megahertz FirstNet technology (Figure 8-3).

The National Public Safety Telecommunications Council[10] published the *EMS Telemedicine Report*. The report is a result of a nationwide questionnaire to EMS providers and directors, hospital ED and trauma center directors, and online EMS medical control physicians

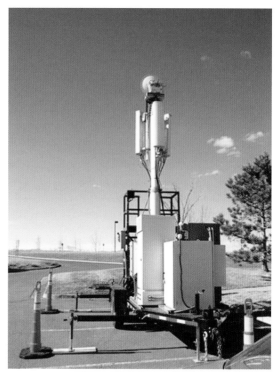

▲ **Figure 8-3.** Easily deployable cellular on wheels to support 700 megahertz public safety networks. (From https://www.nist.gov/programs-projects/public-safety-700-mhz-broadband-deployable-systems.)

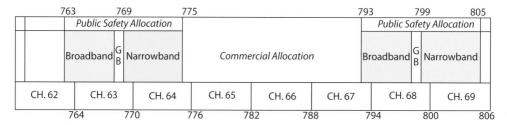

▲ **Figure 8-2.** The so-called "D block" allocated for public safety includes 758 to 763 MHz (far left) and 788-793 MHz. (From https://www.fcc.gov/general/700-mhz-public-safety-spectrum-0.)

and summarized the following applications of telecommunications that seemed most relevant in the EMS environment:

- Real-time transmission of video and still images of the patients, scene environment (eg, crashed vehicle, home setting), specific injuries, and/or other physical assessments
- Bidirectional conferencing between field providers and patients with medical control or consulting staff
- Transmission of diagnostic still and video images (eg, ultrasound, eye/ear/nose/throat images, electronic stethoscope sounds, and multi–vital sign monitoring devices)

When selectively querying EMS medical control physicians, physicians judged that the most important elements included:

- Physician-assisted critical care at the scene (64%)
- Risk management/mitigation and patient refusal scenarios (60.5%)
- Improved decision support (57.3%)

In the following scenario-specific situations:

- 81.4% suggested use in severe injury/motor vehicle trauma
- 81% for physician-assisted assessment for stroke patients
- 79.5% for assistance with pediatric asthma patients
- 76.5% thought two-way audio–video would be helpful in managing mass casualty situations
- 65.1% thought it would help with diabetic patients who refuse care

▶ On-Scene Documentation

To operationalize the video communications, the scene staff have the choice of body cameras, helmet cameras, combination devices, and vehicular cameras.[11] This camera evidence is acquired in real time and can be transmitted and archived for clear documentation of what actually happened.[12–14] Real-time video allows remote staff to observe and advise on the application of complex/unique technology such as the abdominal aortic junctional tourniquet for severe inguinal and pelvic hemorrhage,[15] aid in the interpretation of complex dysrhythmias, advanced cardiac life support (ACLS)

direction, etc. The technology can include audio with the video and be supplemented by GPS positioning.[16]

Vendors are solving the connectivity problems by developing technology that roams between carriers and communication technologies and developing "ruggedized" equipment for the scene incorporating real-time audio and video, which can be linked with SpO2 monitoring, electrocardiogram (ECG), noninvasive BP monitoring, electronic stethoscope, specialized cameras, and screening ultrasonography.

LifeBot technology can be carried to the scene, moved with the patient to the transport vehicle, and travel with the patient into the ED, allowing a virtual physician presence from the scene to the hospital (Figure 8-4).

There are concerns and challenges with real-time recordings that may slow or limit adoption in some jurisdictions. The pros and cons of video recordings include[17]:

Pros:

- Every patient interaction chronicled
- Speech patterns, statements, complaints, skin color, and environmental factors confirmed and considered by remote providers
- Treatments, techniques, and processes chronicled and used for reference and training
- False accusations refuted while mistreatment or misconduct is quickly addressed
- Care providers and patient accountability

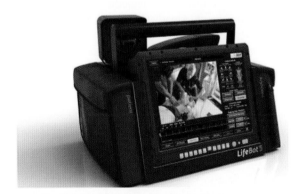

▲ **Figure 8-4.** Commercially available product, self-contained with monitoring and diagnostic equipment incorporated into a portable 700 MHz public safety band–compatible device. (Reproduced with permission of LifeBot, http://www.lifebot.us/lifebot5/.)

Cons:

- Every patient interaction chronicled
- Existence of information begets the disclosure
- Patient privacy compromised
- Fear of disclosure could prevent patients from sharing sensitive medically essential facts
- Delayed unsupported judgment by reviewers and legal community
- Significant expense and logistic challenges

Of note, there have recently been decisions regarding Health Insurance Portability and Accountability Act (HIPAA) confidentiality of patient images, rendering it a punishable offense if identifiable images are posted on any form of public media.[18] The acquisition, transmission, viewing, and storage must meet the HIPAA requirements to protect both patient health information (PHI) and personal identification information.

In summary, there is EMS interest in enhanced, on-scene, high-level medical assistance; there is meaningful and functional bandwidth set aside for the EMS; there is government promotion of technology; the technology is available; and there is private-sector investment in developing it further. Other than technical issues with archiving, the negative concerns and objections are relatively small and manageable.

TELEHEALTH IN TRANSPORT

In an extensive review of telemedicine in the prehospital environment, Amadi-Obi et al.[19] screened 1,279 pertinent articles published between 1970 and 2014, excluding 1,240 from review and focusing on 39 articles. Twenty-five were related to stroke, nine to trauma, and five to myocardial infarction. Summarizing the 25 stroke articles, the application of the National Institute of Health Stroke Score (NIHSS) was as reliable when performed remotely via telemedicine as when done face to face, the number of consults with experts was greater, and the clinical outcomes were equivalent to rapid face-to-face encounters. Summarizing the trauma literature, where local expertise was lacking, teleradiology as part of the trauma diagnosis improved the diagnosis and decreased the rate of expensive transfers. Burn assessment was equally accurate remotely as when performed face to face. In particular, EMS staff

paramedics were able to perform a FAST exam under the guidance of remote emergency medicine physicians and were able to identify key physical signs and better direct medical decision making. Finally regarding myocardial infarction, transfer time to a STEMI center (ST elevation myocardial infarction) for percutaneous coronary intervention (PCI) was shorter with an associated decrease in mortality when the emergency vehicle is equipped with 12-lead ECG telemedicine technology for the transmission of prehospital ECG data. Despite computer and/or paramedic interpretation of ECGs for STEMI being 92.6% sensitive and 85.4% specific,[20] interventional cardiologists may still prefer to have the ECG transmitted directly for decisions to activate the interventional cardiac catheterization lab.

Delivery of critical care services and life-sustaining interventions are essential at the scene and must continue in route to the hospital. In general, the United States has adhered to a "swoop and scoop" philosophy,[21] also referred to as the "Anglo-American" model, where ambulances are staffed with EMTs and paramedics. By contrast, in the German-Franco model, the ambulance is staffed by physicians[22,23] who provide advanced physician skills for stabilizing interventions on the scene. The World Health Association[24] has maintained that prehospital care be:

- Simple, sustainable, practical, efficient, and flexible
- Integrated into a country's existing health care, public health, and transportation infrastructures where available

The meaning and magnitude of integration are undefined, but should include real-time audio–video integration with remote higher-level care providers. On the other hand, The Association of Critical Care Transport,[25] while defining what a critical care transport is (eg, describing the characteristics of a patient needing critical care transport and staffing requirements), has been silent on the place, need, or requirements for a virtual physician presence.

Combining high-level technology with telemedicine, the University of Texas (UT)[26] in consortium with the Cleveland Clinic has launched a mobile stroke unit (MSU): an ambulance equipped with small, relatively portable CT scanners. The telestroke literature indicates that the visual exam enhances accuracy for neurologic diagnosis and increases application of the NIHSS.

When a stroke is suspected, a remote exam is performed, and physicians review the field-generated CT scan of the brain to determine if there is sufficient evidence to administer tissue plasminogen activator (tPA). Preliminary data from the MSUs suggest that patients get tPA about 40 minutes sooner than those receiving usual EMS transport and care once arriving at the ED. Brain tissue is particularly vulnerable to ischemia. Complete interruption of blood flow to the brain for only 5 minutes triggers the death of vulnerable neurons in several brain regions, whereas 20 to 40 minutes of ischemia is required for cardiac myocytes or kidney cell death.[27]

The concept and value of expediting efforts to reperfuse brain tissue related to a thrombotic stroke has been demonstrated multiple times.[28-30] This MSU technology minimizes the brain loss associated with the time of transport. However, the technology is expensive. The Economic Cycle Research Institute (ECRI) estimates that the total fixed and continuing costs over 5 years for the University of Texas's unit will be $1.65 million. That includes a $375,000 mobile CT scanner, a $60,000 retrofit of the vehicle, $30,000 in telemedicine equipment, and other ongoing expenses related to training and certification of personnel and telemedicine network coverage.[31]

Ongoing real-time management is possible with cellular-based communications during the transport with continuous physician management (Figure 8-5). The medical staff performing the transport management could be an ED physician, a specialist consultant, etc., but would be available to provide continuous care in route and a "hand-off" to the next physician receiving the patient with specific details of assessment, interventions, responses, and impressions.

TELEHEALTH IN THE EMERGENCY DEPARTMENT

EDs are under siege. There is a "perfect storm" of shrinking capacity, ever-increasing demand for services, and more Americans relying on EDs for their routine and acute care needs, including aging "Boomers" and people newly enrolled in Medicaid. The American College of Emergency Physicians (ACEP) published the national Emergency Medicine Report card,[32] giving a D+ overall, which is down from a C− 5 years earlier. In specific areas of patient access to care and access to subspecialists, the grade was essentially failing at D−. The general "lay-of-the-land" per the report is shown in Figure 8-6.

The ACEP report provides 11 general recommendations, including the recommendation to "continue to increase the use of systems, standards, and *information technologies* to track and enhance the quality and patient safety environment."[32] This recommendation could be interpreted as support for the growth and expansion of telemedicine to, among other things, enhance access to subspecialists. The Emergency Telemedicine section of the ACEP was established almost 2 decades ago, in 1998, to bring together emergency medicine

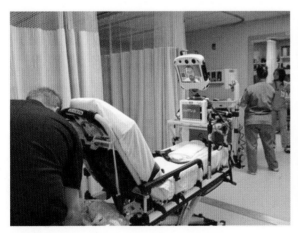
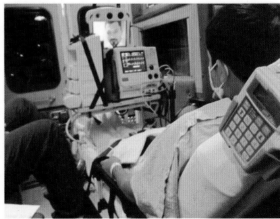

▲ **Figure 8-5.** Continuous real-time remote management of a transport patient with bidirectional audio–video communications. (Reproduced with permission and courtsey of InTouch Health. All rights reserved.)

OVERALL STATE GRADES

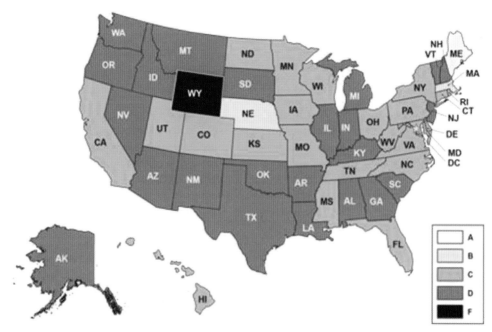

▲ **Figure 8-6.** Overall state grades awarded by the American College of Physicians (ACEP) in the 2014 American Emergency Environment Report. Image downloaded from the public access website for the ACEP. (© 2011-2016, American College of Emergency Physicians. Reprinted with permission.)

practitioners with an interest in telehealth. At that time, the ACEP produced *The Telemedicine in Emergency Medicine Information Paper*[33] outlining status and capabilities to include collaborative patient management, "remote sensing" (ECG and digital radiographs), and decision-making tools accessible online. The section lost membership over time in the mid-2000s and was re-established in 2012. This revived section updated the information paper in the 2014 "primer" of Telemedicine for the Emergency Department[34] and reviewed technology, clinical applications, billing codes, reimbursement, mobile apps, cost, security, and integration with existing electronic medical records.

EMERGENCY DEPARTMENT TELEMEDICINE MODELS

In general, applications of telemedicine within the ED can be categorized into three models:

1. Use of telemedicine to enhance ED processes

2. Extend capabilities outside the local ED

3. Bring specialists or capabilities into the ED from the outside

ENHANCING AN ED PROCESS

The following is not meant to be an exhaustive review of all applications, but rather a review of several important concepts designed to provoke the interested reader to examine new applications.

▶ Patient ED Flow

The University of California San Diego launched a pilot project to virtually bring in an ED physician for triage in the event of a major patient surge. The EDTITRATE study[35] was designed to solve the problem of wasted overstaffing versus the delay of arrival of an on-call back-up physician. During times of patient surges, the back-up MD is called in virtually. The on-call back-up physician meets the patient via telemedicine technology, with the support of an on-site ED-RN, and examines the ear, nose, and throat; listens to lung and heart sounds; remotely reviews laboratory and radiographic data; and either triages to higher expedited care or prescribes care and discharges the patient. Currently, the study is not completed but suggests a creative solution for the surge problem.

▶ Avoiding Unnecessary Transfers

Brennan et al.[36] performed a comparative analysis of traditional face-to-face care with remote care to demonstrate that remote ED care can be performed from an urban to a rural ED without degradation of quality. In a unique cross-over fashion, they demonstrated equivalent quality of care, with similar 72-hour return rate, patient satisfaction, and a 10-minute shorter average ED length of stay with telemedicine. The implication is that urban ED overcrowding could be mitigated by telemedicine by reducing transfers from rural to urban settings.

A Houston-based effort called the Emergency Telehealth and Navigation project (ETHAN)[37] connects emergency physicians with EMS providers who are on scene with the intent of avoiding needless transports to the ED. The process includes real-time communications among EMS, physicians, and the patient. When summoned to see a patient, if the EMS judges the issue not urgent, a video link is established with an ED physician, and an evaluation is performed by an ED physician using a tablet, with the EMS provider performing vital signs and physical assessment under the direction of the remote physician. Early results suggest that up to 40% of EMS transports in Houston did not require acute care, but rather needed referral to primary care for their chronic conditions.[38] The ETHAN project was able to avoid unnecessary transport, ultimately reducing ED overcrowding and reducing wait times for those needing urgent care.

▶ Extend Capabilities Outside the Local Emergency Department

The concept is to take advantage of the unique characteristics of EDs staffed 24/7/ 365 with physicians and advanced practitioners who possess a broad skill set (eg, general medicine, pediatrics, CCM, trauma,

toxicology) and apply the specialty skills remotely outside of the specialty center or ED setting.

Emergency Department Consultations

Sophisticated or specialty centers can reach out to other less resource-rich institutions, extending the capabilities to the more remote ED. As far back as 1996, a Chinese university–based program established ED outreach to an offshore hospital in Taiwan.[39] During a 12-month period, they performed 275 consultations, including 24 specialist/subspecialists spanning more than 100 different members of the medical staff with a very high satisfaction rating. This type of program has been operational at the University of Maryland Medical System since February 2017.

Trauma

Eastern Maine Medical Center[40] Tele-Emergency Department and Trauma Services connects more than 12 hospital centers to the main trauma center. Receiving over 800 patients per year with 50% from rural community hospitals, the program is able to consult immediately, avoid unnecessary transfers, and begin therapy within minutes rather than waiting hours to arrive at distant specialty centers for interventions.

In 2006, the University of Arizona Medical Center joined with the Tucson Fire Department and Tucson Department of Transportation (DOT) to develop a citywide EMS telemedicine system built around the DOT's mesh broadband wireless network.[41,42] At the hospital end there were workstations located in the ED and the "trauma room." On the EMS vehicle, cameras were positioned both inside the ambulance and outside with a 360-degree pan capability with a 19-inch monitor for the patient or EMS personnel to see the remote trauma physician in real time. Although there were limitations to coverage and a full report was not published, the authors did describe remote assistance with endotracheal intubation when onsite providers used the video laryngoscope device Glidescope technology.[43]

Correctional System Health Care

This area suffers from complexity of movement, security risks with prisoner transport, and major public safety issues if a detainee were to become violent or attempt to escape. The ACEP has nicely outlined the issues of correctional care in the ED.[44] As far back as 1997, telemedicine within the correctional system has been shown to be cost and medically effective while minimizing security risk of transport.[45] ED telemedicine programs can serve as an immediate resource for prison-related trauma or general emergency medical services.

Remote Care

A variety of industries and individual adventure travelers require emergency medical support in remote and often austere environments. There are both commercial and university-based providers of on-demand emergency care via telemedicine to oil, gas, aviation, maritime, and remote research stations. Medical support services may be provided directly to patients and in other cases a remote EMT, paramedic, nurse, or physician providing care in consultation with the remote physician. With 24/7 staffing, the ED may be the optimal provider.

Mobile Integrated Health Care with Direct Audio-Visual Patient Contact

Evolution Healthcare in Dallas has implemented an audiovisual connection with EMS providers who go into the homes of at-risk patients and provide a patient–physician real-time, live audio–video interaction.[46] The goal is to avoid EMS responses, ED visits, and medical inpatient admissions. The project has demonstrated a 19% decrease in ED visits per member per month (PMPM) costs, a 21% decrease in ED utilization, a 37% decrease in inpatient PMPM costs, and a 40% decrease in patient utilization (all reaching statistical significance) through this telemedicine-coordinated care program.

▶ Bring Specialists or Capabilities into the Emergency Department from the Outside

"Tele-radiology is one of the oldest, most established, successful, and widely used clinical telemedicine specialties"[47–49] "with on-call emergency reporting being used in over 70% of radiology practices in the US."[50] Teleradiology is of primary value to smaller hospitals with the inability to staff onsite radiologists. From the

perspective of the ED physician, timeliness of reports is paramount. Distant radiologists must be available and work in real time to avoid delayed overreads that can be problematic once the patient has left the ED.[51,52] Currently there are no data regarding the penetration of teleradiology into the ED, but it is presumed high in otherwise uncovered facilities.

Telecardiology

When considering the raw numbers of ECGs transmitted, next to teleradiology, telecardiology may be the second-most used remote technology to support ED physicians and patients. Telecardiology includes remote reading of ECGs, echocardiograms, pacemaker interrogation and monitoring, and review of angiograms. When looking at a prehospital review of electronically transmitted ECGs, there has been a shortened "door to balloon" time.[53] There is little information regarding the development of telecardiology networks as is seen in telestroke networks. Nor has there been much emphasis on the visual examination of the cardiac patient. Certain European programs have evolved to cloud-based 12-lead ECG computing, making the information available to a cardiologist via a handheld device.[54] The University of Maryland telemedicine program is currently providing remote support and management of congestive heart failure (CHF) patients with chronically implanted left ventricular assist devices (personal communication with program director).

Telestroke

It is recognized that tPA improves outcomes for nonhemorrhagic thrombotic stroke. The American Heart Association estimates that only 3% to 5% of patients eligible to receive tPA actually receive it.[55] With the desire to share risk in the administration of tPA, the ED physician may seek a qualified and emergent neurologic opinion. Silva et al.[56] in a Health Resources and Services Administration (HRSA)–supported national study was only able to identify 56 active telestroke programs in the United States as of 2012. Of the programs being interviewed, 100% provide ED consultations. All highlighted limitations or barriers to implementing or maintaining these programs, such as lack of reimbursement, need for state licensure, and lack of sustained funding. Therapeutically, telestroke programs can lead to use of tPA in greater than 50% of the eligible candidates, dramatically better than those without telestroke.[57] Due to remote geographic sites, the shortage of neurologists, and the relative paucity of telestroke systems, stroke patients in rural areas are 10 times *less* likely to receive timely administration of tPA.[58] Of note, the visual examination of the stroke patient was felt to be important and improved the accuracy of diagnosis.

Telepsychiatry

According to the World Health Organization and the American Hospital Association (AHA),[59,60] neuropsychiatric illnesses are now the number-one cause of disability. As many as 40% of ED patients may have a mental illness, with mental illness being the fastest-growing component of emergency medical practice.[61] To confound the situation, the AHA has reported a growing shortage of psychiatrists and mental health care workers in general. The American Psychiatry Association believes that video-based telepsychiatry helps meet patients' needs for convenient, affordable, and readily accessible mental health services, leading to improved outcomes.[62] In 2009, ED telepsychiatry was rare, with only three recognized programs.[63] More recently in 2011, the ACEP[64] reported results of a state-wide telepsychiatry program managing ED psychiatric patients. Six thousand patients seen by telepsychiatry in the ED were compared to equal numbers of patients in nontelepsychiatry EDs. Admission rate was reduced 30% (from 12% to 8%), 30-day outpatient follow-up was increased 36%, and both Medicaid and private payors received smaller bills. By 2015, the South Carolina Department of Mental Health[65] reported that daily telepsychiatry visits had increased from 8.7 to 14.7 during the period 2010 to 2015, and ED length of stay (LOS) had dropped from approximately 48 to 72 hours to 8.5 hours. In telepsychiatry programs, the visual evaluation of the mentally distressed or ill was generally felt to be significant.

Tele-ICU in the Emergency Department

Little is written about tele-ICU in the ED, perhaps because the ED is staffed with physicians trained in acute care and critical illness. There is an increasing interest among ED physicians to continue critical care until the patient actually leaves the ED.[66] The growing concept is that the ED intensivists (EDIs) would staff an ED-ICU. This concept could simply provide an expansion of coverage of a larger resuscitation bay or more bays. A lexicon has developed surrounding the ED-ICU adopted from Weingar et al.[66]:

- **Emergency medicine critical care**—subspecialty of emergency medicine focused on care of the critically ill in the ED
- **EP intensivist**—a physician who has completed a residency in emergency medicine and a fellowship in critical care.
- **ED critical care**—emergency medicine critical care practiced specifically in the ED
- **ED-ICU**—unit within an ED with the same or similar staffing, monitoring, and capability for therapies as an ICU
- **RED-ICU**—hybrid Resuscitation unit in the Emergency Department providing ICU care

If the concept of a second set of eyes is valid, then the application to the ED tele-ICU is logical and would be a mechanism to smooth transition from the ED to the ICU or to provide comprehensive intensive care in the ED in the event of a patient surge.

Telesupervision of Advance Practice Providers

Appropriate distribution for trained human resources in emergency care is a challenge across the United States, but especially in rural areas. Advanced practice providers (nurse practitioners [NPs] and physician assistants) help meet provider needs, but often require consultation with a supervisory physician. Since 2003, the University of Mississippi has been providing trained NPs working in rural EDs remote supervision and collaborative consultation via telemedicine.[67] A decade later Summers et al.[68] reported that the program had expanded to 19 rural hospital EDs, with each NP seeing approximately 200 patients per month. The parent program had conducted over 400,000 teleconsultations (about 40% of patient encounters). Of the patients seen by acute care practitioners, 57% were discharged from the ED and 21% were transferred to a higher level of care. General satisfaction was high, with 93% of patients comfortable or very comfortable with the telemedicine system, 98% could see and hear the remote physician well, 85% rated the combined NP with remote physician care as good or excellent, and 91% said they would return because of the telemedicine system.

THE OPERATIVE SUITE

The Society of American Gastroenterological and Endoscopic Surgeons[69] has noted a multitude of applications for telemedicine, including surgical teleconferencing, teleproctoring (observing and teaching), telemonitoring, telemanagement, and telesurgery (Figure 8-7).

In fact, the first actual remote surgery was performed more than 14 years ago in 2002.[70] In a similar era, despite a 14,000-km virtual round trip and a transmission delay of 155 ms Marescaux et al.[71] were able to successfully perform a remote cholecystectomy from New York with a patient in Strasbourg using robotic-assisted technology. With minimally invasive surgery, tele-OR management has extended into urological and other arenas.[72] In 2014, a newsletter was developed that is dedicated to telesurgery.[73]

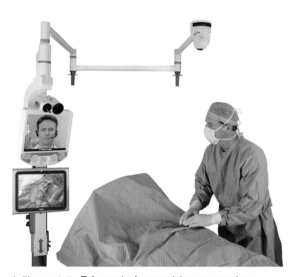

▲ **Figure 8-7.** Telesurgical supervision, mentoring, monitoring, or proctoring. Remote physician has direct eye-to-eye contact with the onsite operating surgeon while peering directly down into the surgical field from a remotely controllable camera. (Reproduced with permission from InTouch Health.)

Doarn and Latifi[74] have conceptually connected telemedicine in trauma and the OR with telemedicine in the ED. With readily available technology, some utilizing open-architecture technology, it is easy to imagine a remote physician observing or just taking "hand-off" from a critically ill patient as they move through the operative suite heading to the ICU. However, at this time, utilization of the technology has not been described. A thorough review of the technology has been provided by Whitten and Mair.[75]

TELEHEALTH IN THE INTENSIVE CARE UNIT

▶ Intensivist Manpower Issues

According to the AHA's 2014 annual survey,[76] the United States has 5,686 hospitals. Essentially all acute care hospitals have at least one ICU with nearly 55,000 critically ill patients cared for each day. From 2006 to 2010, the number of critical care beds in the United States increased 15%, from 67,579 to 77,809.[77,78]

In the late 1990s, the initial primary driving force for the development of the tele-ICU was the shortage of intensivists[79-83] confounded by a maldistribution of the workforce.[84] Recently, the American Association of Medical Colleges (AAMC) posted the 2016 update[85] regarding predicted physician supply and demand. Although not focused on CCM, the estimated shortfall of physicians by 2025 is predicted to range from 61,700 to 98,700 and could be as high as 125,200 under worst-case scenarios. From 2016 to 2025, 41% of the population will be older than 65 years of age, the population known to be the greatest consumers of health care services. Reports in the early 2000s suggested a manpower undersupply of critical care physicians of $+/-30,000$. However, a new trend has evolved with more graduating medical students choosing EM residencies, and many doing an additional critical care fellowship. Data from the National Residency Matching Program (NRMP)[86] indicate that from 2000 to 2015 there has been a near doubling of the EM residencies offered, from 971 to 1,821. With a near 100% match rate, this predicts a near doubling of EM physicians entering the marketplace.

In 2009, the American Board of Internal Medicine (ABIM) and the American Board of Emergency Medicine (ABEM) established a pathway for EM physicians to gain board certification in CCM and emergency medicine.[87] The pathway has subsequently been approved by the American Board of Medical Specialties (ABMS) in 2011. Currently, at least 20 US programs train combined EM and CCM.[88,89] However, it is not clear if this adds to the total number of trained intensivists, as EM-trained residents may just fill positions previously taken by internal medicine–trained residents. Additionally, as reported by the NRMP, the number of pulmonologists seeking combined pulmonary-CCM training has risen 17% a year from 118 to 135. Additional critical care board certification pathways for EM-trained physicians include surgical critical care (boards from the American Board of Surgery [ABS]), neurology critical care (certified by the United Council of Neurologic Subspecialties), and an anesthesia pathway (American Board of Anesthesia [ABA]).

In summary, pathways to achieve CCM certification now include[90]:

• ABEM/ABIM	– Double boarded (EM/CC)
• ABEM/ABA	– Double boarded (EM/Anesthesia)
• ABEM/ABS	– Double boarded (EM/Surgery)
• ABEM/ABIM	– Triple boarded (IM/EM/CC)
• UCNS	– Double boarded (Neurology/Neurocritical care)

The Critical Care Societies Collaborative, a joint effort between the American Association of Colleges of Nursing (AACN), American College of Chest Physicians (CHEST), American Thoracic Society (ATS), and the Society of Critical Care Medicine (SCCM), was established in 1995 to work on common issues in the critical care workforce. A history of the efforts through 2007 to optimize and enhance the critical care workforce is nicely reviewed at http://ccsconline.org/workforce.[84]

OTHER DRIVERS FOR DEVELOPMENT AND HINDRANCE OF THE TELE-ICU

In addition to the early manpower shortage, a variety of quality issues further pushed the advancement of telemedicine in the ICU to include growing evidence of value of intensivists,[91–94] a recognition of the value of structured care to mitigate unwarranted variability,[95–102] an early burst of enthusiastic reports on the tele-ICU,[103–113] and finally, hospital corporate pressure to comply with the so-called Leapfrog Guidelines.[114] However, despite numerous efforts to demonstrate a positive return on investment (ROI), growth of telemedicine in the ICU has plateaued at approximately 12% of all ICU beds in the United States (when considering Philips-Visicu and all other technologies).

As of fall 2012, there were 54 civilian and government tele-ICU monitoring centers in the United States. These monitoring centers were owned and operated by academic medical centers, regional hospitals, certain health plans, the Veterans' Health Administration (VHA), and commercial firms. Most (nearly 90%) of the technologies used by these monitoring centers are virtually identical and designed by a single leading vendor, and to a large extent tele-ICU practice patterns have also been single-vendor driven across users.

The homogeneity of the technology stems from litigation launched by Visicu apparently intended to control the growth of competition in the early 2000s.[115] As a result, there was essentially no growth in competition, allowing Visicu to take a dominant hold of the market. Ultimately, the patent infringement case was dismissed in 2010,[116] but leaving Philips/Visicu with the lead market share. Because of this, most studies of the structured tele-ICU care delivery model employ Philips-Visicu technology. The Sentara Health system was the first to install the Philips-Visicu technology and is the longest-running Philips-Visicu program, currently covering 108 beds.[117] At the project's 10-year point (2010), approximately 1,000,000 patients had been under their tele-ICU management process.[118]

TELE-ICU MODELS

For a detailed comparative discussion of tele-ICU characteristics, see Refs 119–121. The following definitions have been extracted from those references. Note, the definitions imply absolute purity of definition; certain programs may use a hybrid design and not fit into such strict definitions.

▶ Centralized Tele-ICU vs. Decentralized

Centralized Tele-ICU

The "hub-and-spoke" model is one with the medical staff stationed at the hub and providing tele-critical care to a variety of "spoke" hospitals. The hub (or center) is an established "brick-and-mortar" site staffed with combinations of intensivists, nurses, and clerical and technical staff. The hub is connected to one or more medical facilities or one or more ICUs. Staff are physically located in this single facility for a defined number of hours per day. Centralized programs include a discrete site and generally a structured process. The Philips-Visicu model is a centralized program that employs a "continuous," proactive care delivery model that is facilitated by integrated software and is intended to interface with local electronic health records (EHRs), including visualization of the patient remotely and essential laboratory and radiographic information.

Decentralized Tele-ICU

There is no defined or established central monitoring facility. The decentralized model typically involves computers, tablets, smart phones equipped with camera, speakers, and microphones located at sites of convenience for the physician, such as medical offices, homes, or clipped to a belt. The decentralized tele-ICU is not a specific site, but rather a process focused on convenience and flexibility for the care provider whether he or she is the intensivist or a consulting physician.

▶ Communications Technology

Open Architecture

This involves a communications system without dedicated individual transmission lines that supports connectivity from one or many remote sites to one or many originating sites. Open architecture generally implies connectivity via the Internet, permitting a care provider to virtually visit patients from essentially anywhere. When the software includes conferencing capabilities, multiple remote care providers can virtually visit the same patient remotely for simultaneous consultations. There is inherent redundancy in the Internet negating the need for alternative lines but increasing the challenge of assuring system security.

Closed Architecture

This generally has dedicated, point-to-point, hardwired communication lines from the care provider to the patient area—typically a high-speed T1 or T3 line from a hub to a spoke. A single hard wire can be vulnerable to failure, mandating a second alternative pathway for data transmission. Medical care providers outside the system typically are not able to perform virtual evaluations. The dedicated lines exist outside the Internet, although data may be transmitted using Internet Protocol (IP). Presumably, the closed architecture has greater data security.

▶ Care Service Model

Continuous Monitoring and Management

This implies 24/7 real-time monitoring and reactive and pre-emptive management, but some programs may only apply continuous monitoring 12 hours per day. During the "live" hours, the nurse virtually roams from patient to patient, reviewing their status, while the physician focuses on active or unstable patients.

Scheduled Intermittent

Physician staff schedules a particular time to perform routine rounds, such as 6 hours after the daytime intensivist has left. Alternatively, for programs without onsite intensivists, the remote intensivist can perform routine rounds for part of or the entire ICU.

Reactive

In this case the physician responds to a communication requesting support with a certain patient, performing an admission evaluation or a consultation.

THE TELE-ICU LITERATURE, RESEARCH, AND RESEARCH AGENDA

An extensive review of the tele-ICU experience from 2004 through 2013 has been completed by Coustasse et al.[122] and included more than 35 studies. Summarizing the reviews:

- Sixteen studies demonstrated shortened LOS
- Eleven studies showed greater adherence to "best practices" protocols
- Seven studies indicated improved financial performance
- Four studies found greater teamwork
- Five studies described improved patient care without further specification

None of the studies suggested negative impact or worsened outcomes. Because most of these studies were published during the 10 years of tele-ICU litigation, they generally use the Philips/Visicu technology and similar care delivery models.[106] Twenty-two of these studies were pre-post studies, nine literature reviews or meta-analysis, and four surveys. In no case was there a parallel comparative study of different models of the tele-ICU nor a head-to-head study of in-house 24/7 intensivists compared to the tele-ICU (Table 8-1).

Most studies used a before-and-after study design and are subject to numerous biases, including unmeasured changes in case mix, temporal trends, coincident interventions, and random variation.[123] Additionally,

Table 8-1. Review of Tele-ICU Literature by Coustasse et al.

Author, Year	Study Design	Outcome
Aaronson et al, 2006	Literature review	Higher rates of ICU staff adherence to critical care best practices
Badawi et al, 2010	Pre/posttest of tele-ICU implementation	Higher rates of ICU staff adherence to critical care best practices
Badawi and Shemmeri, 2006	Pre/posttest of tele-ICU implementation	Higher rates of ICU staff adherence to critical care best practices
Berenson et al., 2009	Literature review	Improved patient care
Breslow et al., 2004	Pre/posttest of tele-ICU implementation across several hospitals	Improved hospital financial performance, improved ICU financial performance, improved patient care
Chu-Weininger et al., 2010	Pre/posttest of tele-ICU implementation and utilization in 3 ICUs	Improved teamwork and/or safety climate
Coletti et al, 2008	Cross-sectional survey of residents in ICU and tele-ICUs	Improved teamwork and/or safety climate
Dickhaus, 2006	Pre/posttest of tele-ICU implementation and utilization in a multistate hospital system	Lower ICU LOS
Giessel and Leedom, 2007	Pre/posttest of tele-ICU implementation and utilization	Higher rates of ICU staff adherence to critical care best practices
Groves et al, 2008	Literature review	Lower ICU LOS
Howell et al, 2007	Pre/posttest of tele-ICU implementation and utilization	Lower ICU LOS
Howell et al, 2008	Pre/posttest of tele-ICU implementation and utilization	Lower ICU LOS
Ikeda et al, 2009	Pre/posttest of tele-ICU implementation and utilization	Lower ICU LOS
Kohl et al, 2007	Pre/posttest of tele-ICU implementation and utilization	Lower ICU LOS
Kohl et al, 2007	Pre/posttest of tele-ICU implementation and utilization	Improved ICU financial performance, lower ICU LOS
Kohl et al, 2012	Pre/posttest of tele-ICU implementation and utilization	Lower ICU LOS
Kumar et al, 2013	Literature review	Improved ICU financial performance
Khunlertkit and Carayon, 2013	Qualitative study with semistructured interview of tele-ICU staff	Improved ICU staff adherence to evidence-based protocols for sepsis, ventilator-associated pneumonia, and blood transfusion
Lilly et al, 2011	Pre/posttest of tele-ICU implementation and utilization	Higher rates of ICU staff adherence to critical care best practices, lower ICU LOS, improved patient care
Mora et al, 2007	Survey of residents practicing in tele-ICUs	Improved patient care
Norman et al, 2009	Literature review and meta-analysis	Improved ICU financial performance

(continued)

Table 8-1. Review of Tele-ICU Literature by Coustasse et al. (*continued*)

Author, Year	Study Design	Outcome
Patel et al, 2007	Pre/posttest of tele-ICU implementation and utilization of 6 tele-ICUs	Higher rates of ICU staff adherence to critical care best practices, lower ICU LOS
Rincon et al, 2007	Pre/posttest of tele-ICU utilization in prevention of sepsis	Higher rates of ICU staff adherence to critical care best practices: • Antibiotic administration increased from 55% to 74% • Serum lactate measurement increased from 50% to 66% • Central line placements increased from 33% to 50%
Scales et al, 2011	Literature review	Higher rates of ICU staff adherence to critical care best practices
Thomas et al, 2007	Pre/posttest of tele-ICU implementation and utilization	Improved teamwork and/or safety climate
Vespa et al, 2007	Pre/posttest of tele-ICU implementation and utilization	Improved ICU financial performance, lower ICU LOS, improved patient care
Wilcox and Adhikari, 2012	Meta-analysis of 11 studies	Lower ICU LOS
Willmitch et al, 2012	Pre/posttest of tele-ICU implementation and utilization over 3 years	Lower ICU LOS
Youn, 2006	Literature review and meta-analysis	Higher rates of ICU staff adherence to critical care best practices
Young et al, 2011	Meta-analysis of 11 studies	Lower ICU LOS
Zawada et al, 2006	Survey of physicians practicing in remote areas using tele-ICU	Higher rates of ICU staff adherence to critical care best practices, lower ICU LOS
Zawada et al, 2007	Pre/posttest of tele-ICU implementation and utilization	Improved ICU financial performance, lower ICU LOS
Zawada et al, 2008	Pre/posttest of tele-ICU implementation and utilization in a rural health care system	Higher rates of ICU staff adherence to critical care best practices, improved ICU financial performance
Zawada and Herr, 2008	Pre/posttest of tele-ICU implementation and utilization	Improved patient care
Zawada et al, 2009	Pre/posttest of tele-ICU implementation and utilization	Improved hospital financial performance

ICU, intensive care unit; *LOS*, length of stay.
(Reprinted from Coustasse A, Deslich S, Bailey D, Paul D. A business case for tele-intensive care units. *Perm J*. 18(4): 76-84, 2014, with permission from The Permanente Press.)

ICU telemedicine often introduces multiple interventions at the same time, including audiovisual surveillance, staffing changes, decision-support tools, and new electronic medical records. Ultimately, the conclusions of these studies have been questioned. Khan et al.[124] have suggested, in their 2011 "Research Agenda for ICU Telemedicine" that research should have a:

• Standardized approach to assessing the preimplementation ICU environment, including patients, hospital, ICU, community characteristics, and organizational context

• Standardized lexicon for defining the telemedicine intervention and develop a common language defining characteristics, processes, and intentions

This research agenda has proposed a specific framework for assessing telemedicine to include clinical outcomes, technical acceptability, health system interface, costs and benefits, patient/provider acceptability, and access. The research agenda includes a lists of unknowns or knowledge gaps. Khan et al. suggest that the first knowledge gap is: "What is the optimal telemedicine model for different clinical settings?"

To the point of needing better studies and improved quality of care, the New England HealthCare Institute (NEHI)[125] developed the following recommendations for best practices (annotations by the authors in parentheses):

1. Collect 6 months of preimplementation data prior to going live with any tele-ICU program. Consider appointing a clinical manager 6 to 8 months prior to implementation *(better pre/post implementation studies)*.

2. Extend tele-ICU coverage to institutions outside the parent or "home" organization, offsetting staffing and operational costs and establishing referral patterns *(improve the ROI)*.

3. Rotate clinicians from the bedside to the tele-ICU environment: "human glue" to hold together the bedside clinicians with the remote tele-ICU monitoring site, both nursing and MD, and preferably rotate at clinical sites that have the remote monitoring technology *(maintain connection to both the clinical side and remote side)*.

4. Extend coverage to the small and rural hospitals to include critical access hospitals. Essentially, all rural and critical access hospitals suffer from intensivists shortages. As per NEHI. less than 50% of the 54 tele-ICU programs connect to rural sites *(greater chance to demonstrate greater impact)*.

5. Extend tele-ICU coverage outside of the ICU via carts and wireless devices. Most frequent uses include ED-telemonitored bed providing early remote management and monitoring of critically ill patients while awaiting transfer to the ICU and for assistance with Rapid Response Team (RRT) *(greater value to the parent institution)*.

6. Make a business of renting services to other facilities. The *advanced ICU* model includes the following services *(improve ROI)*:

   - Reviewing each ICU admission for appropriateness for ICU care, treatment protocol, and planned discharge
   - MD intensivist rounding on each patient every 12 hours
   - Nurse intensivist rounding on each patient every 12 hours
   - Preparation and review of ICU discharge documents

HUMAN TECHNOLOGY ISSUES

From the perspective of a tele-ICU user and operator, and from the perspective of a clinician at the bedside, there are some low-level, moment-to-moment elements that add to the frustration, as outlined by Lyden[126]:

- Slow/multiple-click log-ins
- Short, security-driven, "on-time" requiring repetitive log-ins
- Frequent rebooting
- Different passwords and usernames for each facility Picture Archiving and Communications System (PACS) systems, computerized physician order entry (CPOE), or legacy systems
- Lack of familiarity with different icons in multiple PACS
- PACS with greater or lesser capability
- Incompatibility or incomplete data exchange and importation between the hospital legacy systems and the proprietary emergency medical record (EMR) of the tele-ICU system
- Laborious transition between the hospital CPOE systems and the tele-ICU technology
- Rigid hunt-and-click systems for creating diagnosis and medical plans embedded in the tele-ICU EMR
- Unintuitive hunt-and-click diagnostic systems embedded in the tele-ICU EMR

GENERAL FINANCIAL ISSUES

The biggest ongoing cost after the initial setup is physician, midlevel, and nursing clinician salaries and benefits. Initial setup costs for a typical complete Philips-Visicu tele-ICU have ranged from $1 million to more than $7 million.[110,122] However, after the one-time setup, ongoing operational costs vary depending on the hours of coverage/support, but may range up to $2.2 million per year. Under the Philips/Visicu model, the yearly cost per bed charged to the facility ranges from $37,500 to $40,000. Under these models, the financial burden is carried by the medical facility receiving the tele-ICU services. The degree of charging fee for service is unknown but believed to be low.

In the past, there has been no Medicare fee-for-service billing for critical care services rendered via telemedicine.[127] However, under pressure from the American Telemedicine Association (ATA), the Centers for Medicare and Medicaid Services (CMS) has proposed several changes in the codes to include a temporary code for critical care telemedicine services[128–130]

CMS did not propose adding critical care evaluation and management (E&M) codes. However, it recognized the potential benefit of critical care telemedicine and has now proposed creating temporary codes GTTT1 and GTTT2. The services would be limited to once per day, per patient, and would be valued relative to existing E&M services. The physician providing tele-ICU care will also have to define the point of service (POS)—the site where the patient is located, not where the provider is located.

Regarding billing commercial payors and Medicaid, the reader is referred to the *State Telemedicine Gaps Analysis: Coverage and Reimbursement* by Thomas and Capistrant.[131] In this document, the ATA has graded reimbursement by commercial and state Medicaid on a scale of A to F based upon state legislation. It should be noted that wording of legislation and functional outcomes after legislation is passed may vary widely. Maryland was given an "A" initially based on apparently good Medicaid legislation. However, the rating was downgraded to a "C" when it became apparent that Maryland state regulators were eager to limit the growth of telemedicine reimbursement. Additional information can be found in the SCCM publication *Coding and Billing for Critical Care: A Practice Tool*, sixth edition.[127]

CONCLUSIONS

- The sources of manpower and supply are changing significantly and could have a long-term impact upon the basic shortage premise driving tele-ICU. The Critical Care Societies Collaborative workforce must continue real efforts and include ACEP, as well as those representing surgery, anesthesia, and neurocritical care, as sources of critical care manpower. It is time to get beyond the limited four-society group.

- New innovative models need to be created and tested with a focus on the economics, particularly with different staffing models.

- Real scientific studies are needed, perhaps including the guidance from Kahn et al. and the NEHI.

- The tele-ICU providers need to look for expanded opportunities to provide greater ROI.

- Perhaps the tele-ICU model needs to expand widely in the spectrum of critical care as discussed earlier in the beginning of the chapter.

- The tele-ICU model should evolve away from proprietary EMRs that are limited to the ICU stay.

REFERENCES

1. Critical Care Statistics. http://www.sccm.org/Communications/Pages/CriticalCareStats.aspx. Accessed October 5, 2016.

2. Toffler A. *Future Shock*. New York: Bantam Publishers; 1970.

3. Scalf PE, Torralbo A, Tapia E, Beck DM. Competition explains limited attention and perceptual resources: implications for perceptual load and dilution theories. *Front Psychol* 2013;4:243.

4. Norri-Sdeerholm T, Paakkonen H, Kurola J, Saranto K. Situational awareness and information flow in prehospital emergency medical care from the perspective of paramedic field supervisors: a scenario-based study. *Scand J Trauma Resuscitation Emerg Med* 2015;23:4.

5. Brice JH, Studnek JR, Bigham BL, et al. EMS provider and patient safety during response and transport: proceedings of an ambulance safety conference. *Prehosp Emerg Care* 2012;16(1):3–19.

6. Goran SF. A second set of eyes: an introduction to tele-ICU. *Crit Care Nurse* 2010;30(4):46–55.

7. *The Four Eyes Principal*. http://whatis.techtarget.com/definition/four-eyes-principle. Accessed October 12, 2016.

8. *700 MHz Public Safety Spectrum*. https://www.fcc.gov/general/700-mhz-public-safety-spectrum-0. Accessed October 10, 2016.

9. *Public Safety 700-MHz Broadband Deployable Systems*. https://www.nist.gov/programs-projects/public-safety-700-mhz-broadband-deployable-systems. Accessed October 10, 2016.

10. *National Public Safety Telecommunications Council EMS Telemedicine Report Prehospital Use of Video Technologies*. http://www.npstc.org/download.jsp?tableId=37&

column=217&id=3612&file=EMS_Telemedicine_Report_Final_20160303.pdf. Accessed September 9, 2016.

11. White D. *Are Cameras in EMS Worth It? There are Three Main Types of Cameras, and Pros and Cons to Using Each One.* January 10, 2014. http://www.ems1.com/ems-products/cameras-video/articles/1646787-Are-cameras-in-EMS-worth-it/. Accessed October 10, 2016.

12. Careless J. *NPSTC Delves into Prehospital Video for EMS as FirstNet Approaches.* August 9, 2016. http://www.ems-world.com/article/12246993/npstc-delves-into-prehospital-video-for-ems-as-firstnet-approaches.

13. Tanner K. *Body Camera Footage from an EMT Shows What Actually Happens during a Heroin Overdose, and It's Horrific.* 2016. http://rare.us/story/body-camera-footage-from-an-emt-shows-what-actually-happens-during-a-heroin-overdose-and-its-horrific/. Accessed October 21, 2016.

14. San Bernadino County Fire Department (SBDCoFD). *Helmet Cam Records Extrication of Calif. Driver.* May 24, 2016. http://www.emsworld.com/video/12213182/helmet-cam-records-extrication-of-calif-driver. Accessed October 21, 2016.

15. *Abdominal Aortic Junctional Tourniquet* (AAJT). 2014. http://www.emsworld.com/video/11290180/aajt-helmet-cam. Accessed October 21, 2016.

16. Burger L. *Firefighters Create Live-Streaming Body Camera with Reliable Solution.* 2014. http://www.firerescue1.com/fire-products/vehicle-equipment/fire-cameras-video/articles/2011337-Firefighter-creates-live-streaming-body-cam-with-reliable-storage-solution/. Accessed October 21, 2016.

17. Givot D. *5 Pros and Cons of Cameras in Ambulances.* September 2014. http://www.ems1.com/ems-products/cameras-video/articles/1989401-5-pros-and-cons-of-cameras-in-ambulances/. Accessed October 10, 2016.

18. *HIPAA: A Twist on a New Problem. Posting EMS Scene Images Could Be Punishable.* http://www.patc.com/weeklyarticles/print/2013_hipaa_varone.pdf. Accessed October 10, 2016.

19. Amadi-Obi A, Gilligan P, Owens N, O'Donnell C. Telemedicine in pre-hospital care: a review of telemedicine applications in the pre-hospital environment. *Int J Emerg Med* 2014;7:29.

20. Trivedi K, Schur JD, Cone DC. Can paramedics read ST-segment elevation myocardial infarction on pre-hospital electrocardiograms? *Prehosp Emerg Care* 2009;13(2):207–214.

21. Smith RM, Conn AK. Prehospital care - scoop and run or stay and play? *Injury* 2009;40(Suppl 4):S23–S26.

22. Page C, Vazquez K, Sibat M, Yalcin ZD. *Worcester Polytechnic Institute Analysis of Emergency Medical Systems across the World.* http://web.wpi.edu/Pubs/E-project/Available/E-project-042413-092332/unrestricted/MQFIQP2809.pdf. Accessed October 10, 2016.

23. Adnet F, Jouriles NJ, Le Toumelin P, et al. Survey of out-of-hospital emergency intubations in the French prehospital medical system: a multicenter study. *Ann Emerg Med* 1998;32(4):454–460.

24. The World Health Organization. *Pre Hospital Trauma Systems.* http://www.who.int/violence_injury_prevention/publications/services/39162_oms_new.pdf. Accessed October 10, 2016.

25. Cody J, McCool S. *Association of critical care transport - The Critical Care Transport Standards Project.* https://www.nasemso.org/Projects/GovernmentAffairs/documents/AACTMedPACSept2012.pdf. Accessed October 10, 2016.

26. *Mobile Stroke Unit: University of Texas Puts CT Scanner in an Ambulance.* https://www.uth.edu/media/story.htm?id=b1485cfc-110f-4a4c-91ea-06b573b3ba6d. Accessed September 29, 2013.

27. Lee JM, Grabb MC, Zipfel GJ, Choi DW. Brain tissue responses to ischemia. *J Clin Invest* 2000;106(6):723–731.

28. Cerejo R, John S, Buletko AB, et al. A mobile stroke treatment unit for field triage of patients for intra-arterial revascularization therapy. *J Neuroimaging* 2015;25(6):940–945.

29. Ebinger M, Winter B, Wendt M, et al. Effect of the use of ambulance-based thrombolysis on time to thrombolysis in acute ischemic stroke: a randomized clinical trial. *JAMA* 2014a;311(16):1622–1631.

30. Fassbender K, Balucani C, Walter S, et al. Streamlining of prehospital stroke management: the golden hour. *Lancet Neurol* 2013;12(6):585–596.

31. Rubenfire A. *UT and Cleveland Clinic Place Mobile CT in Ambulance: Cost and Efficacy.* January 4, 2016. http://www.modernhealthcare.com/article/20160104/NEWS/160109988. Accessed November 5, 2016.

32. American College of Physicians. America's Emergency Care Environment. 2014. http://www.emreportcard.org/Content.aspx?id=388. Accessed October 14, 2016.

33. American College of Emergency Medicine: Telemedicine in Emergency Medicine *Information Paper.* https://www.acep.org/content.aspx?id=8988. Accessed September 29, 2016.

34. Sikka N, Paradise S, Shu M. *Telehealth in Emergency Medicine: A Primer.* June 2014. https://www.acep.org/uploadedFiles/ACEP/Membership/Sections_of_Membership/telemd/ACEP%20Telemedicine%20Primer.pdf. Accessed October 13, 2016.

35. *EDTITRATE (Emergency Department Telemedicine Initiative to Rapidly Accommodate in Times of Emergency).* June 8, 2016. https://health.ucsd.edu/

news/releases/Pages/2013-06-11-pilot-telemedicine-program-in-emergency-department.aspx. Accessed October 13, 2016.

36. Brennan JA, Kealy JA, Gerardi LH, et al. Telemedicine in the emergency department: a randomized controlled trial. *J Telemed Telecare* 1999;5(1):18–22.

37. Begley C, Courtney C, Abbass I, et al. *Houston Hospitals Emergency Department Use Study. 2013. January 1, 2011 through December 31, 2011.* Health Services Research Collaborative, University of Texas School of Public Health. https://sph.uth.edu/research/centers/chsr/hsrc/.

38. Langabeer JR, Gonzalez M, Alqusairi D, et al. Telehealth-enabled emergency medical services program reduces ambulance transport to urban emergency departments. *West J Emerg Med* 2016;17(6):713–720.

39. Chi CH, Chang I, Wu WP. Emergency department-based telemedicine. *Am J Emerg Med* 1999;17(4):408–411.

40. *Tele-Emergency Department and Tele-Trauma Services.* https://www.emmc.org/Telemedicine/Tele-Emergency-Department-and-Tele-Trauma-Services.aspx. Accessed October 13, 2016.

41. Bashford C. *Telemedicine Today: Part 3—System Examples and Lessons Learned.* March 2016. http://www.emsworld.com/article/12184044/telemedicine-today-part-3-system-examples-and-lessons-learned. Accessed October 17, 2016.

42. Latifi R, Weinstein RS, Porter JM, et al. Telemedicine and telepresence for trauma and emergency care management. *Scand J Surg* 2007;96(4):281–289.

43. Sakles JC, Mosier J, Hadeed G, et al. Telemedicine and telepresence for prehospital and remote hospital rracheal intubation using a GlideScope™ videolaryngoscope: a model for tele-intubation. *Telemed J E Health* 2011;17(3):185–188.

44. ACEP Public Health Committee. *Recognizing the Needs of Incarcerated Patients in the Emergency Department.* April 2006. https://www.acep.org/Clinical---Practice-Management/Recognizing-the-Needs-of-Incarcerated-Patients-in-the-Emergency-Department/. Accessed October 17, 2016.

45. National Commission on Correctional Health Care. *Telemedicine Technology in Correctional Facilities.* 1997. http://www.ncchc.org/telemedicine-technology-in-correctional-facilities. Accessed October 17, 2016.

46. Castillo DJ, Myers JB, Mocko J, Beck EH. Mobile integrated healthcare: preliminary experience and impact analysis with a medicare advantage population. *JHPOR* 2016;4(2):172–187.

47. Thrall JH, Teleradiology. Part I. History and clinical applications. *Radiology* 2007;243(3):613–617.

48. Thrall JH. Teleradiology. Part II. Limitations, risks, and opportunities. *Radiology* 2007;244(2):325–328.

49. Silva E3rd, Breslau J, Barr RM, et al. ACR white paper on teleradiology practice: a report from the Task Force on Teleradiology Practice. *J Am Coll Radiol* 2013;10(8):575–585.

50. Krupinski EA. Teleradiology: current perspectives. *Reports in Medical Imaging.* January 2014;2014(7):5–14.

51. Seay T, Davis SM, Burrell TA, et al. *Clinical Practice and Management Statement of the American College of Emergency Physicians, 2006: Radiologic Imaging and Teleradiology in the Emergency Department.* https://www.acep.org/clinical---practice-management/radiologic-imaging-and-teleradiology-in-the-emergency-department/. Accessed October 15, 2016.

52. Gunn AJ, Mangano MD, Pugmire BS, et al. Toward improved radiology reporting practices in the emergency department: a survey of emergency department physicians. *J Radiol Radiat Ther* 2013;1(2):1013.

53. Afolabi BA, Novaro GM, Pinski SL, et al. Use of the prehospital ECG improves door-to-balloon times in ST segment elevation myocardial infarction irrespective of time of day or day of week. *Emerg Med J* 2007;24(8):588–591.

54. Hsieh JC, Hsu MW. A cloud computing based 12-lead ECG telemedicine service. *BMC Med Inform Decis Mak* 2012;12:77.

55. Adeoye O, Hornung R, Khatri P, Kleindorfer D. Recombinant tissue-type plasminogen activator use for ischemic stroke in the United States: a doubling of treatment rates over the course of 5 years. *Stroke* 2011;42:1952–1955.

56. Silva GS, Farrell S, Shandra E, Viswaathan A, Schwamm LH. The status of telestroke in the United States: a survey of currently active stroke telemedicine programs. *Stroke* 2012;43(8):2078–2085.

57. Bladin CF, Cadilhac DA. Effect of telestroke on emergent stroke care and stroke outcomes. *Stroke* 2014;45(6):1876–1880.

58. Demaerschalk BM, Raman R, Ernstrom K, Meyer BC. Efficacy of telemedicine for stroke: pooled analysis of the Stroke Team Remote Evaluation Using a Digital Observation Camera (STRokE DOC) and STRokE DOC Arizona telestroke trials. *Telemed J E Health* 2012;18:230–237.

59. World Health Organization. *Global Burden of Disease.* http://www.who.int/healthinfo/global_burden_disease/2004_report_update/en/index.html. Accessed October 15, 2016.

60. The American Hospital Association. *The State of the Behavioral Health Workforce: A Literature Review.* http://www.hpoe.org/Reports-HPOE/2016/aha_Behavioral_FINAL.pdf. Accessed October 15, 2016.

61. Larkin GL, Beautrais AL, Spirito A, et al. Mental health and emergency medicine: a research agenda. *Acad Emerg Med* 2009;16(11):1110–1119.

62. American Psychiatry Association. *Telepsychiatry.* https://www.psychiatry.org/psychiatrists/practice/telepsychiatry. Accessed October 15, 2016.

63. Williams M. Pfeffer M, Boyle J. *Telepsychiatry in the Emergency Department: Overview and Case Studies.* 2009. http://www.chcf.org/~/media/MEDIA%20LIBRARY%20Files/PDF/PDF%20T/PDF%20TelepsychiatryProgramsED.pdf. Accessed October 15, 2016.

64. Otto MA. *Telepsychiatry Cuts Admissions, Saves Money.* July 2011. https://www.acep.org/content.aspx?id=80804. Accessed October 15, 2016.

65. South Carolina Department of Mental Health. *DMH Emergency Department Telepsychiatry Program.* 2015. http://www.state.sc.us/dmh/telepsychiatry/.

66. Weingart SD, Sherwin RL, Emlet LL, et al. ED intensivists and ED intensive care units. *Am J Emerg Med* 2013;31(3):617–620.

67. Galli RL, Keith JC, McKenzie K, Hall GS, Henderson K. TelEmergency: a novel system for delivering emergency care to rural hospitals. *Ann Emerg Med* 2008;51(3):275–284.

68. Summers RL, Henderson K, Isom K, Galli RL. The anniversary of TelEmergency. *J Miss State Med Assoc* 2013;54(12):340–341.

69. Society of American Gastroenterological and Endoscopic Surgeons (SAGES). *Guidelines for the Surgical Practice of Telemedicine.* 2010. http://www.sages.org/publications/guidelines/guidelines-for-the-surgical-practice-of-telemedicine/. Accessed October 12, 2016.

70. Eadie LH, Seifalian AM, Davidson BR. Telemedicine in surgery. *Br J Surgery* 2003;90(6):647–658.

71. Marescaux J, Leroy J, Rubino F, et al. Transcontinental robot-assisted remote telesurgery: feasibility and potential applications. *Ann Surg* 2002;235(4):487–492.

72. Bove P, Stoianovici D, Micali S, et al. Is telesurgery a new reality? Our experience with laparoscopic and percutaneous procedures. *J Endourol* 2004;17(3):137–142.

73. Baram-Clothier E. *Surgical Telementoring News.* 2014. http://www.medicalfoundation.org/wp-content/uploads/2012/04/Surgical-Telementoring-News-2014e.pdf. Accessed November 6, 2016.

74. Doarn C, Latifi R. Telementoring and teleproctoring in trauma and emergency care. *Curr Trauma Rep* 2016;2(3):138–143.

75. Whitten P, Mair F. Telesurgery versus telemedicine in surgery--an overview. *Surgical Technology Int* 2004;12:68–72.

76. Health Forum, LLC. *American Hospital Association Hospital Statistics, 2015 (2014 Survey Data).* Chicago, IL: American Hospital Association; 2015.

77. *Critical Care Statistics.* http://www.sccm.org/Communications/Pages/CriticalCareStats.aspx. Accessed October 5, 2016.

78. Wallace DJ, Angus DC, Seymour CW, Barnato AE, Kahn JM. Critical care bed growth in the United States. A comparison of regional and national trends. *Am J Respir Crit Care Med* 2015;191(4):410–416.

79. Angus DC, Kelley MA, Schmitz RJ, White A, Popovich J. Current and projected workforce requirements for care of the critical ill and patients with pulmonary disease: can we meet the requirements of an aging population? *JAMA* 2000;284:2762–2770.

80. *Health Resources and Services Administration Report to Congress: The Critical Care Workforce: A Study of the Supply and Demand for Critical Care Physicians.* Requested by: Senate Report 108-81. http://bhpr.hrsa.gov/healthworkforce/reports/criticalcare/default.htm. Accessed September 2006.

81. Kelly MA, Angus DC, Chalfin DB, et al. The critical care crisis in the United States: a report from the profession. *Crit Care Med* 2004;32:1219–1222.

82. Grover A. Critical care workforce: a policy perspective. *Crit Care Med* 2006;34(Suppl):S7–S11.

83. Krell K. Critical care workforce. *Crit Care Med* 2008;36:1350–1353.

84. *Critical Care Wokforce.* http://ccsconline.org/workforce. Accessed October 5, 2016.

85. Dall T, West T, Chakrabarti R, Iacobucci W. *The Complexities of Physician Supply and Demand: Projections from 2014 to 2025.* 2016. https://www.aamc.org/download/458082/data/2016_complexities_of_supply_and_demand_projections.pdf. Accessed October 3, 2016.

86. *National Residency Matching Program.* http://www.nrmp.org/match-data/nrmp-historical-reports/. Accessed October 4, 2016.

87. *EM-CCM Fellowships.* http://emccmfellowship.org/. Accessed October 4, 2016.

88. Emergency Medical Residents Association. *Critical Care Division.* https://www.emra.org/committees-divisions/critical-care-division/. Accessed October 4, 2016.

89. *ABIM Offers Opportunity for Triple Board Certification in IM, EM, and CCM.* https://www.abim.org/certification/policies/combined-training/internal-medicine-emergency-medicine-critical-care-medicine/overview.aspx. Accessed October 4, 2016.

90. *ACEP 5 Alternative Pathways to Board Certification in Critical Care Medicine.* https://www.acep.org/critical-care-faq/. Accessed October 4, 2016.

91. Reynolds HN, Haupt MT, Carlson R. Impact of critical care physician staffing on patients with septic shock in a university medical care unit. *JAMA* 1988;260(33) 3446–3450.

92. Li TC, Phillips MC, Shaw L, et al. On site physician staffing in a community hospital intensive care unit: impact on test and procedure use and on patient outcome. *JAMA* 1984;252:2023–2027.

93. Young M, Birkmeyer J. Potential reduction in mortality rates using an intensivist model to manage intensive care units. *Eff Clin Pract* 2000;3:284–289.

94. Engoren M. The effect of prompt physician visits on intensive care unit mortality and cost. *Crit Care Med* 2005;33:727–732.

95. Patel B, Kao L, Thomas E, et al. Improving compliance with surviving sepsis campaign guidelines via remote electronic ICU monitoring. *Crit Care Med* 2007;35:A275.

96. Giessel GM, Leedom B. Centralized, remote ICU intervention improves best practices compliance. *Chest* 2007;132:444a.

97. Youn BA. ICU process improvement: using telemedicine to enhance compliance and documentation for the ventilator bundle. *Chest* 2006;130:226S.

98. Badawi O, Shemmeri E. Greater collaboration between remote intensivists and on-site clinicians improves best practice compliance. *Crit Care Med* 2006;34(12):A20.

99. Rincon T, Bourke G, Ikeda D. Centralized, remote care improves sepsis identification, bundle compliance and outcomes. *Chest* 2007;132:557S–558S.

100. Aaronson M, Zawada ET, Herr P. Role of a telemedicine intensive care unit program (TISP) on glycemic control (GC) in seriously ill patients in a rural health system. *Chest* 2006;130(Suppl):226S.

101. Youn BA. Utilizing robots and an ICU telemedicine program to provide intensivist support for rapid response teams. *Chest* 2006;130(4_MeetingAbstracts):102S. doi:10.1378/chest.130.4_MeetingAbstracts.102S-a.

102. Latif A, Romig M, Barasch N, Pronovost P, Sapirstein A. A consultative tele-ICU service improves compliance with best practice guidelines in a highly staffed ICU. Presented at the 40th Society of Critical Care Medicine Symposium, San Diego, CA, 2011.

103. Breslow MJ, Rosenfeld BA, Doerfler M, et al. Effect of a multiple-site intensive care unit telemedicine program on clinical and economic outcomes: an alternative paradigm for intensivist staffing. *Crit Care Med* 2004;32:31–38.

104. Rosenfeld BA, Dorman T, Breslow MJ, et al. Intensive care unit telemedicine: alternate paradigm for providing continuous intensivist care. *Crit Care Med* 2000;28:3925–3931.

105. Breslow MJ. Remote ICU care programs: current status. *J Crit Care* 2007;22(1):66–76.

106. McCambridge M, Jones K, Paxton H, et al. Association of health information technology and teleintensivist coverage with decreased mortality and ventilator use in critically ill patients. *Arch Int Med* 2010;170(7): 648–653.

107. New England Healthcare Institute. *Tele-ICUs: Remote Management in Intensive Care Units.* Cambridge, MA: Massachusetts Technology Collaborative and Health Technology Center; 2007.

108. Garingo A, Friedlich P, Tesoriero L, et al. The use of mobile robotic telemedicine in the neonatal intensive care unit. *J Perinatol* 2012;32(1):55–63.

109. Vespa PM, Miller C, Hu X, et al. Intensive care unit robotic telepresence facilitates rapid physician response to unstable patients and decreased costs in a neuro-intensive care. *Surg Neurol* 2007;67(4):331–337.

110. Lilly CM, Cody S, Zhao H, et al. Hospital mortality, length of stay, and preventable complications among critically ill patients before and after tele-ICU reengineering of critical care processes. *JAMA* 2011;301(21):2175–2183.

111. Chu-Weininger MY, Wueste L, Lucke JF, et al. The impact of tele-ICU on provider attitudes about team work and safety climate. *Qual Safe Healthcare* 2010;19(6):1–5.

112. Young LB, Chan PS, Cram P. Staff acceptance of tele-ICU coverage. A systemic review. *Chest* 2011;139(2):279–288.

113. Forni A, Skeham N, Hartman CA, et al. Evaluation of the impact of a tele-ICU pharmacist on the management of sedation in critically ill mechanically ventilated patients. *Ann Pharmacother* 2010;44(3):432–438.

114. Leapfrog: Four Leaps in Hospital Quality, Safety and Affordability. http://www.leapfroggroup.org. Accessed August 27, 2011.

115. *Cerner Sues Firm, Alleges Patent Misuse.* November 17, 2004. http://www.bizjournals.com/kansascity/stories/2004/11/15/daily24.html.

116. *Cerner Wins Law Suit with VISICU.* February 26, 2010. https://www.santarosaconsulting.com/SantaRosaTeamBlog/post/2010/02/26/Healthcare-e28093-The-Newest-Technology-Battlefield.aspx.

117. Janathi A. *Checking In on the Country's First Tele-ICU: 15 Years Later.* December 2015. http://www.beckershospitalreview.com/healthcare-information-technology/checking-in-on-the-country-s-first-tele-icu-15-years-later.html. Accessed October 2, 2016.

118. *Sentara Marks 10-Year Anniversary of Groundbreaking eICU System.* June 23, 2010. www.sentara.com/News/NewsArchives/2010/Pages/Sentara-marks-10-year-anniversary-of-groundbreaking-eICU-system.aspx.

119. Reynolds HN, Bander J, McCarthy M. Different systems and formats for tele-ICU coverage. Designing a tele-ICU system to optimize functionality and investment. *Crit Care Nurs Q* 2012;35(4):1–14.

120. Reynolds HN, Rogove H, Bander J, et al. A working lexicon for the tele-ICU: we need to define tele-ICU to grow and understand it. *Telemed J E Health* 2011;17(10):773–783.

121. Reynolds HN, Bander JJ. Options for tele-intensive care unit design: centralized vs decentralized and other considerations: it is not just a another black sedan. *Crit Care Clin* 2015;31(2):335–350.

122. Coustasse A, Deslich S, Bailey D, Paul D. A business case for tele-intensive care units. *Perm J* 2014;18(4):76–84.

123. Koepsell TD, Weiss NS. *Epidemiologic Methods: Studying the Occurrence of Illness.* New York: Oxford University Press; 2003.

124. Khan J, Hill N, Lilly C, et al. The research agenda in ICU telemedicine: a statement from the Critical Care Societies Collaborative. *Chest* 2011;140(1):230–238.

125. New England Healthcare Institute, Massachusetts Technology Collaborative. *Critical Care, Critical Choices: The Case for Tele-ICUs in Intensive Care.* Westborough, MA: Massachusetts Technology Park Corporation; 2010.

126. Lyden C. Technical barriers with the tele-ICU. From paper to computer documentation: one easy step? *Online J Nurs Inform* 2008;12(3):1–20.

127. Reynolds HN. Remote critical care services. In: Dorman T, Britton F, Brown D, Munro N, eds. *Coding and Billing for Critical Care: A Practice Tool.* 6th ed. Mount Prospect, IL: Society of Critical Care Medicine; 2014:49–61.

128. *Medicare Program; Revisions to Payment Policies Under the Physician Fee Schedule and Other Revisions to Part B for CY 2017; Medicare Advantage Pricing Data Release; Medicare Advantage and Part D Medical Low Ratio Data Release; Medicare Advantage Provider Network Requirements; Expansion of Medicare Diabetes Prevention Program Model.* https://www.federalregister.gov/documents/2016/07/15/2016-16097/medicare-program-revisions-to-payment-policies-under-the-physician-fee-schedule-and-other-revisions. Accessed October 19, 2016.

129. Linkous J. *American Telemedicine Response to CMS Proposed Revisions to Physician Fee Schedule.* https://higherlogicdownload.s3.amazonaws.com/AMERICANTELEMED/3c09839a-fffd-46f7-916c-692c11d78933/UploadedImages/Policy/ATA%20comments%20on%202017%20fee%20schedule.pdf. Accessed October 19, 2016.

130. *CY 2017 Proposed Physician Fee Schedule (CMS-1654-P) Summary of Key Provisions.* July 15, 2016. http://www.amga.org/wcm/Advocacy/Tools/cy2017PFSSummary.pdf. Accessed October 19, 2016.

131. Thomas L, Capistrant G. *State Telemedicine Gaps Analysis: Coverage and Reimbursement.* Washington, DC: American Telemedicine Association; 2014.

Teledermatology[*]

Hon Pak, MD, Ivy A. Lee, MD and John D. Whited, MD, MHS

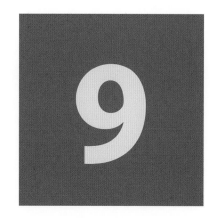

"Around 2001, teleconsultation of a 17 days old child from Louisiana with a red patch on the face was performed with dermatologists at Brooke Army Medical Center (see Figure 9-1). Given the association of hemangiomas on lips with upper respiratory involvement, the dermatologists requested additional information and confirmed some respiratory symptoms that the pediatrician was attributing to potential asthma. The mother drove 8 hours and brought her child to San Antonio, Texas for an in person evaluation the next day where the child was found to have increasing respiratory difficulty. Ear, nose, and throat (ENT) consultation revealed a significant hemangioma in the upper airway. A few days later, the patient had surgery and left the hospital in great condition. We saved a life."

Teledermatology is the practice of dermatology using information communication technologies. Teledermatology has experienced an explosive growth in the last several years as health care reform accelerates. As technologies continue to evolve, teledermatology will also evolve as digital skin imaging advances. Teledermatology is well suited for telehealth given the visual nature of the specialty, and it is one of the most mature and well-studied telemedicine applications. Use of teledermatology was first published by Murphy and Bird using a two-way audiovisual microwave circuit at Massachusetts General Hospital to 1,000 patients 2.7 miles away at the Logan International Airport.[1] Teledermatology is now widespread in its use, as documented by an American Telemedicine Association (ATA) *Current Active Teledermatology Programs* survey[2] (survey is being updated; personal communication with Dr. April Armstrong et al.). Teledermatology is being used by many health care organizations, including federal and state entities (eg, Department of Veterans Affairs [VA], Department of Defense [DoD], Federally Qualified Health Center [FQHC]), academic medical centers, and private/group practices and is being reimbursed by many payors. Although Medicare reimbursement for teledermatology has not changed, state and commercial reimbursement is rapidly evolving to cover teledermatology. Recent health care reforms emphasize value-based care. As virtual care becomes more integrated into mainstream medicine, there is also a shift of focus to a) education of providers and patients, b) quality assessments, and c) resource utilization as part of the value-based care. Finally, direct to patient/consumer teledermatology has had exponential growth, and it will likely increase in demand.

This chapter will review the different modalities used in the practice of teledermatology and the different models of implementation, such as teleconsultation and teletriage. The current status of legislation and its impact on the practice of teledermatology, credentialing and privileging, prescribing, and licensure will be discussed. The challenges facing teledermatology

[*] The views expressed in this chapter are those of the author (JDW) and do not necessarily represent the views of the United States Department of Veterans Affairs or the United States government.

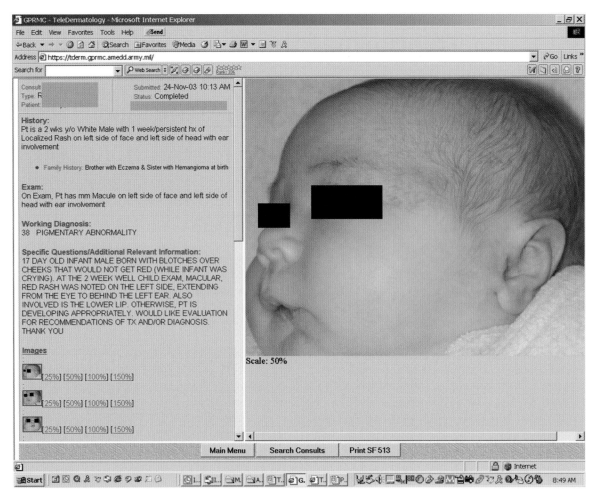

▲ Figure 9-1. Child with infantile hemangioma.

will be addressed, including reimbursement, quality management, and electronic health record (EHR) integration. Existing practice guidelines and other teledermatology resources will be presented. The chapter will conclude with a brief review of teledermatology's evidence base and resources.

TELEDERMATOLOGY MODALITIES

▶ Live Video (Synchronous)

Live two-way interaction between a person and a provider using audiovisual telecommunications technology. This type of service is also referred to as "real-time"

or "synchronous." Live video can be used for both consultative and diagnostic and treatment services.

▶ Store-and-Forward (Asynchronous)

Transmission of recorded health information (eg, history, digital photos, pre-recorded videos) through a secure electronic communications system to a practitioner, usually a specialist, who uses the information to evaluate the case and render a diagnosis or disposition. As compared to a real-time visit, this asynchronous service provides access to data after they have been collected and involves communication tools such as a secure website, mobile application, or email.

Hybrid

A combination of store-and-forward and live interactive modalities can be used to leverage the strengths of each modality. However, it suffers from the live video limitation of scheduling scalability.

We do not consider mobile health a separate modality because it can support any of the three modalities. It typically involves the use of mobile communication devices such as cell phones and tablet computers. Applications range from self-education, self-referrals, and on-demand care or as part of traditional teledermatology programs specifically to increase convenience and access to patients.

MODELS OF TELEDERMATOLOGY

Teleconsultation

A referring provider (commonly primary care but could be any specialty, including dermatology) sends a consult to a dermatologist for diagnostic review and/or management recommendation. In this model, the consultant's recommendation is returned to the referring provider for all management and follow-up. The referring provider takes full ownership of the patient. There is usually a history and data capture from the referring site.

Telereferral

In this model, the referring provider sends the patient as is done with traditional referral to a dermatologist, but the dermatologist who is evaluating the patient virtually takes control over managing the patient.

Teletriage

A variant of the telereferral model, a virtual dermatologist typically evaluates each case being referred for triaging and disposition purposes with the goal of improving access to appropriate conditions requiring urgent evaluation. Typically, this model is used by an organization to optimize resources to route patients to the most appropriate level of care (eg, Kaiser Permanente).

Direct to Patient

We are proposing new terminology to differentiate direct to patient (DTP) and direct to consumer (DTC).

Although many feel that this differentiation is subtle, we believe that this new proposed categorization will help inform regulatory policy; but most importantly, it will bring clarity and transparency to patients utilizing teledermatology. We propose that in this model, a provider either has an established relationship with a patient or has access to necessary medical records and is able to provide appropriate follow-up. This can be done most easily within the VA, Kaiser Permanente, or other large integrated delivery systems that have integrated EHRs.

Direct to Consumer

We are proposing that we limit this term to interactions without an established provider–patient relationship and/or without an integrated delivery system and available EHR. This is largely on-demand teledermatology where the information submitted (via smart phone, laptop, or personal computer) is provided by the consumer and used for the convenience of the consumer. Separating DTC from DTP reflects how teledermatology is being conducted and its implications related to quality and safety.

Miscellaneous

Given the rise of urgent clinics now using EHRs and telemedicine, teledermatology in this setting could be seen as a teleconsultation or telereferral. Mobile apps are not a separate model, but rather a technology that can enable any modality or that can support any of the models. Mobile apps are increasingly used for self-help or education. In the future, imaging diagnostics may be supported via mobile apps; however, at this time, we are not aware of any validated apps that allow patients to accurately auto-diagnose skin conditions.

CHALLENGES

Policy

There are numerous policy challenges. Providers must be licensed in the state where the patient is located. Full and unrestricted licenses are required with rare exceptions. Few states allow reciprocity with neighboring states or conditional telemedicine licenses. Interstate licensure for telemedicine continues to be a barrier to wider adoption and will not be discussed in detail here. However, the Federation of State Medical Boards (FSMB) Interstate Medical Licensure Compact was originally adopted in 2015 by legislators in Alabama, passing the threshold of seven states needed to enact the compact.[3] Eighteen states have enacted the compact to date. The compact simplifies the licensing procedure and will enable more physicians to treat people in more states through the use of telemedicine. Updates on the compact are available. This compact aims to expedite physician licensure in the states that have adopted it. Licensees would still need to be licensed in each state where they treat patients, either in person or using telemedicine. Physicians also need to comply with the law of each state in which they provide care, and states retain disciplinary authority. The compact does not create reciprocity or a single multistate license. Participation in the compact is voluntary for both states and physicians.

▶ Electronic Health Record Integration

With the Health Information Technology for Economic and Clinical Health (HITECH) Act of 2009 and Medicare Access and CHIP Reauthorization Act of 2015 (MACRA), whose final rule was released in October 2016 by the Centers for Medicare & Medicaid Services (CMS), EHR adoption has substantially increased.[4] In 2015, 96% of all nonfederal acute care hospitals possessed certified health information technology (HIT). Small rural and small urban hospitals had the lowest rates at 94%. Ninety-six percent of critical access hospitals (CAHs) had certified HIT, whereas 98% of large hospitals and 97% of medium hospitals had certified HIT—the highest rates among these hospital types.

EHR certification did not include a telehealth requirement or, importantly, the interoperability needed to support telemedicine. Most telemedicine services in use today are not present or fully integrated into EHRs. There are exceptions, such as the VA, which is using its EHR to support store-and-forward teledermatology capability. Furthermore, the large EHR vendors do not have integrated telehealth capabilities (store-and-forward or real-time), which renders the use of telemedicine burdensome to providers. Some existing and new EHR vendors have begun offering telemedicine capability, but do not support interoperability outside the system. As an example, most EHRs cannot send a virtual consult order from the existing consult module to an outside network provider who can answer and return the consult back to the originating provider in the EHR where the consult was generated. We believe that there is a significant opportunity, especially through Fast Healthcare Interoperability Resources (FHIR) and Health Information Exchanges (HIEs), to support teledermatology portability and interoperability.

▶ Maintaining Quality

The ATA and the American Academy of Dermatology (AAD) have established a set of guidelines for teledermatology. Although many programs are using these guidelines, there is currently no concrete measure of the level of compliance for quality and patient safety. The ATA offers an accreditation program to address the growing issue of quality, especially for virtual health or DTC or DTP telemedicine service providers who are seeing rapid growth.

In a recent study, Resneck and colleagues noted that DTC teledermatology is expanding rapidly but has not been well studied.[5] To test some of these DTC sites, the researchers posed as patients with skin-related symptoms. They received responses from 16 DTC sites for 62 online visits in February and March 2016. The hypothetical patients submitted photos of various cancerous, inflammatory, and infectious skin conditions to teledermatology websites offering services to California residents. They claimed to be uninsured and paid fees using Visa gift cards. Incorrect diagnoses, inappropriate treatments, lack of information about possible side effects and risks, and lack of transparency about a doctor's credentials were among the concerns raised in the study. No sites asked for proof of identification, and licensing information was provided in only about a quarter of cases. Some of the sites used foreign physicians without California licenses. In less than a quarter of cases did the sites ask the name of the patient's primary care physician. In only 10% of cases did they offer to send medical records. Furthermore, if patients would need in-person care because their condition worsens or they have a medication side effect, many teledermatology clinicians do not have local contacts and cannot facilitate an appointment. Quality assessment and improvement programs are a focus for gap analysis in telemedicine, and many stakeholders, including the National Quality Forum, are convening specific workgroups to tackle this practice gap.[6]

LEGISLATION AND REIMBURSEMENT

Regulations and reimbursement for telemedicine are quickly evolving to keep pace with patient demand and technology. This section reviews the core concepts that providers should be cognizant of when practicing teledermatology.

▶ Legislation

Credentialing and Privileging

Credentialing and privileging refers to the assessment of a provider's qualifications and competence. In 2011, CMS issued a Final Rule that included two components that promoted telemedicine adoption in hospitals and CAHs. The Final Rule allowed providers to deliver telemedicine services to patients through written agreements with a distant-site hospital or a distant-site telemedicine entity. The Final Rule also streamlined credentialing and privileging for telemedicine providers and allowed hospitals and CAHs to rely, when granting telemedicine privileges, upon the privileging decisions of a distant-site hospital or telemedicine entity where they have a written agreement that meets Medicare requirements. This aligned CMS with the privileging by proxy standards initially set forth by The Joint Commission.[7]

Online Prescribing

Regulation of prescriptions obtained virtually varies significantly with state legislation, as well as by state medical and pharmacy boards. Policies have been created to protect patients from online "pill mills." At the time of this publication, 12 states allowed electronic means to establish the patient–physician relationship and exam. Few states require an in-person follow-up appointment after a telemedicine encounter. There are no requirements to obtain patient information regarding underlying past medical history, allergies, drug adverse effects, other medications and potential drug interactions, contraindications, and safety in pregnancy or lactation. Patient safety and ethical concerns arise from whether an appropriate patient–provider relationship is established; the adequacy of the physical exam; patient education on the diagnosis, risks, benefits, and alternatives of treatment and follow-up if adverse events occur; and continuity and coordination of care with the patient's other health care providers.

Medicolegal Liability

Telemedicine possesses the same duty of care as traditional in-person medicine does. To date, there have been no legal actions concerning teledermatology. There is much debate surrounding clinical and quality standards of care in telemedicine and whether it should or should not differ from that of traditional in-person medicine. Prior to practicing teledermatology, it is prudent to contact one's liability carrier to discuss specific plans (technical modality, patient populations, prescription capacity, etc.) and whether current or supplemental coverage is sufficient.

Reimbursement

In traditional fee-for-service models, reimbursement has expanded with the passage of parity laws that apply to private insurers and self-pay with the emergence of DTP/DTC care. Parity laws can include coverage parity that mandates telemedicine services be covered to the same extent and in the same manner as in-person services and/or payment parity that requires the same rate of payment for services delivered via telehealth. Twenty-nine states have parity laws for private insurers, and there is a trend towards removing eligible provider, technology, and patient setting restrictions for reimbursement. With the explosive growth in direct care teledermatology services and prevalence of high-deductible insurance plans, many patients are paying out of pocket or using flexible spending accounts for their teledermatology care. In a recent study by Fogel and Sarin, asynchronous, store-and-forward teledermatology consultations typically range from $25 to $100 per encounter.[8]

Reimbursement by federal payors such as Medicare and Medicaid lags behind private payors and has significant room for improvement. Medicare currently reimburses live interactive teledermatology encounters with geographic restrictions to health professional shortage areas (HPSAs) and only reimburses store-and-forward teledermatology in Alaska and Hawaii. In addition to geographic restrictions, Medicare limits the type of eligible providers and eligible facilities that it will reimburse. Medicaid coverage resembles Medicare coverage in its preference for live interactive modalities, and only nine states reimburse for store-and-forward technologies. Medicaid is even more restricted than that of Medicare with significant geographic restrictions, limited eligible patient populations, eligible providers, authorized technologies, and patient consent. Forty-eight state Medicaid programs have some type of coverage for telemedicine, which includes a number of states covering store-and-forward teledermatology (as of 2016). One area of expanded coverage is reimbursement for telemedicine under state employee health plans. Twenty-four states now (as of 2016) have some type of coverage for telehealth under one or more state employee health plans.[9]

With the enactment of MACRA in 2015, there is an increasing focus on value-based reimbursement models and alternative payment models such as capitation, bundled payments, shared savings, medical home model, or pay for performance. A recent study by Rosen et al. demonstrates the feasibility and viability of such business models as well as traditional reimbursement schemes in teledermatology.[10]

Legislative Landscape

With an increasing focus on population health management and value-based care, telehealth will continue to be a popular topic for state and federal legislation in the foreseeable future. The definition, appropriate use, licensure, and reimbursement of telehealth are quickly evolving in an attempt to catch up with the pace of practice.

PRACTICE GUIDELINES

Because of dermatology's early role in telemedicine and extensive experience, both the ATA Teledermatology Special Interest Group and the AAD have created guidelines to promote appropriate, high-quality teledermatology practice. Although not specific to teledermatology, the American Medical Association (AMA) and the ATA offer general guidelines for implementing and practicing telemedicine.

▶ Dermatology Specific

American Academy of Dermatology Position Statement

Revised in 2016, the AAD Position Statement defines live interactive and store-and-forward teledermatology and outlines the pertinent benchmarks for technology, credentialing and privileging, privacy and confidentiality, licensing, reimbursement, responsibility, and liability. Most importantly, the position statement specifies criteria for delivering high-quality teledermatology.[11]

American Telemedicine Association Practice Guidelines for Teledermatology

Updated in 2016 after an extensive review of the evidence base, the *ATA Practice Guidelines for Teledermatology* comprehensively cover clinical practice and technological and administrative processes.[12] The clinical practice guidelines highlight important preliminary considerations before engaging in teledermatology practice, management recommendations, and quality and ethical suggestions. The technical guidelines review the communication modes and applications, devices and equipment, image quality, display, and privacy. The administrative guidelines include security, licensing and credentialing, and liability recommendations.

American Telemedicine Association Quick Guide for Store-and-Forward and Live Interactive Teledermatology

Created in 2012, the *ATA Quick Guide for Store-and-Forward and Live Interactive Teledermatology* includes concise, practical information on clinical workflows, technical specifications, and insightful tips on optimizing image quality.[13]

▶ Dermatology Nonspecific

American Medical Association Telemedicine Guidelines

Created in 2014 and accessible to AMA members only, the *AMA's Telemedicine Guidelines* offers safeguards and standards on the practice of high-quality telemedicine, reimbursement, and coverage concerns.[14]

American Medical Association Steps Forward

The AMA's *Steps Forward* program includes straightforward, concrete steps to consider prior to creating and implementing a telemedicine program. This includes online resources as potential continuing medical education (CME) credits.[15]

TELEDERMATOLOGY'S EVIDENCE BASE

A comprehensive review of the teledermatology literature is beyond the scope of this book, but an excellent review was recently carried out by Bashshur et al.[16] It should be noted, however, that teledermatology is one of the most studied disciplines in telehealth. The following briefly summarizes research findings for some clinically relevant aspects of delivering telehealth care via teledermatology. Most of the data are from provider-to-provider teleconsultation because data from DTC/DTP are limited.

▶ Diagnostic Agreement

Diagnostic agreement refers to whether two or more clinicians can agree on a diagnosis. Although agreement does not predict whether the clinicians have provided a correct or accurate diagnosis, it is nonetheless an important diagnostic feature. Diagnostic disagreement occurs in all medical disciplines and with all modes of health care delivery. The most important question to answer is: How does diagnostic disagreement rendered by teledermatology compare to disagreement found among different clinicians examining patients during an in-person encounter? A few studies have addressed that issue for store-and-forward teledermatology.[17-19]

Diagnostic agreement among teledermatologists has been comparable to diagnostic agreement recorded among different in-person dermatologist examiners. Likewise, one study that assessed live interactive teledermatology found comparable diagnostic agreement among teledermatologists compared to examinations performed by in-person dermatologists.[20]

▶ Diagnostic Accuracy

Diagnostic accuracy refers to whether a particular diagnosis is correct or not. Ideally, accuracy is measured against a gold standard, when one is available or

can be applied. For example, the presumptive diagnosis of a skin lesion as a squamous cell carcinoma can be measured against the gold standard test: histopathological review of biopsied tissue. For store-and-forward teledermatology, accuracy studies have yielded varying results. Most studies have demonstrated comparable diagnostic accuracy when compared to in-person diagnoses.[17,21-24] However, other studies have demonstrated inferior diagnostic accuracy, in particular for pigmented skin lesions.[25,26] In general, store-and-forward teledermatology is considered an accurate means of diagnosing of skin conditions, but teledermatologists should be cognizant of the evidence to date that suggests diagnostic inferiority when evaluating pigmented skin lesions with store-and-forward teledermatology. This is an area that would benefit from further research to add clarity. No definitive data on the accuracy of live interactive teledermatology diagnoses currently exist.

▶ Clinical Outcomes

Clinical course refers to the clinical outcome that patients experience through their interaction with a health care system and any treatment they may receive. Two studies have compared the clinical course experienced between patients receiving conventional referrals with clinic-based evaluations and store-and-forward teledermatology interventions in a randomized trial study design.[27,28] Both studies found no evidence for a difference in clinical course experienced by patients who received a teledermatology referral compared to the conventional referral process and in-person visit. In both studies and in both referral groups, the majority of patients were rated as having an improvement and/or resolution of their referred condition at the study endpoints. A wide range of ambulatory skin conditions were represented among the patient populations assessed. Studies with a similar design have not been conducted using real-time interactive teledermatology.

▶ Economic Outcomes

The conclusions drawn from economic analyses often depend on the type of analysis used and the economic perspective(s) taken by those analyses. For example, a cost analysis only considers the costs involved with teledermatology implementation, whereas cost effectiveness considers both costs and the chosen measure(s) of effectiveness with the intent of generating incremental cost-effectiveness ratios. The most common economic perspectives represented in the teledermatology literature are societal and the health care system. The conclusions drawn are varied. This reflects, in part, differences in the health care system under review, the population and geographic areas being served, and the economic perspective(s) considered. In various settings, teledermatology has been found to be both more economical and more costly when compared to conventional dermatology referrals and care. When effectiveness measures have been analyzed, teledermatology is generally considered to be a cost-effective intervention.[29] As an example, prior evidence that clinical course (effectiveness) was not found to differ between store-and-forward teledermatology and conventional referrals[27] was the basis for a cost minimization analysis of those two referral systems.[30] Cost data revealed that from the economic perspective of the U.S. DoD health care system, teledermatology was the more costly alternative, with an average cost per patient of $294 versus $283 for conventional referrals. From the more comprehensive societal economic perspective, teledermatology was less costly at $340 per patient versus $372 for conventional care. Thus, with similar effectiveness, costs were lower with teledermatology from a societal perspective and were incrementally higher by $11 per patient from the health care system perspective. Teledermatology would be the favored economic strategy from a societal perspective and may be considered cost effective from the health care perspective, particularly if the implementation of teledermatology accrues other benefits such as improved access to care or shorter wait times.

▶ Quality of Life

Quality of life is an important metric in all aspects of health care and is arguably the most important one in dermatologic health care. A study that compared quality of life between patients undergoing a store-and-forward teledermatology referral and a conventional referral with a clinic-based visit found no difference in quality of life between the two referral groups.[31] Patients in both groups experienced an improvement in quality of life at the study's endpoint, indicating that quality of life improved with both store-and-forward teledermatology and the conventional referral process. Although no comparison group was included, when real-time teledermatology was used, quality of life improved between baseline and the end of the study period.[32] Because of its importance in dermatology, further research and other applications of quality-of-life assessments would make important contributions to our knowledge base.

TELEDERMATOLOGY RESOURCES

▶ American Telemedicine Association (www.americantelemed.org/home)

The ATA is a leading source of telemedicine information. The association's Teledermatology Special Interest Group (http://www.americantelemed.org/main/membership/ata-members/ata-sigs/teledermatology-sig) is the repository for teledermatology-specific information. Resources that can be found at the Teledermatology Special Interest Group site include the *Quick Guide to Store-and-Forward and Live Interactive Teledermatology for Referring Providers*, *Practice Guidelines for Teledermatology*, *Current Active Teledermatology Programs* (which is a compendium of health care entities that engage in teledermatology), and a *Summary of the Status of Teledermatology Research* providing an updated overview of teledermatology research publications on select topics.

▶ American Academy of Dermatology (www.aad.org)

The AAD hosts a teledermatology site and *Teledermatology Toolkit* at www.aad.org/practice-tools/running-a-practice/teledermatology. The site includes a summary of modalities, links to educational and policy resources, and a description of AccessDerm. AccessDerm is a teledermatology initiative for the provision of dermatology care to underserved populations. The policy links include the AAD's *Position Statement on Teledermatology*. A video tutorial, *Introduction to Store-and-Forward Teledermatology*, is another educational resource found at this site.

▶ Center for Connected Health Policy (www.cchpca.org)

The Center for Connected Health Policy (CCHP) is a national resource supported by funding from the Office for the Advancement of Telehealth, Health Resources and Service Administration, Department of Health and Human Services. The site covers the broad spectrum of telemedicine and includes a link to the other telehealth resource centers that provide telehealth advice at the state level (www.telehealthresourcecenter.org). The Telehealth Resource Center site provides information related to features common to all aspects of telemedicine, such as reimbursement, legal and regulatory issues, and marketing issues, among others. The consortia of telehealth resource centers are listed, many of which include information specific to teledermatology. For example, the Mid-Atlantic Telehealth Resource Center includes a site dedicated to teledermatology (www.matrc.org/teledermatology).

▶ **Other Resources**

- The British Association of Dermatologists (www.bad.org.uk) includes *Quality Standards for Teledermatology Using "Store and Forward" Images*. Although the document is written for practice within the United Kingdom's National Health Service, much of the text includes useful information relevant to teledermatology implementation in any setting.

- The Center for Telehealth and e-Health Law (www.ctel.org) provides information and expertise on legal and regulatory aspects of telemedicine.

- Two journals are dedicated to publishing telemedicine-related content. The *Journal of Telemedicine and Telecare* is published by Sage Publications Limited (http://jtt.sagepub.com/), and *Telemedicine and e-Health* is published by Mary Ann Liebert, Incorporated (www.liebertpub.com/overview/telemedicine-and-e-health/54/).

- Dermatology-specific journals that publish teledermatology research and other teledermatology-specific content include:
  - *JAMA Dermatology* published by the AMA (http://jamanetwork.com/journals/jamadermatology)
  - *Journal of the American Academy of Dermatology* published by Elsevier, Incorporated (www.jaad.org)
  - *International Journal of Dermatology* (www.onlinelibrary.wiley.com/journal/10.1111/(ISSN)1365-4632) published by John Wiley and Sons, Incorporated

  - *British Journal of Dermatology* (www.onlinelibrary.wiley.com/journal/10.1111/(ISSN)1365-2133) published by John Wiley and Sons, Incorporated

- Books dedicated to teledermatology include:
  - *Teledermatology: A User's Guide* (Pak, Edison, & Whited, eds.) published by Cambridge University Press, 2008
  - *Teledermatology* (Wootton & Oakley, eds.) published by The Royal Society of Medicine Press, Limited, 2002
  - *Telemedicine in Dermatology* (Soyer, Binder, Smith, & Wurm, eds.) published by Springer, 2012
  - *Telemedicine and Teledermatology* (Burg, ed.) published by Karger Medical and Scientific Publishers, 2003

- Another important resource is the U.S. Department of Veterans Affairs Health Services Research and Development Evidence Synthesis Program report titled *Teledermatology for Diagnosis and Management of Skin Conditions* (http://www.hsrd.research.va.gov/publications/esp/telederm.cfm). This document is a systematic review of the literature related to teledermatology's use in the diagnosis and management of dermatologic conditions.

CONCLUSION

As the case report at the beginning of this chapter illustrates, the goal of teledermatology is to deliver timely, effective, and high-quality care that, in some cases, may not be available without the use of telemedicine technology. The evidence base for teledermatology suggests that it is a reliable and accurate means of making diagnoses, and it results in comparable clinical and quality-of-life outcomes. It is an economically viable method of delivering dermatology care and can even be a cost-saving strategy. There are many sources of guidance on teledermatology that are ever expanding and constantly undergoing refinement. However, teledermatology is not without its challenges. Licensure as it relates to interstate practice, EHR-related issues such as support of telehealth technology and "out-of-network" communication, and quality assurance in teledermatology settings are among the most pressing of challenges. Other matters such as online prescribing, medicolegal liability, and reimbursement are evolving areas of interest to the teledermatology community. Perhaps the area of greatest current controversy is the application of DTC and DTP teledermatology, areas that have experienced tremendous growth in recent years—likely fueled in part to the ubiquitous use of smart phones coupled with consumer demand. Because of its achievements and in spite of its challenges, teledermatology is widely practiced and continues to grow because at its core, it is simply a way for patients to get the timely dermatology care that they need and a way for clinicians to efficiently serve those patients.

REFERENCES

1. Murphy RL, Bird KT. Telediagnosis: a new community resource. Observations on the feasibility of telediagnosis based on 1000 patient transactions. *Am J Public Health* 1974;64:113–119.

2. *Current Active Teledermatology Programs.* 2016. http://www.americantelemed.org/main/membership/ata-members/ata-sigs/teledermatology-sig.

3. *Interstate Medical Licensure Compact.* 2016. http://www.licenseportability.org/.

4. *Center for Medicare and Medicaid Services.* 2016. https://www.cms.gov/Medicare/Quality-Initiatives-Patient-Assessment-Instruments/Value-Based-Programs/MACRA-MIPS-and-APMs/MACRA-MIPS-and-APMs.html.

5. Resneck JS, Abrouk M, Steuer M, et al. Choice, transparency, coordination, and quality among direct-to-consumer telemedicine websites and apps treating skin disease. *JAMA Dermatol* 2016;152(7):768–775.

6. *National Quality Forum.* 2016. http://www.qualityforum.org/Home.aspx.

7. *The Joint Commission.* 2016. https://www.jointcommission.org/.

8. Fogel AL, Sarin KY. A survey of direct-to-consumer teledermatology services available to US patients: explosive growth, opportunities and controversy. *J Telemed Telecare* 2017;23(1):19–25.

9. *Center for Connected Health Policy.* 2016. http://cchpca.org/.

10. Rosen AR, Littman-Quinn R, Kovarik CL, et al. Landscape of business models in teledermatology. *Cutis* 2016;97(4):302–304.

11. *Position Statement on Teledermatology.* 2016. https://www.aad.org/Forms/Policies/Uploads/PS/PS-Teledermatology.pdf.

12. *ATA Practice Guidelines for Teledermatology.* 2016. http://www.americantelemed.org/main/membership/ata-members/ata-sigs/teledermatology-sig.

13. *ATA Quick Guide for Store-and-Forward and Live-Interactive Teledermatology.* 2016. http://www.americantelemed.org/main/membership/ata-members/ata-sigs/teledermatology-sig.

14. *AMA Telemedicine Guidelines.* 2016. https://www.ama-assn.org/.

15. *Steps Forward.* 2016. https://www.stepsforward.org/modules/adopting-telemedicine.

16. Bashshur RL, Shannon GW, Tejasvi T, et al. The empirical foundations of teledermatology: a review of the research evidence. *Telemed J E Health* 2015;21(12):953–979.

17. Whited JD, Hall RP, Simel DL, et al. Reliability and accuracy of dermatologists' clinic-based and digital image consultations. *J Am Acad Dermatol* 1999;41:693–702.

18. Ribas J, da Graca Souza Cunha M, Schettini APM, et al. Agreement between dermatological diagnoses made by live examination compared to analysis of digital images. *An Bras Dermatol* 2010;85(4):441–447.

19. Lamel SA, Haldeman KM, Ely H, et al. Application of mobile teledermatology for skin cancer screening. *J Am Acad Dermatol* 2012;67:576–581.

20. Lesher JL, Davis LS, Gourdin FW, et al. Telemedicine evaluation of cutaneous diseases: a blinded comparative study. *J Am Acad Dermatol* 1998;38:27–31.

21. Krupinski EA, LeSueur B, Ellsworth L, et al. Diagnostic accuracy and image quality using a digital camera for teledermatology. *Telemed J* 1999;5(3):257–263.

22. Moreno-Ramirez D, Ferrandiz L, Bernal A, et al. Teledermatology as a filtering system in pigmented lesion clinics. *J Telemed Telecare* 2005;11:298–303.

23. Oakley AMM, Reeves F, Bennett J, et al. Diagnostic value of written referral and/or images for skin lesions. *J Telemed Telecare* 2006;12:151–158.

24. Rios-Yuil JM. Correlation between face-to-face assessment and telemedicine for the diagnosis of skin disease in case conferences. *Actas Dermosifiliogr* 2012;103(2):138–143.

25. Warshaw EM, Lederle FA, Grill JP, et al. Accuracy of teledermatology for nonpigmented neoplasms. *J Am Acad Dermatol* 2009;60:579–588.

26. Warshaw EM, Lederle FA, Grill JP, et al. Accuracy of teledermatology for pigmented lesions. *J Am Acad Dermatol* 2009;61:753–765.

27. Pak H, Triplett CA, Lindquist JH, et al. Store-and-forward teledermatology results in similar clinical outcomes to conventional clinic-based care. *J Telemed Telecare* 2007;13:26–30.

28. Whited JD, Warshaw EM, Kapur K, et al. Clinical course outcomes for store and forward teledermatology versus conventional consultation: a randomized trial. *J Telemed Telecare* 2013;19:197–204.

29. Snoswell C, Finnane A, Janda M, et al. Cost-effectiveness of store-and-forward teledermatology: a systematic review. *JAMA Dermatol* 2016;152(6):702–708.

30. Pak HS, Datta SK, Triplett CA, et al. Cost minimization analysis of a store-and-forward teledermatology consult system. *Telemed J E Health* 2009;15(2):160–165.

31. Whited JD, Warshaw EM, Edison KE, et al. Effect of store and forward teledermatology on quality of life: a randomized trial. *JAMA Dermatol* 2013;149(5):584–591.

32. Al Quran HA, Khader YS, Ellauzi ZM, et al. Effect of real-time teledermatology on diagnosis, treatment, and clinical improvement. *J Telemed Telecare* 2015;21(2):93–99.

Telepsychiatry

Maryann Waugh, MEd, Peter Yellowlees, MD,
Rachel Dixon and Jay H. Shore, MD, MPH

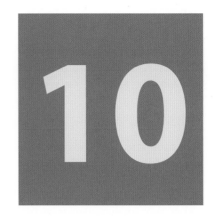

CASE STUDY

A psychiatrist is providing a weekly telepsychiatry clinic for a small rural community mental health center in the intermountain west. She evaluates a new patient, John a 74-year old recently widowed rancher whose children have brought him out of their concern of his increasing isolation. John reports that since his wife passed three months ago he has been having difficulty sleeping, leading to increasing fatigued during the day. He has lost his appetite and motivation to engage in ranch work or socialize with others. Although he denies current or history of suicidality, he feels that he has no reason to go on living and has access to firearms at home. The psychiatrist works with the clinic's onsite social worker to develop a treatment plan, which includes an antidepressant and sleep medication along with grief-focused supportive therapy. The psychiatrist educates John and his adult children about depression and loss and engages in a candid discussion about firearm safety in the context of a depressive episode and risks for suicide. The family agrees until the depression has resolved to hold John's firearms for him. Over the next 8 to 12 weeks through medication management and therapy John's depression begins to resolve, with the psychiatrist following John's progress in their follow-up video sessions and through contact with the clinic's social worker.

INTRODUCTION

Technological advances have led to significant changes in psychiatric service delivery models.[1] As broadband and wireless Internet access become widely available, and smart phones, tablets, and other small, portable devices allow convenient, mobile access to the Internet, virtual care options are expanding. These virtual options have emerged not only because of improved technological ability, but also because of an increasing recognition of the need to maximize the ability of a limited number of psychiatric providers to serve a larger patient population; a growing consumer demand for patient-centered, convenient care options; and payor demand for more cost-effective care.[2] The American Medical Association (AMA) aptly notes that "[i]nnovation in technology, including information technology, is redefining how people perceive time and distance. It is reshaping how individuals interact with and relate to others, including when, where, and how patients and physicians engage with one another."[3] Virtual modalities lend themselves particularly well to the field of psychiatry where providers need no peripheral devices or instruments for patient assessment or treatment. Through an increasingly diverse set of modalities and treatment models, telepsychiatry—defined broadly as leveraging audio and video technology to provide services from a distance[4]—is changing the nature of the traditional psychiatrist–patient relationship to a collaborative experience. This chapter is designed to describe the current treatment modalities and models that support the evolving practice, summarize the evidence for efficacy, and provide an overview of the pragmatic considerations related to telepsychiatry implementation across a variety of care settings.

MODALITIES/MODELS

Telepsychiatry uses two primary service delivery modalities, real time, also known as synchronous, and store-and-forward, also known as asynchronous. Synchronous modalities leverage audio and/or video technology for live, two-way interactive communication. This includes phone or video conferencing, both of which mimic in-person services and have the advantage of immediate response as part of real-time interaction.[5] In asynchronous applications, digital information, whether audio, video, or document format, is sent via email or other web applications to a specialist for later review. The sending and receiving parties do not need to be present at the same time.[5,6]

Telepsychiatry is implemented via direct and indirect consultation across a variety of models. Psychiatrists can directly prescribe medications, carry out psychotherapy, and maintain full responsibility for psychiatric treatment via televideo in any setting with appropriate privacy and connectivity. Psychiatrist expertise can be further maximized across a continuum of increasing indirect consultation with primary care providers (PCPs) and decreasing direct patient consultation. This continuum ranges from collaborative care models where virtual behavioral health teams apply population-based care within a primary care team, to consultation-liaison models where the psychiatrist consults directly with patients for diagnosis/evaluation and provides diagnostic and treatment recommendations to PCPs, to curbside consultations/case reviews with PCPs and no direct patient consultation.[7] Many integrated care models include both direct and indirect consultation. A well-known and well-researched collaborative care model is the IMPACT model (Improving Mood-Promoting Access to Collaborative Treatment) where psychiatrists participate in multidisciplinary primary care teams to provide feedback and treatment planning suggestions to PCPs. IMPACT's telepsychiatrists use electronic health record (EHR) messaging and provide phone/email curbside consultations for real-time advice on diagnoses, treatment plans, and medications.[8]

Asynchronous applications still face reimbursement challenges, but have the potential to increase efficiencies across the continuum of models. Store-and-forward allows a more diverse and potentially less expensive pool of clinic staff to collect patient interview data using a semistructured, recorded format in settings like primary care medical homes, which are already convenient to patients. Recordings and patient medical records are sent to a psychiatrist for later review so psychiatrists can maximize smaller segments of unscheduled time.[6,9–11] Emerging research shows this is more cost effective than either in-person or synchronous telepsychiatry service when economies of scale exceed 250 consultations per provider per year.[10]

TECHNOLOGIES

Historically, videoconferencing technology had a variety of logistical and financial obstacles. It demanded challenging audiovisual connections (including early microwave technology and closed-circuit television) and bulky fixed hardware, required dedicated technology support, and had high capital and labor demands.[12,13] Because the hardware and transmission technology was so large and expensive, teleoptions were limited primarily to large academic medical institutions.[12] Now, wireless Internet-based solutions make streaming audio and video for virtual psychiatric care feasible using secure, mobile, integrated, electronic platforms on laptops, cell phones, and tablets. The American Telemedicine Association (ATA) notes that Internet-based video conferencing needs a bandwidth of at least 500 Kbps in each of the downlink and uplink directions and a minimum of 640 × 480 resolution at 30 frames per second for all televideo applications, which applies equally to telepsychiatry.[14]

Currently, most mobile devices include high-resolution video cameras and displays, Internet connectivity, audio inputs and outputs, and the processing power to support a variety of applications (apps) for patient data collection, patient monitoring, and treatment through synchronous and asynchronous modalities.[1,15] Technological advances/apps already take advantage of accelerometers, technology embedded in smart phones to estimate WiFi activity and allow a global position system (GPS) to locate the device to track general user activity (eg, fitness "steps"). Research is underway to assess the utility of this existing technology to collect user activity data that may help assess for depression,[16] mania,[17] and psychotic disorders.[18] Other researchers are looking into the potential for avatar therapists, or virtual animations trained to respond therapeutically to patients' movements and language.[19]

Technologic advances in audio solutions, such as interactive voice response (IVR), have furthered the ability of both PCPs and psychiatric providers to support patient engagement in behavioral health treatment. Using IVR, primary care providers have been able to screen patients for alcohol abuse and engage them in brief alcohol intervention. Patients randomized to IVR-enhanced intervention had higher rates of substance use disclosure and higher rates of treatment engagement, and received more informed behavioral and medication recommendations compared to those receiving intervention with no follow-up-call enhancement.[20]

SUMMARY EVIDENCE/LITERATURE

Telemental health has been characterized as having more randomized controlled trials than any other medical discipline area.[21] The telepsychiatry literature shows a growing consensus regarding the efficacy, feasibility, and acceptability of virtual psychiatric services.[21,22] Telepsychiatry has demonstrated efficacy along the continuum of services—from psychoeducation, to assessment, diagnosis, and treatment.[22] It has been used to treat a wide variety of behavioral health diagnoses, including depression, anxiety, bipolar, posttraumatic stress disorder, eating disorders, and schizophrenia, and is associated with increased treatment engagement and adherence, improved symptoms, fewer hospital admissions, and shorter hospital stays.[22] In a comprehensive review of telemental health, Bashshur and colleagues[21] noted consistent evidence that virtual psychiatric and other mental health services are linked to improved quality of life and symptomology indicators across demographically and diagnostically diverse groups of patients. Virtual treatment modalities have had a significant impact upon psychiatric care access, particularly for historically underserved populations such as rural residents, college students, veterans, native

populations, and incarcerated persons.[2] Acceptance rates show that patients and providers comfortably use telehealth platforms[5] with some subgroups of patients (ie, patients who are younger, immobile, elderly, worried about stigma, or on the autism spectrum) reporting a preference for virtual over in-person care.[15,23,24]

As previously noted, telepsychiatry is showing particular success in improving care access through integrated care models. Virtual care platforms enable workforce multiplication, through which one psychiatric provider can provide consultation to primary care and other medical providers, thereby improving their ability to manage psychiatric symptoms and medication across their entire patient population. Team-based, primary-care depression care models with virtual psychiatry are associated with measures of patients' treatment satisfaction and adherence, symptom reduction, and quality of life that exceed usual care treatment outcomes.[21] Future research will move beyond measures of feasibility and efficacy and inform effective means of telepsychiatry implementation into health care systems.[25]

REIMBURSEMENT AND REGULATORY ISSUES

With the ever-increasing evidence base for efficacy, feasibility, and acceptability, reimbursement and other regulatory issues may represent the final challenge to telepsychiatry expansion.[2] Although Medicare, Medicaid, and increasing numbers of third-party payors reimburse for telepsychiatry treatment, constraints on reimbursable activities, originating (patient location) site, and the ability to reimburse at subsets of federally designated provider sites (ie, rural health centers) still challenge providers and systems in developing and sustaining telepsychiatry. As of late 2016, 46 states allow Medicaid reimbursement for telemental health services provided via live video (to approved originating sites) and 24 states have mandated that telehealth be covered by third-party payors—but uniform coverage for telepsychiatry and other virtual mental health modalities is lacking.[12] Some home-based telepsychiatry is occurring, but is often only delivered through self-pay options and by private telepsychiatry companies. This form of payment and care is especially suited to those who want enhanced privacy and may not even want their insurance companies to know that they are seeking psychiatric treatment.

As previously noted, asynchronous telepsychiatry options may have a particularly high potential to increase care access and decrease costs. This is especially so in capitated systems of care. Asynchronous telepsychiatry is likely part of the future world of accountable care organizations and with the payment models being introduced in 2018–2019 in the United States through the Medicare Access & CHP Reauthorization Act of 2015 (MACRA) and the Merit-Based Incentive Payment System (MIPS) and Alternative Payment Models (APMs), all of which will substantially reform Medicare, and consequently all private insurance programs. It is highly likely that these reforms will lead to dramatically more telepsychiatry in general, both synchronous and asynchronous.

Originating Medicaid sites can bill for a facility fee (currently, a $25 reimbursement for providing the physical and administrative structures needed for the patient visit), which provides some telepsychiatry-related income. However, the inability to bill for services beyond direct patient treatment still minimizes the ability of providers and systems to realize the full efficacy and cost efficiency of telepsychiatry solutions. The majority of reimbursement challenges are not specific to telepsychiatry and represent general telehealth obstacles. Given the particular shortage of psychiatric providers, the huge burden of untreated mental illness,[21] and the significant opportunity to increase psychiatric care access through workforce multiplication using virtual means, these challenges are particularly critical.

CARE IMPROVEMENT

Telepsychiatry has great potential to improve care quality and health outcomes. The change in the power structure of the doctor–patient relationship makes consumer engagement more likely, both through the more personal and flexible interactions with providers and through the opportunities for behavior modification using a number of psychotherapeutic approaches that have become solidly evidence based.[21] Telepsychiatry is also improving clinical efficiency, especially in integrated care systems, by easing the impact of provider shortages—in particular, psychiatrists—as well

as improving care coordination, increasing staff efficiency, and speeding up access to appointments with experts. As noted later, the research evidence shows improvements in both patient symptoms and outcomes (ie, emergency department use), all of which can contribute to improved care, financial savings, and a clear return on investment.[7]

POTENTIAL PITFALLS

Telepsychiatry is, by definition, dependent upon technology, making technology glitches a significant potential pitfall. The stability and strength of Internet connections vary from clinic to clinic, as do the quality of computers, webcams, speakers, and other hardware. Some sites may have IT support, some may not. Conducting a baseline technological assessment at the outset of a telepsychiatry program allows for early identification and resolution of technology issues.[25] Technological requirements are determined primarily by the platform used and are often associated with minimum standards set forth by the service provider.[26] Baseline technology assessments at newly implementing clinics should include a full complement of both technological and workflow questions (see Table 10-1).

Table 10-1. Questions to Address Prior to Telepsychiatry Service Implementation

Ensure Affirmative Answers Prior to Virtual Care Delivery:

- Does the clinic's Internet bandwidth meet the minimum required standards for the telemedicine video platform being used?
- Does the designated telemedicine device (iPad, computer, mobile cart unit) meet the recommended criteria set forth by the videoconferencing platform for minimum CPU capacity, processing speeds, and RAM requirements?
- Who will respond to technical support questions?
- Who will set up the technology in advance of a virtual psychiatrist visit?
- Is there a phone available to continue sessions if there are videoconferencing technology glitches?
- Is the room adequate in terms of ambient lighting, privacy, ambient noise levels, and lack of distracting background materials?

Introducing a virtual medium into a physical clinic, such as a community mental health center or a primary care clinic, also includes pragmatic workflow challenges. Scheduling patients across both virtual and in-person visit types creates opportunity for potential pitfalls that can be avoided through strong communication and planning. Including front desk/receptionist team members as early telepsychiatry "champions" or early adopters can be particularly helpful. These staff members often hold key insights regarding workflow components that make the most sense within current clinic practices and that are likely to optimize the patient—and the provider—experience. Well-trained front desk staff improves the likelihood that technology will be set up accurately and consistently, telepsychiatry providers will be scheduled appropriately, and patients will be receptive to telemedicine modalities due to a positive and smooth experience. Further, ensuring that the staff responsible for scheduling patients have established communication channels with, and up-to-date availability information for the virtual psychiatrist, can avoid an underutilized psychiatrist.[27]

QUALITY IMPROVEMENT

As telepsychiatry is implemented across increasing numbers of diverse settings, there are lessons to be learned about the best ways to improve and maintain the quality of telepsychiatry service delivery. Practitioners who have embarked on this virtual modality cite communication as a critical focus for improving the quality of telepsychiatry workflows. Unlike in traditional psychiatry settings, members of originating and distant telepsychiatry site teams do not see, or even communicate with, each other every day. Virtual teams can work as efficiently as traditional teams with a program design that fosters clear communication channels and ongoing quality improvement.[25] Establishing systematic processes for regular ongoing communication can maintain a focus on quality. It is recommended that telepsychiatry implementation teams create a venue, such as monthly telehealth team meetings, to quickly identify and troubleshoot workflow issues to prevent escalation.[25] Clearly articulating, reviewing, and refining clinic workflow to include scheduling, patient referral, and documentation improves the implementation experience. Implementation success is much more likely when all clinic staff members, from front desk administrative assistants to medical directors, understand their role in the process.[25]

ETHICAL PRACTICE IN TELEMEDICINE

Although a virtual medium does not change the practice or ethical responsibilities of psychiatry, it does expand the patient population and types of care settings in which a psychiatrist may practice. Further, the opportunities for team-based care may mean that a psychiatrist has varying levels of accountability for different patients on her or his caseload. Psychiatrists are responsible for maintaining an appropriate level of cultural competency across all patients served and for being accountable for participating appropriately within a variety of clinical workflow models. In addition, there are ethical considerations specific to telepsychiatry. Patient security and information privacy considerations are at the forefront of virtual care. According to the AMA, physicians, including psychiatrists, are responsible for confirming that their telemedicine service/platform comes with appropriate protocols to prevent unauthorized access and to protect the security and integrity of patient health information during transmission and at both patient and provider ends of the electronic encounter.

They note that ethically sound care via virtual mediums include:

1) Informing patients about the limitations of the provider/patient relationship and virtual services

2) Confirming each patient's identity and that telepsychiatry is an appropriate medium for the patient's individual situation and medical needs

3) Tailoring the informed consent process for patients (or their surrogates) to include information about the virtual medium, in addition to standard medical and treatment information

4) Demonstrating proficiency with relevant technologies and comfort with virtual interaction

5) Recognizing any limitations of the technologies used and taking appropriate steps to overcome those limitations (ie, having a phone call back-up plan for videoconferencing outages)

6) Advising patient and other provider users about how to arrange for needed follow-up care as indicated

7) Appropriately documenting the clinical evaluation and outcomes

8) Taking steps to support continuity of care by making records accessible to patients and encouraging sharing with patients' primary care providers

Other ethical practices include disseminating information about both positive and negative treatment outcomes associated with the medium and advocating for policies that promote greater health care access such as through telepsychiatry.

Patient consent, in particular, is addressed in state legislation and in the ATA's Core Operational Guidelines. These state that "[o]rganizations shall have a mechanism in place for ensuring that patients and health professionals are aware of their rights and responsibilities with respect to accessing and providing health care via telehealth technologies (whether within a healthcare institution or other environment such as the home, school or work), including the process for communicating complaints."[26] Specific to telemental health, the ATA notes the best practices include reviewing confidentiality, emergency plans, process by which patient information will be documented and stored, potential for technical failure, and the procedure for coordination of care with other health professionals. Processes for patient safety and emergency management, such as in the case of suicidal ideation, must be established with the originating site staff in advance of any patient session. Any such protocols should be aligned with all pertinent professional guidelines and should also be aligned with the originating site emergency and safety management protocols.[26] Finally, providers have a fiduciary obligation to disclose any financial or other interests associated with the telehealth/telemedicine application or service and to make a reasonable effort to manage or eliminate any potential conflicts of interest.[3]

STANDARDS/GUIDELINES

Two very influential clinical guidelines have been published by the ATA. The first, published in 2009,[28] focused mainly on telepsychiatry performed in a hub-and-spoke format to and from clinics and hospitals. This guideline has been adopted widely around the world in many telepsychiatry programs and provides detail with respect to clinical, administrative, technical, and regulatory issues. In 2013 a follow-up guideline was published that focused on the provision of telepsychiatry into the home environment. These guidelines are likely to be updated in 2017 to take account of the increasing use of mobile environments and the use of telepsychiatry in team-based care, especially in integrated primary care systems, as neither of the current published guidelines has enough of a focus on these areas. The core guidelines are supported by generic operational guidelines, an evidence-based review, and a lexicon of relevant assessment and outcome measures of relevance. ATA guidelines are accessible online. They include the following: 1) Core Operational Guidelines for Telehealth Services Involving Provider-Patient Interactions; 2) A Lexicon Assessment and Outcome Measurements for Telemental Health; 3) Practice Guidelines for Video-Based Online Mental Health Services; 4) Practice Guidelines for Videoconferencing-Based Telemental Health; and 5) Evidence-Based Practice for Telemental Health.

SUMMARY

In summary, technological advances have enabled a diverse set of virtual psychiatric and integrated care models. Videoconferencing technology is increasingly being used to not only increase access to care, but also increase care quality and efficiencies through models that leverage both direct and indirect care in a variety of care settings. With a strong evidence base to support assessment, diagnosis, and treatment across a wide variety of mental health problems and across a wide variety of models, remaining challenges include policy and reimbursement and implementation efficacy and quality improvement. The ATA has a variety of web-based guidelines and resources that provide pragmatic help with implementation, and the AMA's recently published ethical considerations for telehealth support diffusion in a manner that is consistent with patient-centered values.

REFERENCES

1. Chan S, Parish M, Yellowlees P. Telepsychiatry today. *Curr Psychiatry Rep* 2015;17(11):89.

2. Deslich SA, Stec B, Tomblin S, Coustasse A. Telepsychiatry in the 21st century: transforming healthcare with technology. *Perspect Health Inf Manag* 2013;10(1f):1–17.

3. American Medical Association: Ethical Practice in Telemedicine H-140.839. https://searchpf.ama-assn.org/SearchML/searchDetails.action?uri=/AMADoc/HOD-140.839.xml. Accessed September 22, 2016.

4. National Center for Telehealth and Technology (T2) US Department of Defense, Defense Centers of Excellence for Psychological Health and Traumatic Brain Injury. *Introduction to Telemental Health.* http://t2health.dcoe.mil/sites/default/files/cth/introduction/intro_telemental_health_may2011.pdf. Accessed April 7, 2016.

5. Malhotra S, Chakrabarti S, Shah R. Telepsychiatry: promise, potential, and challenges. *Indian J Psychiatry* 2013;55(1):3–11.

6. Odor A, Yellowlees P, Hilty D, et al. PsychVACS: a system for asynchronous telepsychiatry. *Telemed J E Health* 2011;17(4):299–303.

7. Fortney JC, Pyne JM, Turner EE, et al. Telepsychiatry integration of mental health services into rural primary care settings. *Int Rev Psychiatry* 2015;27(6):525–539.

8. Unützer J, Katon W, Callahan CM, et al. IMPACT investigators. Improving mood-promoting access to collaborative treatment. Collaborative care management of late-life depression in the primary care setting: a randomized controlled trial. *JAMA* 2002;288(22):2836–2845.

9. Yellowlees P, Odor A, Patrice K, et al. Disruptive innovation: the future of healthcare? *Telemed J E Health* 2011;17(3):231–234.

10. Butler TN, Yellowlees P. Cost analysis of store-and-forward telepsychiatry as a consultation model for primary care. *Telemed J E Health* 2012;18(1):74–77.

11. Yellowlees PM, Odor A, Parish MB. Cross-lingual asynchronous telepsychiatry: disruptive innovation? *Psychiatr Serv* 2012;63(9):945.

12. Lambert D, Gale J, Hartley D, et al. Understanding the business case for telemental health in rural communities. *J Behav Health Serv Res* 2016;43(3):366–379.

13. Waugh M, Voyles D, Thomas R. Telepsychiatry: benefits and costs in a changing health-care environment. *Int Rev Psychiatry* 2015;27(6):558–568.

14. American Telemedicine Association. *Core Guidelines for Telemedicine Operations.* http://www.americantelemed.org/home. Accessed October 12, 2016.

15. Chan S, Torous J, Hinton L, et al. Towards a framework for evaluating mobile mental health apps. *Telemed J E Health* 2015;21(12):1038–1041.

16. Ben-Zeev D, Young MA, Depp CA. Real-time predictors of suicidal ideation: mobile assessment of hospitalized depressed patients. *Psychiatry Res* 2012;197(1-2):55–59.

17. Torous J, Powell AC. Current research and trends in the use of smartphone applications for mood disorders. *Internet Intervent* 2015;2(2):169–173.

18. Ben-Zeev D. Mobile technologies in the study, assessment, and treatment of schizophrenia. *Schizophr Bull* 2012;38(3):384–385.

19. Yellowlees PM, Holloway KM, Parish MB. Therapy in virtual environments: clinical and ethical issues. *Telemed J E Health* 2012;18(7):558–564.

20. Rose GL, Badger GJ, Skelly JM, et al. A randomized controlled trial of IVR-based alcohol brief intervention to promote patient-provider communication in primary care. *J Gen Intern Med* 2016;31(9):996–1003.

21. Bashshur RL, Shannon GW, Bashshur N, et al. The empirical evidence for telemedicine interventions in mental disorders. *Telemed J E Health* 2015;21(5):321–354.

22. Hilty DM, Ferrer DC, Parish MB, et al. The effectiveness of telemental health: a 2013 review. *Telemed J E Health* 2013;19(6):444–454.

23. Pakyurek M, Yellowlees PM, Hilty DM. The child and adolescent telepsychiatry consultation: can it be a more effective clinical process for certain patients than conventional practice? *Telemed J E Health* 2010;16(3):289–292.

24. Rogers EM. Diffusion of innovations: modifications of a model for telecommunications. In: Stoetzer MW, Mahler DA, eds. *Die Diffusion von Innovationen in der Telekommunikation.* Berlin: Springer, 1995:25–38.

25. California Telehealth Resource Center. *Telehealth Program Developer Kit, A Roadmap for Successful Telehealth Program Development.* 2014. http://www.telehealthresourcecenter.org/sites/main/files/file-attachments/complete-program-developer-kit-2014-web1.pdf. Accessed September 16, 2016.

26. American Telemedicine Association. *Core Operational Guidelines for Telehealth Services Involving Provider-Patient Interactions.* 2014. http://www.americantelemed.org/home. Accessed October 12, 2016.

27. Broderick A, Lindeman D. Case studies in telehealth adoption: scaling telehealth programs: lessons from early adopters. The Commonwealth Fund 2013;1654(1):1–9.

28. Yellowlees P, Shore J, Roberts L. American Telemedicine Association. Practice guidelines for videoconferencing-based telemental health. *Telemed J E Health* 2010;16(10):1074–1089.

Remote Patient Monitoring and Care Coordination

Amy L. Tucker, MD, MHCM, FACC

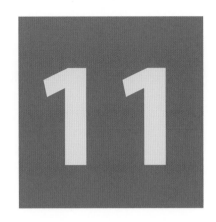

L.H. is a 76-year-old man with a history of coronary artery disease and multiple myocardial infarctions for which he received several stents prior to having coronary artery bypass surgery. He had a history of aortic stenosis and had undergone aortic valve replacement. His prior myocardial infarctions left him with an ischemic cardiomyopathy with an ejection fraction of 20% to 25%. His cardiovascular risk factors included hypertension and hyperlipidemia. In the 2 months following his coronary artery bypass surgery, Mr. H. was admitted to the hospital three times for congestive heart failure. He lived alone and ate fast food most of the time; he also had a friend who cooked high-sodium Southern favorites for him, such as biscuits and gravy. He endorsed adherence to his medications and attended all of his scheduled follow-up visits. He was seen by a nutritionist during his first readmission.

Mr. H. participated in a remote patient monitoring program and was seen in an advanced heart failure clinic. He expressed frustration with his frequent readmissions and monitored his daily weights with his nurse care coordinator very closely. During one conversation with his nurse care coordinator regarding a 3-pound weight gain from the previous day, the nurse asked him to do a 24-hour food recall. When she asked about his sodium and fluid restrictions, the nurse discovered that Mr. H. had a knowledge deficit about hidden sources of sodium. He had eaten a sandwich at a fast food establishment the previous day containing 1500 mg of sodium, although he thought he was making a heart-healthy choice. After the nurse coordinator told him that one 6-inch sandwich contained three-fourths of the sodium he should eat in an entire day, Mr. H. became more vigilant about tracking the sodium in the foods he ate.

The nurse care coordinator and the nurse practitioner in the heart failure clinic worked closely with Mr. H. to optimize his outpatient diuresis, to help him recognize symptoms of fluid overload, and to teach him to monitor his daily fluid intake and sodium consumption. Mr. H.'s weight and symptoms stabilized, and he became highly engaged in tracking his weight, fluid intake, and the sodium content in his food. On more than one occasion when his nurse care coordinator called him to discuss a mild weight gain, he answered the phone with "I knew you were going to call; let me explain."

Mr. H. finished his remote patient monitoring program without being readmitted again. He called his nurse care coordinator about a month after finishing the program and stated he was meeting friends at Cracker Barrel for lunch and that their website was down so he wasn't sure what to order. He asked the nurse, "What should I do?" After joking, "Don't go to Cracker Barrel," the nurse gave him general guidance for high-sodium "key words" and for healthier options.

Mr. H. follows up with his providers regularly, still weighs himself daily, and hasn't been admitted for heart failure for over a year and a half.

INTRODUCTION

Innovative disruption of the status quo in U.S. health care delivery is widely recognized as an imperative. Our current system is neither effective nor financially sustainable. The crucible of our health care crisis is formed from the convergence of four primary drivers:

- Rising health care costs
- Increased demand associated with an epidemiologic shift in our population
- Inadequate supply of health care providers
- Poor outcomes on health metrics

In order to optimize the value equation in our health care system, it is clear that we must find ways to do much more with much less. More of the same will not work. Disruptive innovation is required. Remote patient monitoring (RPM)–enabled care coordination is among the telehealth applications that promise to support high-value redesign in health care delivery. As the case earlier illustrates, when most effective, RPM often enhances, rather than replaces, the personal interactions in effective care coordination.

Health care spending in the United States reached $3.2 trillion in 2015, approximately 17.8% of the gross domestic product (GDP)[1] and is expected to exceed 20% by 2025.[2] In 2013, the cost of health care in the United States was $9,086 per capita and exceeded $10,000 per person in 2015.[3,4] The United States spends nearly 50% more than the next highest spending system; however, our financial investment is not reflected in better health outcomes. In its World Health Report 2000, the World Health Organization ranked the U.S. health care system 37th among its 191 member countries.[5] Among the 13 high-income countries analyzed in 2013 by the Organisation for Economic Co-operation and Development (OECD), the United States ranked last, with gaps in key health indicators such as life expectancy and access to care.[3] Given that the United States was the only country among the 13 analyzed without publicly funded universal health coverage, it is not surprising that private health care spending in the United States was the highest in the world. However, even prior to the enactment of the major insurance provisions of the 2010 Affordable Care Act (ACA), with only 34% of the population covered by public programs, public spending on U.S. health care was still higher than in all but two countries. Americans also spent more out-of-pocket for health care than any other country except Switzerland.[3,4]

Higher health care spending in the United States has not translated into improved access to care or outcomes. The United States invests less than other developed nations in population health and social services. In fact, as a percentage of GDP, the US spent less than any of the other wealthy countries on social services. As of 2011, the United States had the lowest life expectancy (78.8 years versus an OECD median of 81.2) and the highest infant mortality (6.1 deaths/1,000 births versus the OECD median of 3.5) of any of the countries in the OECD study. Epidemiologically, the U.S. population is aging, which, coupled with unhealthy lifestyles, is increasing the burden of chronic disease. Among the 13 OECD countries, the United States bears the highest burden of chronic diseases, with 25% of all Americans[6] and 68% of those over the age of 65 carrying the diagnosis of two or more chronic conditions. In the 2013 OECD analysis, the burden of chronic conditions for the other 12 countries ranged between 33% and 56%.

The demand for health care associated with this high burden of chronic diseases is one of the major drivers of health care costs in the United States. Currently, an estimated 86% of health care expenditures are for treatment of chronic diseases,[7] up from 75% several years ago. Notwithstanding the high burden of disease and costs of care, Americans do not enjoy greater access to or engagement in care. Higher costs appear to be driven by greater use of expensive technologies and higher prices for services and pharmaceuticals rather than investments in access and care delivery. The OECD analysis demonstrated that Americans had, on average, fewer ambulatory visits (4 per year compared to the OECD mean of 6.5) than the citizens of other wealthy nations and have fewer physicians per capita (2.6 versus 3.2 per 1,000 population).[3,4] To compound the issue, the health care needs of the growing and aging population are expected to increase by 17% between 2013 and 2025, creating a projected provider shortage of 46,000 to 90,000 physicians by 2025.[8] Health care must be redesigned to reduce costs, improve access to care, and more effectively manage chronic medical conditions across the entire population.

The prevailing model of U.S. health care is fragmented. Delivery is characterized by isolated episodes of ambulatory care occurring at arbitrary, low-frequency intervals, often determined by the availability of the provider. Care is further punctuated by exorbitantly expensive emergency and inpatient care for acute illness or deterioration of chronic conditions. The fragmented, reactive delivery system lends itself poorly to providing the education, coaching, and monitoring across the care continuum that promotes optimal management of chronic medical conditions. Additionally, when unchecked, the fee-for-service payment model creates demand for services rather than compensating for quality or incentivizing cost containment. The ACA has created some levers for change through the introduction of payment models that promote cost reduction and apply penalties for substandard outcomes.

Although the ACA provides incentives to accelerate the pace of change, the blueprint for our current national quality initiative predates it, having been galvanized in response to the call to action report *To Err Is Human* published by the Institute of Medicine in 2000[9] and its follow-up article *Crossing the Quality Chasm* in 2001.[10] *Crossing the Chasm* outlines six redesign imperatives for the health care system with an eye toward achieving the six aims of safe, effective, patient-centered, timely, efficient, and equitable health care. The six imperatives are reengineered care processes; effective use of IT; knowledge and skills management; development of effective teams; and coordination of care across patient conditions, services, and sites of care over time.[10] Improved care coordination is specifically enumerated as one of the imperatives to "close the quality chasm" in health care.[10]

Care coordination, particularly for transitional care and comprehensive management of chronic conditions, is front and center in health care reform. A growing body of research indicates that care coordination can improve outcomes and reduce costs. Analysis of effective care coordination models, including the Medicare Coordinated Care Demonstration (MCCD), Care Management Plus (CMP), and others, has identified common practices that distinguish effective care coordination[11,12]:

- Targeting high-risk patients
- Improving communication between patients and providers

- Working with providers to identify and correct areas in which care is not consistent with evidence-based guidelines
- Monitoring patients' symptoms, well-being, and adherence between clinic visits
- Advising patients to seek appropriate follow-up
- Notifying primary care providers of status changes

Similarly, Schraeder and Shelton[11] have identified practices shared among effective transitional care programs, such as the Transitional Care Model (TCM) and the Care Transitions Initiative (CTI):

- Target high-risk patients while hospitalized to prepare them for successful transition
- Follow patients for a limited, intense period after discharge
- Teach and coach patients about their medications, self-care, symptom recognition, and management
- Remind, encourage, and assist patients to attend follow-up appointments with primary care providers

Many of the processes central to effective care coordination for chronic disease management and transitional care lend themselves to telehealth. Health care IT (information technology) will play a central role in scaling care coordination across large patient populations of individuals with different medical conditions, each of which has specific needs. IT can be leveraged to identify patients at risk, automate data collection, identify concerning trends, prioritize tasks, facilitate communication, incorporate evidence-based guidelines and practices into workflow, and amplify patient engagement. Coye et al.[13] have enumerated six aspects of chronic care that can be facilitated by RPM:

- *Early intervention* to detect deterioration and intervene before unscheduled and preventable services are needed
- *Integration of care* for exchange of data and communication across multiple providers and complex disease states
- *Coaching* via motivational interviewing and other techniques to encourage patient behavioral change and self-care
- *Increased trust*, patient satisfaction, and feelings of "connectedness" with providers

- *Workforce changes* with shifts to lower-cost and more plentiful health care workers, including medical assistants, community health workers, and social workers
- *Increased productivity* resulting from decreased home visit travel time and automated documentation

DEFINITIONS

What Is RPM?

The Center for Connected Health Policy divides telehealth into four distinct domains that have been explained in detail in other chapters: live video, store-and-forward, remote patient monitoring, and mobile health.[14] RPM uses digital technology to securely collect and transmit health data from patients to health care providers in a different location for analysis and recommendation, including, but not limited to, physiologic measurements, answers to survey questions, and information about adherence. Data can be transmitted to care coordination centers, off-site case management programs, specialty and primary care practices, hospitals, skilled nursing facilities, or intensive care units (ICUs) for analysis and initiation of appropriate interventions. RPM is shifting patient care from expensive locations such as emergency departments, hospitals, rehabilitation centers, and skilled nursing facilities, into lower-cost locations such as the patient's home. Home telehealth is sometimes used synonymously with RPM, but home telehealth encompasses other services, such as simple telephone support, telemedicine provider encounters, telerehabilitation, and mental health/behavioral counseling.

RPM is a rapidly growing sector that extends patient management beyond conventional clinical settings and across the care continuum. Integrated RPM-care coordination strategies have been shown to improve management of chronic medical conditions. RPM delivered into a patient's home can promote engagement, education, and self-management skills to improve outcomes for those burdened with chronic diseases.[15] RPM has been used in patients with complex medical problems, such as home dialysis, to provide patients and their families with a greater sense of empowerment and security, knowing that they have access to support should problems arise.[15] RPM increases care efficiency

and improves access to care.[16] Trend analysis of physiologic measurements and patient symptoms can enable early detection of clinical deterioration, allowing timely intervention, reducing emergency department visits, hospitalizations, or undesired clinical outcomes.[17–20] RPM can allow some elderly or disabled patients who would otherwise require institutional care to preserve their independence.[21] By preventing complications, reducing hospital readmissions, and preserving patient independence, RPM can decrease medical costs.[15,18,21]

In an increasingly technological society for which the market expectation is continuous connectivity, immediate access, affordability, and prompt service, health care is a straggler. RPM is one of a growing armamentarium of tools with the potential to promote controlled disruption of the health care status quo. The definition of the large-scale Veteran's Administration Care Coordination/Home Telehealth (CCHT)[18] initiative summarizes the aims that effective RPM can help achieve:

> "The use of health informatics, disease management, and home telehealth technologies to enhance and extend care and case management to facilitate access to care and improve the health of designated individuals and populations with the specific intent of providing the right care in the right place and the right time."

REMOTE PATIENT MONITORING SYSTEMS: TECHNOLOGY, MODELS, MARKET, FINANCIAL MODELS, AND REGULATIONS

Overview

RPM systems can be standalone devices to monitor data for a specific condition, such as implantable cardiovascular devices (ICDs) used to treat cardiac arrhythmias and monitor heart failure, glucometers to guide the treatment of diabetes, and chronic positive airway pressure (CPAP) machines that treat sleep apnea. RPM can also be integrated into comprehensive care management programs that rely on multiple data streams, including physiological data from multiple peripheral devices and patient-entered responses to queries. Both the standalone and integrated RPM models follow the same process flow (Figure 11-1): acquire, transmit, analyze, notify, and intervene.

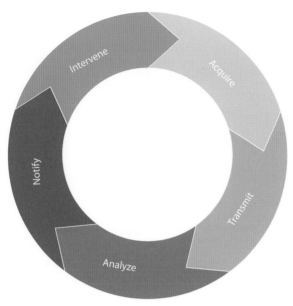

▲ Figure 11-1. The remote monitoring process.

Acquisition of Patient Data

Data can be acquired from peripheral devices and new applications actively or passively through patient-initiated interaction. Examples include blood pressure, pulse, temperature, oxygen saturation, weight, blood glucose, peak flows, medication adherence, location, position, frequency of activity, heart rhythm, nocturnal oxygen desaturations, intravascular fluid status, pro-times/international normalization ratios (INRs), cardiac auscultation, electroencephalograph, photographs (wounds, rashes, retinas), and the metamorphopsia of macular degeneration. Although some RPM programs may require patients to enter data from peripheral devices, in most systems the peripheral devices plug into or wirelessly connect to a hub. Hubs can be dedicated remote monitoring telestations (a commercial device with a screen and simple keypad) or a tablet, computer, or mobile device loaded with applications specific to monitoring. As connectivity becomes increasingly robust, systems are being designed in which peripherals wirelessly transmit directly to cloud-based monitoring software, combining the acquisition and transmission processes.

Patient response data (eg, condition-specific health questions regarding symptoms, perceptions of well-being, health-related behaviors, disease management skills, educational needs, medication adherence, health literacy, and mental health) can be presented and answered on a telestation or pulled or pushed from cloud-based software onto a patient's tablet, desktop, or mobile device. Some platforms enable two-way audio and/or video communication, allowing real-time interaction between patients and providers or care coordinators. Some devices include libraries of educational content.

Analysis of Patient Data

Patient data are generally triaged through patient-specific algorithms to categorize risk and alert providers and caregivers when the data exceeds predetermined parameters. Data can be presented to providers and care navigators on a dashboard sorted and designated by risk level. It is imperative that providers and patients understand the accuracy and reliability of these systems, as the false alarm rates may be high.

Notification and Intervention

When data trends suggest elevated risk, standalone RPM systems typically send alerts directly to providers or caregivers who initiate interventions. In comprehensive, integrated RPM programs, such as those that manage chronic medical conditions or transitional care, algorithms may be used to determine which among several interventions should be taken. Depending on the level of risk, interventions include coaching and education, home health visit, expedited ambulatory visit, or instructions to contact emergency medical services (EMS).

Integrated Systems

Large-scale, integrated RPM programs require seamless integration of a committed team with well-defined roles, multiple technologies, and standardized processes and responses (Figure 11-2). Later-generation commercial monitoring devices incorporate software that processes incoming data, applies clinical decision and risk assessment algorithms, and generates output in the form of a workflow dashboard and patient-specific trended reports that are displayed to care coordinators or providers in an easily actionable format. Companies

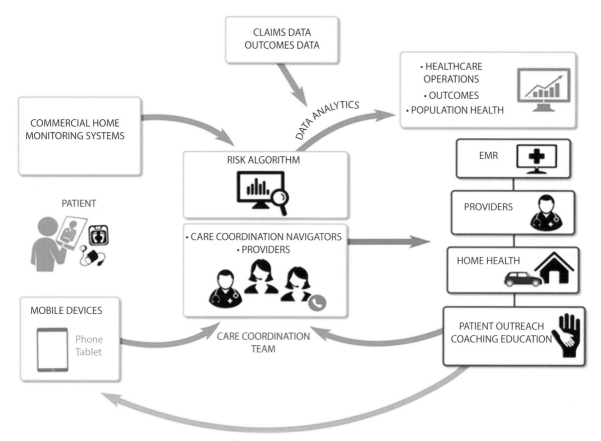

▲ **Figure 11-2.** Processes of an integrated remote patient monitoring program.

that provide care coordination and analytic services for large-scale populations train teams of providers, often nurses and social workers, in best practices of care coordination. They also develop standard processes for monitoring practices, patient coaching and education, intervention, outcomes analysis, and improvement. Strategies that successful scalable RPM programs have in common include an active working relationship with a corporate partner, in-home telehealth units, a database server that integrates physiologic and other data, integration with the electronic medical record (EMR), and outcome data.[18,22–24]

▶ Leveraging Technology to Promote a Continuum of Care

Technological advancements in biosensors, connectivity, and services in RPM-enabled care coordination can drive transformation away from episodes of care separated by care chasms and toward a smooth care continuum. Innovations are creating the ability to continuously monitor physiology and other metrics. Currently, the standard for most RPM applications is still frequent, but episodic, care (Figure 11-3). The standard for the future will be technology-enabled continuous monitoring, extending the right care, at the right time, from any location.

▶ Standards and Regulations

All new medical devices must be either approved or cleared by the Food and Drug Administration (FDA). Approval and clearance follow two distinct paths. Premarket approval (PMA) is the more stringent pathway, requiring extensive testing with documentation of Good Laboratory Practice (GLP). Premarket

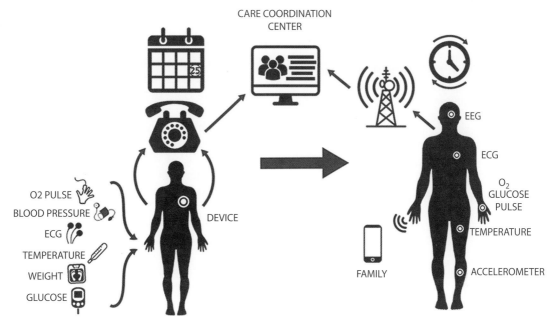

▲ Figure 11-3. Use of remote monitoring systems to promote a care continuum. Technological advances in biosensors and connectivity enable the transition from manual, episodic, location-dependent care to automatic, continuous, location-independent care.

notification (PMN), the second pathway, is also referred to as a 510(k). The 510(k) process was intended to reduce the time and costs associated with a PMA in cases for which the risk to health and safety is not an issue, such as when a new medical device is similar to one that has been previously approved or when modifications have been made to a preexisting design. The majority of remote monitoring devices enter the U.S. marketplace via the 510(k) process. Those used strictly for promotion of health and wellness are excluded from the requirement for PMA or 510(k) clearance; such devices can make claims about sustaining or improving the general state of health, but cannot make reference to diseases or conditions. Examples include devices promoting weight management, physical fitness, stress management, mental acuity, self-esteem, sleep management, and sexual function.[25]

The data stored and transmitted by RPM devices is generally accessed by entities covered by the Health Insurance Portability and Accountability Act of 1996 (HIPAA) and is therefore considered protected health information (PHI) and is subject to patient privacy constraints outlined by the HIPAA. Provisions must be made to ensure security of data transmitted from patients to providers.

RPM systems should comply with Health Level-7 (HL7) standards for transfer of clinical and administrative data between software applications used by various health care providers. Platforms should be designed to integrate a variety of functionalities and services, bringing together physiologic monitoring, mobile, tablet, desktop, and cloud technologies.

Meaningful Use Stage 3, which applies standards for the use of EMRs in clinical practice, may provide more of an opportunity than a barrier for RPM device and service providers. The Coordination of Care through Patient Engagement objective within the Stage 3 Meaningful Use rule requires that over 15% of unique patient records include "patient-generated health data," which provides monitoring device manufacturers with strong incentives to collaborate with EMR vendors to allow RPM data to flow into EMRs.

Demand for Remote Patient Monitoring Is Increasing

The past few years have seen rapid expansion in both the clinical application and financial importance of RPM.[26] According to market analysis by Grand View Research, RPM equipment was the fastest-growing application of medical electronics in 2015,[27] with the market valued at $546.8 million and projected to grow at a compound annual growth rate of 13.4% between 2014 and 2025.[28] Demand for telemedicine is increasing globally, with North America—the United States in particular—seeing the most rapid expansion, followed by Western Europe.[27] Cardiovascular diseases were the leading application segment in 2014, accounting for nearly 30% of the market.[28] Other dominant applications included cancer, sleep disorders, diabetes management, and weight management[28] (Figure 11-4). The opportunity RPM presents is well appreciated by the health care technology industry; the remote monitoring platform market is dominated by health care device and technology giants, including Philips, GE-Intel, and Honeywell in chronic care management (Table 11-1), and Medtronic, St. Jude, Biotronik, and Boston Scientific in cardiovascular implantable devices. Although most of the industry leaders are enjoying growth in the RPM sector, Bosch Healthcare, an early industry leader supplying the Health Buddy system used extensively by the Veterans Health Administration (VHA), shut down in 2015.

Some of the major drivers for and barriers to adoption have been discussed (Table 11-2), including escalating health care costs, the needs of an aging population, increased chronic disease burden, and provider shortages. Other drivers include the need to improve health care efficiency, the need to reduce geographical and socioeconomic health care disparities, and technological advancements. The shift in payment models from volume-based to value-based has had a significant impact on adoption as well.

As previously described, the traditional episodic, fee-for-service system of U.S. health care has resulted in a fragmented care cycle, including discrete episodes of inpatient and ambulatory care, with large chasms in care between. In fact, inpatient and ambulatory care encounters account for a very small fraction of a

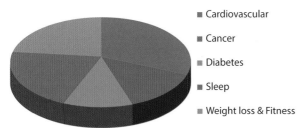

- Cardiovascular
- Cancer
- Diabetes
- Sleep
- Weight loss & Fitness

▲ **Figure 11-4.** U.S. remote monitoring device market by condition. (Adapted from Grand View Research. http://grandviewresearch.com/industry/medical-devices.)

Table 11-1. Examples of Integrated Home Telemonitoring Devices

Device	Company	Features
Telestation	Philips	• Patients answer survey questions presented on telestation screen • Data are transmitted wirelessly from peripherals to the telestation • Data transmitted to providers by phone line • Peripherals: scale, blood pressure cuff, pulse oximeter, thermometer, glucometer
Genesis	Honeywell	• Web-based survey questions for patients, condition-specific • Two-way audio between patients and providers • Peripherals: stethoscope, scale, blood pressure meter, glucometer, pulse oximeter, thermometer, PT/INR meter, peak flow meter
Health Harmony	GE-Intel	• In-home device with cloud-based format and library of educational materials • Two-way audio and video between patients and providers • Wireless peripherals: blood pressure meter, scale, glucometer, pulse oximeter, peak flow meter

Adapted from New England Healthcare Institute. Detailed Technology Analysis: Home Telehealth: New England Healthcare Institute, 2009.

Table 11-2. Drivers and Barriers to Adoption of Remote Patient Monitoring

Drivers for RPM Adoption	Barriers to RPM Adoption
• Increased costs • Aging population • Increased burden of chronic disease • Provider shortages • Access disparities • Need to reduce inefficiency • Technological advances • Readmission penalties • Payment models rewarding cost containment/risk sharing	• Implementation costs • Lack of third-party reimbursement • Concerns about privacy • Cultural resistance • Need for more robust evidence of benefit • Lack of EMR integration

patient's time. Operating in what are now lengthy care chasms between encounters, RPM has the potential to support successful transitions between inpatient and ambulatory episodes and to provide a more continuous cycle of health care for patients with chronic medical conditions. RPM can be used to maximize the time patients spend on the lower-cost segments of the care continuum. RPM empowers patients through increased engagement and health literacy. When employed strategically, RPMs can serve to delegate some tasks from overstretched providers to care coordinators. RPM can be used to monitor and support providers as well as patients. It has been used in ICUs to improve patient safety by reducing provider errors and in nursing homes to ensure adherence to best practices. RPM is one of the tools in a growing armamentarium designed to achieve the Institute for Healthcare Improvement's "triple aim" of health care—improving patient outcomes, increasing access to care, and reducing health care costs.[29]

Significant barriers to RPM implementation remain, however, the most formidable among them being financial.[13,30,31] The capital and operational costs required to establish and run a scalable RMP are considerable. A 2016 systematic review of 13 studies found the combined intervention costs, reflecting equipment, servicing, and monitoring, ranged between $275 and $7,963 per patient per year[32]; although, between 2004 and 2015, adjusted costs were found to be falling with increasingly affordable technology. Prior to

committing the resources required to launch and operate an integrated RPM program, organizations require convincing evidence that it will improve outcomes and reduce costs, especially because most RPM applications are not reimbursed by Medicare or third-party payors. There is now a large and expanding body of evidence showing that RPM improves outcomes and reduces costs. Furthermore, the ACA has introduced cost reduction incentives into payment models that may catalyze further adoption.

Cultural factors can significantly affect the adoption of RPM. Patient and provider resistance can undermine the success of RPM programs. Both providers and patients have concerns about security and privacy. Some patients find remote monitoring intrusive and inconvenient. Additionally, providers, already stretched thin, resist further demands on their time. This may improve as more patient monitoring platforms integrate trended reports within the EMR, making it more convenient for providers to access and act on monitoring data.

▶ Current Financial Models for Remote Patient Monitoring

The costs of program implementation are steadily falling with advances in technology, but reimbursement is another matter. With a few notable exceptions, even in states with telehealth parity laws, RPM is not reimbursed by Medicare or private U.S. carriers. Some covered exceptions include focused applications, such as remote interrogation of implantable cardiac pacemakers and defibrillators; at-home studies for sleep disorders; and the ForeseeHome (Notal Vision, Manasses, VA) daily home telemonitoring program for age-related macular degeneration, coverage for which was approved by Centers for Medicare & Medicaid Services (CMS) in January 2016. If passed, the CONNECT for Health bill (H.R. 4442) presented to Congress February 3, 2016, could expand Medicare payment for telehealth services, including RPM. RPM has enjoyed higher penetration among patients with Medicaid; currently, 19 states fund RPM for Medicaid patients.[33]

The predominant financial driver among early adopters of RPM has been reduction of health care costs by driving care away from expensive inpatient, procedural, and emergency care and toward the lower-cost portions of the care continuum. RPM can also reduce costs by serving as a work force multiplier, shifting some roles away from more expensive providers to less costly ones. It is not surprising that single-payor systems that operate under a model of cost containment rather than revenue generation are among the most notable early adopters of RPM.[23,24,34,35] Likewise, managed care organizations and self-insured employers with incentives to reduce overall costs have also been among early adopters for large-scale chronic care management programs employing RPM.

The passage of the ACA in 2010 introduced strong cost reduction incentives across the U.S. health care system, disrupting a financial structure previously driven almost exclusively by generation of volume-dependent revenues. The Hospital Readmission Reduction Program (HRRP) imposes costly penalties on systems with 30-day risk-adjusted readmission rates in excess of the national benchmark. HRRP has been a major lever in the establishment of transitional care programs, some of which use RPM. Likewise the introduction of performance measures, risk assumption, and cost accountability in new payment models, such as accountable care organizations (ACOs) and patient-centered medical homes (PCMH), provide incentives to improve management of chronic medical conditions.

Another cost reduction lever for adoption of RPM is independent elder care. As the population ages, more elderly people are requiring costly institutional care. According to the 2016 Cost of Care Survey by Genworth, Inc.,[36] the national median monthly cost for a one-bedroom unit in an assisted living facility was $3,628 ($43,536 per year) and for a semiprivate skilled nursing bed was $6,844 ($82,128). These costs are rising by an average of 4.29% per year and can rapidly deplete the retirement savings of elderly individuals. Finding ways to remain safely independent at home for as long as possible has been the impetus behind the development of sophisticated home monitoring systems for the elderly.

Finally, self-insured employers with a vested interest in reducing not only employee health care expenditures, but absenteeism as well, are beginning to use RPM in workforce wellness programs to allow scalability and convenience.

APPLICATIONS AND EVIDENCE

The applications for RPM have exploded over the past decade, and potential applications continue to expand. There is now a substantial body of research examining the effectiveness of RPM to improve outcomes and decrease costs, including systematic reviews and meta-analyses.

▶ An Overview of Evidence through Systematic Reviews

Although drivers for adoption of RPM-facilitated care coordination are pushing it forward, the capital required for robust RPM-enabled care coordination is significant, and health systems want to see that the impact from pilot studies persists when programs are scaled to larger populations. The body of research on RPM-facilitated care coordination is extensive; however, the model is in its infancy, and the majority of the clinical trials published to date are proof-of-principle studies performed in small patient populations. The level of evidence in many circumstances is not yet strong enough to catalyze universal adoption in practice or change in policy. However, the field is in rapid evolution, and large randomized controlled trials (RCTs); systematic reviews; and meta-analyses are emerging to provide stronger evidence regarding the effectiveness of RPM-facilitated care for specific uses.[37-39]

In June 2016, AHRQ mapped the strength of evidence for patient outcomes[37] by segmenting telehealth studies by clinical condition (Figures 11-5, 11-6, and 11-7). The most commonly reported clinical applications were cardiovascular diseases, mixed chronic conditions, diabetes, and behavioral health. They also segmented their findings by modality, one of which was RPM[40] (Figure 11-6). Of the 58 systematic reviews identified, 17 focused on RPM, collectively including 48,321 patients. An additional five assessed multiple telehealth functions, including RPM. RPM was the most frequently represented telehealth modality, accounting for 29% of the single-modality reviews (Figure 11-6), with most using RPM in the context of one or more chronic diseases.[37] Of the 22 reviews involving RPM, 10 concluded that RPM led to positive benefits, 6 that benefits were possible, 2 were inconclusive, and 4 showed no benefit. The 16 that showed clear or possible benefit used RPM for chronic diseases.

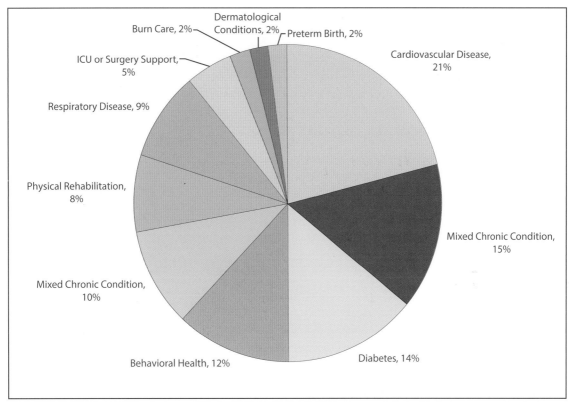

▲ **Figure 11-5.** Distribution of clinical focus for telehealth services represented in systematic reviews analyzed by AHRQ. (Reprinted from Totten AM. *Telehealth: Mapping the Evidence for Patient Outcomes*; with permission of the Agency for Healthcare Research and Quality, Rockville, MD.)

Three of the four reviews showing no benefit were for unusual RPM applications, including uterine monitoring of pregnant women to prevent preterm births, the addition of real-time video to home care, and parental monitoring for babies in the neonatal ICU showing no change in length of stay. The AHRQ analysis supports the application of RPM as a potentially transformative adjunct for management of chronic illness.[37]

INTEGRATED REMOTE PATIENT MONITORING APPLICATIONS

▶ RPM in Chronic Disease Management

The increasing burden of chronic diseases has been a major driver for RPM programs.[38] RPM allows providers to deliver care in nontraditional health care settings.[38] It is beginning to reach the burden of proof

required to catalyze large-scale adoption for specific indications.[38] The strongest evidence comes from the experiences of early large-scale adopters, from a few larger RCTs, and from meta-analyses and systematic reviews.

▶ Lessons from Early Adopters

Kaiser Permanente was one of the early pioneers using home telehealth for chronic disease management. The Tele-Home Health Research Project was one of the earliest RCTs in home telehealth, enrolling 102 intervention and 110 control patients in 1996–1997. Patients with congestive heart failure, chronic obstructive pulmonary disease, cerebrovascular accident, cancer, diabetes, anxiety, or chronic wounds were eligible for randomization. Intervention patients received usual

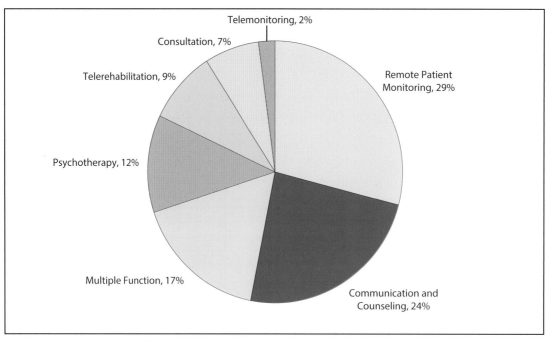

▲ **Figure 11-6.** Distribution of telehealth modality among systematic reviews analyzed by AHRQ. (Reprinted from Totten AM. *Telehealth: Mapping the Evidence for Patient Outcomes*; with permission of the Agency for Healthcare Research and Quality, Rockville, MD.)

care (which included home visits), plus monitoring services that included peripheral devices to assess cardiopulmonary status and video equipment providing two-way interaction with home health providers 24/7. The outcomes measured included three quality indicators (medication adherence, knowledge of disease, and ability for self-care); service utilization; and patient satisfaction. There were no differences between usual care and home telehealth in the quality indicators or patient satisfaction. However, patients receiving home telehealth had total mean costs, excluding home health services, of $1,948, compared to $2,674 for the usual care group. Home health services were higher in the intervention group, but the study group concluded that RPM could potentially substitute for some of the in-person home services provided to both groups.[41]

Faced with increasing demands for chronic disease management by an aging population of veterans, the VHA was another early adopter of RPM, and did so on a large scale. Following a successful Community

Care Coordination Service (CCCS) pilot from 2000–2003, the VHA launched their Care Coordination/Home Telehealth (CCHT) program in 2003 using a first-generation commercially available system called Health Buddy (incorporated videophones, messaging devices, biometric devices, digital cameras, and telemonitoring devices).[18] The goals were to coordinate care of veterans with chronic conditions and reduce unnecessary admissions to long-term institutional care through the systematic implementation of health informatics, home telehealth, and disease management technologies.[18] CCHT leveraged RPM technology to scale its home services to care for a large population while carefully preserving the components shown to be important for successful care coordination and chronic disease management.[11] The study population included patients with diabetes mellitus (48.4%), hypertension (40.3%), congestive heart failure (24.8%), chronic obstructive pulmonary disease (11.6%), depression (2.3%), post-traumatic stress disorder (1.1%), and/or a mental health

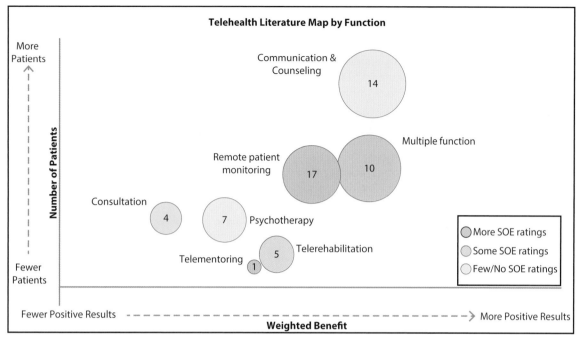

▲ **Figure 11-7.** Evidence map of telehealth literature by modality. A. Bubble size reflects the unduplicated number of individual studies included in the systematic reviews about that clinical focus. The number label on each bubble is the number of systematic reviews. Smaller bubbles indicate fewer studies; larger bubbles indicate more studies. The color of the bubble represents how many systematic reviews included strength of evidence assessment. B. Weighted relative benefit is calculated by weighting the overall conclusion of each review by the number of studies in the review. Bubbles to the right indicate more positive findings, and bubbles to the left represent findings that are unclear or found no benefit. SOE, strength of evidence. (Reprinted from Totten AM. *Telehealth: Mapping the Evidence for Patient Outcomes*; with permission of the Agency for Healthcare Research and Quality, Rockville, MD.)

condition other than depression or posttraumatic stress disorder (2.3%).

Care was coordinated by a dedicated team of trained health care professionals, usually nurses or social workers. Patients were formally assessed by their care coordinator, who selected the appropriate home health technology, provided coaching and training to patients and family members, monitored patient data, coordinated services, and communicated with the patient's provider. Care coordinators selected biometrics to be tracked based on patient-specific medical conditions.

Messaging devices installed with disease management protocols (DMPs) texted questions to patients to assess their health status and educational needs. Based on preset thresholds for biometric data and survey questions, the telemonitoring device risk stratified

patients daily and provided color-coded alerts for care coordinators concerning changes in status, allowing for immediate intervention. The census for CCHT expanded from 2,000 patients in 2003 to 31,570 in 2007, for a total of 43,430 patients. Analysis of care utilization between 2003 and 2007 showed a 25% reduction in days of inpatient care, 19% reduction in hospital admissions, and a patient satisfaction score of 86%. The annual cost of CCHT was $1,600/patient compared to $13,121 for the VHA's home-based primary services.

The Whole System Demonstrator (WSD) launched by the National Health Service (NHS) in England in 2008 was an RCT of the impact of home telemonitoring on utilization and outcomes among 3,230 patients with diabetes, chronic obstructive lung disease, or heart failure spread among 179 general practices in three areas of England over a 12-month period. The cohort with telemonitoring had 18% lower rates of hospitalization and 46% lower mortality rates than did patients in the control arm.[23] Although enrollment is slower than they had hoped, based on the WSD results, England planned to expand RPM to 3 million lives between 2012 and 2017.

The Ontario Telemedicine Network's Telehomecare initiative observed a 46% reduction in emergency department visits, 53% reduction in hospital admissions, and 25% shorter length of stay among 466 patients after enrollment in RPM.[24] Canada is also expanding its remote monitoring programs based on early successes.

Excepting ICDs and glucometers, RPM for chronic diseases typically relies on physiologic information from noninvasive biosensors and from patient survey. A 2016 review of RCTs by Vegesna et al. identified 62 studies on health outcomes.[38] Seventy-one percent were RCTs, and the number of patients varied from 30 to 730. The mostly common conditions were respiratory (22.6% of studies), cardiovascular (17.7%), obesity (17.7%), and diabetes/metabolic syndrome (16.1%). RPM has also been used in psychiatric illness, substance abuse, neurologic diseases, and cancer. Positive health outcomes were reported in 74.2% of the studies, whereas 25.8% were neutral. None identified negative outcomes compared to usual care. Although much of the available literature on the impact of RPM for chronic disease management comes in the form of small RCTs focused on specific conditions, the body of evidence for congestive heart disease, chronic obstructive pulmonary disease, and stroke is more substantive.

In a 2014 review, Bashshur et al. reviewed the empirical evidence of telemedicine for chronic disease management focusing on congestive heart failure, chronic obstructive pulmonary disease, and stroke.[39] The review included studies on RPM between 2000 and 2014 with a robust research design and a sample size of at least 150 patients. For each of the conditions studied, the preponderance of evidence supported benefit from RPM. In general, the benefits were from reductions in service use, including hospitalizations and emergency department visits, but there were often reductions in mortality as well. Few of the studies were mixed or failed to show a benefit. Economic analysis supported the benefits of RPM compared to usual care.

Several meta-analyses and systematic reviews confirm the conclusions reached by Bashshur et al. A 2010 systematic review by Inglis et al. focused on the impact of telemonitoring and structured telephone support in patients with congestive heart failure, analyzing 11 RCT RPM trials with a total of 2,710 patients. Telemonitoring was associated with 34% lower all-cause mortality and 21% fewer heart failure–related hospitalizations,[42] although the studies were small and of low to moderate quality. A 2015 review by the same investigators included nine new trials,[43] for a total of 3,860 patients. RPM was associated with a 20% reduction in all-cause mortality and 15% reduction in heart failure–related hospitalizations, with additional improvements in health-related quality of life, heart failure knowledge, and self-care behaviors. A third systematic review also focused on patients with congestive heart failure, analyzing 12 RCTs and nine observational studies comprising 3,082 patients.[44] The analysis demonstrated a 36% lower all-cause mortality and fewer hospitalizations among patients using RPM.[44]

A systematic review of nine studies using telemonitoring or telephone support versus usual care in 858 patients with chronic obstructive pulmonary disease demonstrated that telemonitoring was associated with lower numbers of hospitalizations and emergency department visits, fewer scheduled visits, and a lower number of home visits.[45] A systematic review and meta-analysis of 26 studies (5,069 patients) on home telehealth (telemonitoring or telephone support) for management of diabetes, 21 of which used telemonitoring, found that telemonitoring was associated with lower glycosylated hemoglobin levels and fewer hospitalizations compared to usual care.[46]

▶ The Impact of Remote Patient Monitoring in Transitional (Postacute) Care

The HRRP outlined in section 3025 of the ACA stimulated the application of several effective transitional care strategies to reduce hospital readmissions, among them Project RED,[47] BOOST,[48] CTI,[49] and Transitional Care Model (TCM).[50] Successful transition programs share the following elements:

- Medication support/reconciliation

- Patient education and coaching on self-management and symptom recognition

- Follow-up planning and reminders
- Coordination of information between providers/settings
- Short-term intensive postdischarge follow-up

In theory, RPM should lend itself nicely to the core components of effective translational care programs and could optimize the efficiency and scaling of these services across large populations. Several health care systems are incorporating RPM into their translational/postacute care strategies.

Several early adopters of RPM into transitional care describe success. Geisinger integrated AMC Health's (New York, NY) telemonitoring platform into its complex care heart failure program in 2008. Examination of claims data from enrolled Medicare patients showed they had a 33% reduction in all-cause hospitalization, 44% lower 30-day readmission rates, 38% lower 90-day readmission rates,[51] and 11.3% lower care costs than when they were not enrolled. The return on investment (ROI) was estimated to be 3.3.

The University of Virginia, in partnership with Locus Health (Charlottesville, VA), incorporated RPM into a comprehensive care coordination strategy for postacute care patients over age 65.[52] Launched in 2013, it initially enrolled only patients admitted with one of the CMS readmission penalty diagnoses and demonstrated a 46% reduction in 30-day readmission rates across all diagnoses with condition-specific reductions ranging from 20% to 50%. As a result of its success, the program expanded to include all diagnoses hospital-wide and uses RPM as one tool in a multicomponent postacute care strategy that includes each of the elements common to successful programs, such as CTI and TCM. Enrollment of eligible patients approaches 80%, and completion rates are 90%.

Early RCTs using RPM for postacute care have reached disparate conclusions. Comparison of negative and positive studies provides some insights about possible drivers for successful implementation of RPM in transitional care coordination.

In 2004, a collaborative of New England health systems tested the impact of the Specialized Primary and Networked Care in Heart Failure (SPAN-CHF) disease management program to reduce readmission among 200 patients discharged with congestive heart failure.[53] The nurse-run intervention used weekly coaching telephone calls for 90 days after discharge. The SPAN-CHF intervention reduced hospitalizations for heart failure by 52% and all cardiac admissions by 43%. In 2010, a follow-on study, SPAN-CHF II,[54] had 188 patients randomized to receive the original SPAN-CHF intervention or SPAN-CHF plus automated home monitoring (AHM) with an interactive scale, blood pressure cuff, text messaging system, and the Bosch Health Buddy. Adding AHM further reduced readmissions, with heart failure admissions reduced by 72% (compared to 52% in SPAN CHF I) and all cardiac readmissions by 63% (compared to 43%).

Similar outcomes were reported by Davis et al., using the Cardiocom device (Chanhassen, MN) in a postacute transitional care program for underserved patients discharged to home from the hospital with a diagnosis of heart failure or chronic obstructive pulmonary disease.[55] In addition to daily biometric monitoring, the program included an interactive educational component and communication with physician providers if concerning trends were identified. Care coordinators performed medication reconciliation, helped the patient develop a care plan, and coached patients to set up regular follow-up appointments. There were 149 intervention patients and 1,028 controls. The duration of the intervention was 90 days. Patients in the intervention arm enjoyed a 50% reduction in 30-day readmission rates and 13% to 19% reduction in 180-day readmission rates. There was no difference in emergency department utilization. Program completion rates were 85%, and adherence to daily monitoring averaged 70%.

The BEAT-HF trial[56] was designed to evaluate the effectiveness of a care transition intervention using RPM to reduce readmission rates in patients aged 50 or older who were discharged after receiving care for heart failure. The intervention consisted of predischarge education; remote monitoring of weight, blood pressure, and heart rate; and nine telephone coaching calls over the 6-month study period. The study found no difference in 30-day or 180-day readmissions between the intervention and control groups. However, intention to treat analysis was used, and only 57% of enrolled patients completed the study; among those who did, adherence to telemonitoring >50% of days was only 55%, and only 61.4% of enrollees completed >50% of the scheduled coaching calls. The low compliance and completion rates make it difficult to draw firm conclusions about the effectiveness of the intervention.

Intensive Care Unit Monitoring of Providers

RPM can support providers as well as patients. Tele-ICU, also known as eICU, refers to the use of an offsite command center staffed by intensivists and critical care nurses connected to inpatients at distant ICUs via real-time video, audio, and electronic means to support care rendered by onsite providers.[57] The concept was originally introduced in the 1970s as a video link and evolved with digital and Internet capabilities into a fully integrated system with continuous access to patient monitoring data and electronic records that provides a safety net of supplemental critical care expertise for onsite caregivers.[57,58,59] Contrary to the overall trend for inpatient units to downsize and shift more care to the ambulatory setting, ICUs are expanding. The Leapfrog Group found that, on average, length of stay was 3 days shorter and ICU mortality rates 40% lower in ICUs staffed by intensivists[60] and have made adequate staffing by intensivists one of the metrics by which hospital performance is measured.[57,61] In 2015, 44% of reporting hospitals met the Leapfrog ICU physician staffing metric, up from 10% in 2007.[60] However, a shortage prevents some hospitals from hiring enough intensivists to manage their ICUs full time. The demand for intensivists is expected to increase by 38% between 2000 and 2020,[62] and current training programs are not turning out providers in numbers sufficient to meet the demand.

The tele-ICU model is one way ICUs can stretch the available workforce to cover demand. The first integrated tele-ICU model was launched by the Sentara Hospital System in 2000 in Norfolk, Virginia, using a platform developed by Visicu (Philips; Amsterdam, Netherlands).[58] Since then Visicu was acquired by Philips, and Cerner and iMDsoft have joined the U.S. tele-ICU market. The average tele-ICU covers 138 beds across 4.6 hospital systems staffed by one critical care nurse for every 30 to 35 beds and one intensivist for every 100 to 130 beds.[62,63] In 2003, 16 (0.4%) hospitals used tele-ICUs. By 2010 the number had increased to 213 (4.6% of total).[64] During the same timeframe, the number of ICU beds covered by telemedicine increased from 598 (0.9% of total) to 5,799 (7.9% of total).[64] Despite penetration of tele-ICU support across the country, reported outcomes have been mixed. Proponents have reported reductions in length of stay, hospital and ICU mortality, and overall costs.[58,62] According to Mackintosh et al., most of the studies reported suffer from significant methodologic shortcomings.[65] They identified only two studies of sufficient rigor to be included in their review. One of the best before and after studies included 6,290 adult patients admitted to one of seven ICUs on two campuses of an 834-bed academic medical center over a 2-year period and showed that implementation of tele-ICU was associated with a 60% reduction in hospital mortality.[66] Following implementation of the tele-ICU there was also reduced ICU mortality, shorter length of stay, lower rates of preventable complications, and lower overall costs.[66] The second study included 118,990 adult patients from 56 ICUs in 32 hospitals from 19 U.S. health systems and observed a 16% reduction in hospital mortality, 26% reduction in ICU mortality, and reduced hospital and ICU lengths of stay following the implementation of the tele-ICU.[67] The aspects of the tele-ICU intervention associated with improved mortality and/or reduced length of stay included review of each case by the intensivist within an hour of admission, timely use of performance data, adherence to ICU best practices, and quicker alert response times.[67]

Tele-ICUs have not worked in every health system and have been deactivated in some. Limitations include high start-up costs, inconsistent interoperability between the onsite EMR and established commercial tele-ICU platforms, unclear impact on patient outcomes in certain cases, and initial resistance and skepticism on the part of some care teams.[62] It is estimated that it costs approximately $30,000 to $50,000/ICU bed in one-time or capital costs to implement a tele-ICU program and an additional $30,000 to 40,000/year/bed in staffing costs for offsite tele-ICU providers.[58,62,63,68] Currently third-party payors, including CMS, do not reimburse tele-ICU intensivists and critical care nurses operating offsite. The limited financial analyses available from systems that have implemented tele-ICU programs indicate that the model is profitable; however, more data are needed to draw general conclusions. In some instances, the impact of the tele-ICU cannot be dissected from that of other quality improvements in the ICU.[63]

Among systems reporting profitability, factors driving the improved margin include decreased lengths of stay allowing increased volumes of new admissions, onsite retention of patients at community hospital sites with tele-ICU coverage, and increased occupancy rate of ICU beds which more than offset the capital and operational costs of the tele-ICU.[58,62] In one system analyzed, the breakeven point was achieved within a year, subsequent to which the combination of the increased contribution margin per case and the increased case volume resulted in a higher total contribution margin.[58] Although payors do not currently reimburse tele-ICU staff, they stand to benefit financially from the decreased lengths of stay and decreased complications experienced by those whose lives they cover. In summary, although some studies show that the tele-ICU model dramatically improves patient outcomes, stretches resources, and reduces costs, taken as a whole, the available data are mixed. Most of the published peer-reviewed studies suffer from limitations in design, and most well-designed studies have been assessed as being at some risk for bias. Notwithstanding these limitations, the tele-ICU model holds considerable promise and is now operational in 11% of the nonfederal ICU beds in the United States.[58]

ICUs are not the only venues providing RPM support for providers. RPM is increasingly being used to monitor the provider performance in postacute facilities that provide rehabilitation and skilled nursing services.

STANDALONE REMOTE PATIENT MONITORING SYSTEMS

▶ Implantable Cardiovascular Devices

RPM has been used for over 15 years for ICDs. One of the earliest applications was remote analysis of the function of pacemakers and ICDs. RPM of invasive cardiac devices is perhaps the most widely adopted RPM strategy, and its benefits have been clearly demonstrated by RCTs. Guidelines recommend that patients with pacemakers should be followed up every 3 to 12 months and those with ICDs every 3 to 6 months. Until remote monitoring of pacemakers and ICDs was launched in 2001 by Biotronik (Berlin, Germany), follow-up had to occur in a clinic. Currently each of the major ICD companies offers RPM technology. Initial systems

required active acquisition by the patient at prespecified intervals. Newer technologies transmit real-time data wirelessly to care coordination centers, which alert providers of high-risk events.

Remote pacer monitoring reduces costs and is more convenient for patients, but new studies now strongly indicate that it improves survival. A large 2015 study of 269,471 patients with implanted cardiac rhythm devices, including pacemakers, implantable defibrillators, and resynchronization devices, demonstrated improved survival among the patients who participated in RPM.[69] Furthermore there was incremental improvement associated with increasing levels of compliance with remote monitoring recommendations, with patients not participating in RPM dying at twice the rate of those having at least 75% compliance.[69] Several other studies, including IN-TIME[70] and ALTITUDE,[71] have also demonstrated decreased mortality associated with regular RPM. Patients with congestive heart failure often receive implantable devices that have volume sensors to allow hemodynamically guided management of heart failure. A 2016 meta-analysis of five major clinical trials including 1,296 patients demonstrated a 38% reduction in heart failure hospitalizations with monitoring.[72]

RPM is being increasingly used for diagnostics and monitoring that previously required in-hospital or in-clinic testing, such as sleep apnea and macular degeneration. Although not appropriate for all patients, at-home sleep studies have reduced wait times to diagnosis and have reduced the costs for sleep apnea management.[73] Recent evidence suggests that daily RPM using the ForeseeHome monitoring system may be sight sparing for patients with macular degeneration. The HOME study demonstrated that neovascularization detected through daily monitoring using the device was associated with less vision loss than that detected by symptoms or routine office follow-up.[74] For each new standalone application, research will be needed to define the most appropriate clinical circumstances in which RPM can substitute for what is now standard care.

▶ Patient Safety and Eldercare

Increasingly sophisticated, yet affordable, monitoring technologies are being developed to prolong independent living and monitor health status. Some applications are targeted to a specific issue, such as MedMinder (Needham, MA), a pill dispenser that reminds patients to take their medications and wirelessly transmits status alerts to family members. More sophisticated applications include "smart homes" in which networks of sensors, monitors, and/or cameras are installed in an elderly person's home. The smart home system sends wireless updates to family, allowing them to monitor location, activity, appliance use, health biometrics, and door use of their elderly relative. A systematic review on smart home technology concluded that there was evidence that elderly adults maintained physical and cognitive status, function in their activities of daily living, and mobility when a smart home system for functional monitoring was installed in their home.[75] The data were conflicting on whether smart home health monitoring technologies have an impact on falls or outcomes associated with heart failure or chronic obstructive pulmonary disease.[75]

SUMMARY

RPM is a rapidly expanding segment of telehealth, with the potential to promote the transformation of ambulatory and transitional care from episodes of reactive care to a care continuum, delivering the right care to the right patient at the right time at any location. Although more work needs to be done to determine the most effective clinical applications and delivery models for RPM, there is a growing body of evidence showing that RPM-facilitated care can improve outcomes and reduce costs. In the cases of chronic disease management and transitional care, RPM also serves as a workforce multiplier, off-loading time-consuming activities such as coaching, monitoring, and education from primary care providers and specialists to teams of trained care coordinators.

ACKNOWLEDGMENT

The author wishes to thank Nicolas Damiani and David Caraway, Jr. for assistance with proofing and editing, Kayleigh Warburton for assistance with graphic design, and Patti Dewberry for assistance with the patient case.

REFERENCES

1. Centers for Medicare & Medicaid Services. *Health Care Expenditure Statistics*. https://www.cms.gov/research-statistics-data-and-systems/statistics-trends-and-reports/nationalhealthexpenddata. Accessed October 26, 2016.

2. Keehan SP, Poisal JA, Cuckler GA, et al. National health expenditure projections, 2015-25: Economy, prices, and aging expected to shape spending and enrollment *Health Aff (Millwood)* 2016;35(8):1522–1531.

3. Organisation for Economic Co-Operation and Development. *Health at a Glance 2013: OECD Indicators.* http://dx.doi.org/10.1787/health_glance-2013-en.

4. Commonwealth Fund. *U.S. Health Care from a Global Perspective.* http://www.commonwealthfund.org/publications/issue-briefs/2015/oct/us-health-care-from-a-global-perspective. Accessed October 26, 2016.

5. The World Health Organization. *WHO World Health Report 2000.* http://www.who.int/whr/2000/en/whr00_en.pdf?ua=1. Accessed October 26, 2016.

6. Ward BW, Schiller JS. Prevalence of multiple chronic conditions among US adults: estimates from the National Health Interview Survey, 2010. *Prev Chronic Dis* 2013;10:E65.

7. Gerteis J, Izrael D, Deitz D, et al. *Multiple Chronic Conditions Chartbook.* AHRQ Publications No. Q14-0038. Rockville, MD: Agency for Healthcare Research and Quality; 2014.

8. Association of Medical Colleges. *Physician Supply and Demand Through 2025: Key Findings.* https://www.aamc.org/download/426260/data/physiciansupplyanddemandthrough2025keyfindings.pdf. Accessed December 12, 2016.

9. Kohn LT, Corrigan JM, Donaldson MS. *To Err Is Human: Creating a Better Health System.* National Academies Press: Institute of Medicine (US) Committee on Quality of Health Care in America; Washington (DC): National Academies Press (US); 2000.

10. Institute of Medicine, Committee on the Quality of Health Care in America. *Crossing the Quality Chasm: A New Health System for the 21st Century*; Institute of Medicine (US) Committee on Quality of Health Care in America. Washington (DC): National Academies Press (US); 2001.

11. Schraeder CS, Shelton P. Effective care coordination models. In: Lamb G, ed. *Care Coordination: The Game Changer—How Nursing Is Revolutionizing Quality Care* Silver Spring, MD: Nursesbooks.org; 2014:57–79.

12. Brown RS, Peikes D, Peterson G, et al. Six features of Medicare coordinated care demonstration programs that cut hospital admissions of high-risk patients. *Health Aff (Millwood)* 2012;31(6):1156–1166.

13. Coye MJ, Haselkorn A, DeMello S. Remote patient management: technology-enabled innovation and evolving business models for chronic disease care. *Health Aff (Millwood)* 2009;28(1):126–135.

14. Center for Connected Health Policy. http://www.cchpca.org. Accessed September 11, 2016.

15. Caffazzo JA, Leonard K, Easty AC, et al. Bridging the self-care deficit gap: remote patient monitoring and hospital at home. Electronic Healthcare: First International Conference, *eHealth 2008*. London, UK, 2009.

16. Baig MM, Antonescu-Turcu A, Ratarasarn K. Impact of sleep telemedicine protocol in management of sleep apnea: a 5-year VA experience. *Telemed J E Health* 2016;22(5):458–462.

17. Ladapo JA, Turakhia MP, Ryan MP, et al. Health care utilization and expenditures associated with remote monitoring in patients with implantable cardiac devices. *Am J Cardiol* 2016;117(9):1455–1462.

18. Darkins A, Ryan P, Kobb R, et al. Care Coordination/Home Telehealth: the systematic implementation of health informatics, home telehealth, and disease management to support the care of veteran patients with chronic conditions. *Telemed J E Health* 2008;14(10): 1118–1126.

19. Darkins A, Kendall S, Edmonson E, et al. Reduced cost and mortality using home telehealth to promote self-management of complex chronic conditions: a retrospective matched cohort study of 4,999 veteran patients. *Telemed J E Health* 2015;21(1):70–76.

20. Au DH, Macaulay DS, Jarvis JL, et al. Impact of a telehealth and care management program for patients with chronic obstructive pulmonary disease. *Ann Am Thorac Soc* 2015;12(3):323–331.

21. De San Miguel K, Smith J, Lewin G. Telehealth remote monitoring for community-dwelling older adults with chronic obstructive pulmonary disease. *Telemed J E Health* 2013;19(9):652–657.

22. Noel HC, Vogel DC, Erdos JJ, et al. Home telehealth reduces healthcare costs. *Telemed J E Health* 2004;10:170–183.

23. Steventon A, Bardsley M, Billings J, et al. Effect of telehealth on use of secondary care and mortality: findings from the whole system demonstrator cluster randomised trial. *BMJ* 2012;344:e3874.

24. Mierdel S, Owen K. Telehomecare reduces ER Use and hospitalizations at William Osler Health System. *Stud Health Technol Inform* 2015;209:102–108.

25. Food and Drug Administration. *General Wellness: Policy for Low Risk Devices. Guidance for Industry and Food and Drug Administration Staff*. http://www.fda.gov/ucm/groups/fdagov-public/@fdagov-meddev-gen/

documents/document/ucm429674.pdf. Access date December 17, 2016.

26. Settles C. Remote patient monitoring in healthcare. *Technology Advice*. http://technologyadvice.com/blog/healthcare/remote-patient-monitoring/Technology Advice June 15, 2015. Accessed October 26, 2016.

27. Grand View Research. Medical Electronics Market Analysis by Application; Therapeutics; Patient Monitoring and Segment Forecasts to 2024. September 2016.

28. Grand View Research. *Remote Patient Monitoring Devices Market Analysis by Product, By End Use, By Application, and Segment Forecasts, 2014–2025*. http://www.grandviewresearch.com/industry-analysis/remote-patient-monitoring-devices-market. Accessed November 25, 2016.

29. Institute for Healthcare Improvement. http://www.ihi.org/engage/initiatives/tripleaim/pages/default.aspx. Accessed November 25, 2016.

30. emids. *Understanding Barriers to Telehealth Adoption*. http://www.emids.com/understanding-barriers-to-telehealth-adoption/. Accessed December 18, 2016.

31. Mohammadzadeh N, Safdari R. Patient monitoring in mobile health: opportunities and challenges. *Med Arch* 2014;68(1):57–60.

32. Peretz D, Arnaert A, Ponzoni N. Determining the cost of implementing and operating a remote patient monitoring programme for the elderly with chronic conditions: a systematic review of economic evaluations. *J Telemed Telecare*. pii: 1357633X16669239. Accessed Sep 19, 2016. [Epub ahead of print]

33. Chiron Health. http://www.chironhealth.com/telemedicine/reimbursement/medicaid/. Accessed December 2016.

34. Darkins A. The growth of telehealth services in the Veterans Health Administration between 1994 and 2014: a study in the diffusion of innovation. *Telemed J E Health* 2014;20(9):761–768.

35. Godleski L, Darkins A, Peters J. Outcomes of 98,609 U.S. Department of Veterans Affairs patients enrolled in telemental health services, 2006–2010. *Psychiatr Serv* 2012;63:383–385.

36. Genworth. https://www.genworth.com.

37. Totten AM, Womack DM, Eden KB, et al. *AHRQ Comparative Effectiveness Technical Briefs*. https://effectivehealthcare.ahrq.gov/search-for-guides-reviews-and-reports/?pageaction=displayproduct&productID=2254. Accessed December 4, 2016.

38. Vegesna A, Tran M, Angelaccio M, Arcona S. Remote patient monitoring via non-invasive digital technologies: a systematic review. *Telemed J E Health* 2017;23(1): 3–17.

39. Bashshur RL, Howell JD, Krupinski EA, et al. The empirical foundations of telemedicine interventions in primary care. *Telemed J E Health* 2016;22(5):342–375.

40. Totten AM, Womack DM, Eden KB, et al. *AHRQ Comparative Effectiveness Technical Briefs. Telehealth: Mapping the Evidence for Patient Outcomes From Systematic Reviews.* Technical Brief No 26 (Prepared by the Pacific Northwest Evidence-based Practice Center under Contract No 290-2015-00009-I) AHRQ Publication No 16-EHC034-EF. Rockville, MD: Agency for Healthcare Research and Quality (US); 2016.

41. Johnston B, Wheeler L, Deuser J, Sousa KH. Outcomes of the Kaiser Permanente Tele-Home Health Research Project. *Arch Fam Med* 2000;9(1):40–45.

42. Inglis SC, Clark RA, McAlister FA, et al. Structured telephone support or telemonitoring programmes for patients with chronic heart failure. *Cochrane Database Syst Rev* 2010;8:CD007228.

43. Inglis SC, Clark RA, Dierckx R, et al. Structured telephone support or non-invasive telemonitoring for patients with heart failure. *Cochrane Database Syst Rev* 2015;10:Cd007228.

44. Polisena J, Tran K, Cimon K, et al. Home telemonitoring for congestive heart failure: a systematic review and meta-analysis. *J Telemed Telecare* 2010;16(2):68–76.

45. Polisena J, Tran K, Cimon K, et al. Home telehealth for chronic obstructive pulmonary disease: a systematic review and meta-analysis. *J Telemed Telecare* 2010;16(3):120–127.

46. Polisena J, Tran K, Cimon K, et al. Home telehealth for diabetes management: a systematic review and meta-analysis. *Diabetes Obes Metab* 2009;11(10):913–930.

47. Jack BW, Chetty VK, Anthony D, et al. A reengineered hospital discharge program to decrease rehospitalization: a randomized trial. *Ann Intern Med* 2009;150(3):178–187.

48. Society of Hospital Medicine. *Essential First Steps in Quality Improvement, Project BOOST Implementation Tool.* http://www.hospitalmedicine.org/Web/Quality_Innovation/Implementation_Toolkits/Project_BOOST/Web/Quality___Innovation/Implementation_Toolkit/Boost/Overview.aspx. Accessed December 2016.

49. Coleman EA, Parry C, Chalmers S, Min SJ. The care transitions intervention: results of a randomized controlled trial. *Arch Intern Med* 2006;166(17):1822–1828.

50. Naylor MD. Transitional care for older adults: a cost-effective model. *LDI Issue Brief* 2004;9(6):1–4.

51. Maeng DD, Starr AE, Tomcavage JF, et al. Can telemonitoring reduce hospitalization and cost of care? A health plan's experience in managing patients with heart failure. *Popul Health Manag* 2014;17(6):340–344.

52. Locus Health. http://locus-health.com/. Accessed November 25, 2016.

53. Kimmelstiel C, Levine D, Perry K, et al. Randomized, controlled evaluation of short- and long-term benefits of heart failure disease management within a diverse provider network: the SPAN-CHF trial. *Circulation* 2004;110(11):1450–1455.

54. Weintraub A, Gregory D, Patel AR, et al. A multicenter randomized controlled evaluation of automated home monitoring and telephonic disease management in patients recently hospitalized for congestive heart failure: the SPAN-CHF II trial. *J Card Fail* 2010;16(4):285–292.

55. Davis C, Bender M, Smith T, Broad J. Feasibility and acute care utilization outcomes of a post-acute transitional telemonitoring program for underserved chronic disease patients. *Telemed J E Health* 2015;21(9):705–713.

56. Ong MK, Romano PS, Edgington S, et al. Effectiveness of remote patient monitoring after discharge of hospitalized patients with heart failure: the better effectiveness after transition-heart failure (BEAT-HF) randomized clinical trial. *JAMA Intern Med* 2016;176(3):310–318.

57. Kumar S, Merchant S, Reynolds R. Tele-ICU: efficacy and cost-effectiveness of remotely managing critical care. *Perspect Health Inf Manag* 2013;10:1f.

58. New England Healthcare Institute and Massachusetts Technology Collaborative. *Critical Care, Critical Choices: The Case for Tele-ICUs in Intensive Care.* http://masstech.org/sites/mtc/files/documents/2010 TeleICU Report.pdf. Accessed November 2016.

59. New England Healthcare Institute, Massachusetts Technology Collaborative, and Health Technology Center. *Tele-ICU: Remote Management in Intensive Care Units.* http://www.nehi.net/writable/publication_files/file/tele_icu_final.pdf. Accessed November 2016.

60. The Leapfrog Group. http://www.leapfroggroup.org/sites/default/files/Files/IPS Fact Sheet.pdf. Accessed November 2016.

61. Pronovost PJ, Angus DC, Dorman T, et al. Physician staffing patterns and clinical outcomes in critically ill patients: a systematic review. *JAMA* 2002;288(17):2151–2162.

62. The Advisory Board. *Telehealth Primer: TeleICU.* https://www.advisory.com. Accessed February 2016.

63. Berenson RA, Grossman JM, November EA. Does telemonitoring of patients—the eICU—improve intensive care? *Health Aff (Millwood)* 2009;28(5):w937–w947.

64. Kahn JM, Cicero BD, Wallace DJ, Iwashyna TJ. Adoption of ICU telemedicine in the United States. *Crit Care Med* 2014;42(2):362–368.

65. Mackintosh N, Terblanche M, Maharaj R, et al. Telemedicine with clinical decision support for critical care: a systematic review. *Syst Rev* 2016;5(1):176.

66. Lilly CM, Cody S, Zhao H, et al. Hospital mortality, length of stay, and preventable complications among critically ill patients before and after tele-ICU reengineering of critical care processes. *JAMA* 2011;305(21):2175–2183.

67. Lilly CM, McLaughlin JM, Zhao H, et al. A multicenter study of ICU telemedicine reengineering of adult critical care. *Chest* 2014;145(3):500–507.

68. Kumar G, Falk DM, Bonello RS, et al. The costs of critical care telemedicine programs: a systematic review and analysis. *Chest* 2013;143(1):19–29.

69. Varma N, Ricci RP. Impact of remote monitoring on clinical outcomes. *J Cardiovasc Electrophysiol* 2015;26(12):1388–1395.

70. Hindricks G, Taborsky M, Glikson M, et al. Implant-based multiparameter telemonitoring of patients with heart failure (IN-TIME): a randomised controlled trial. *Lancet* 2014;384(9943):583–590.

71. Saxon LA, Hayes DL, Gilliam FR, et al. Long-term outcome after ICD and CRT implantation and influence of remote device follow-up: the ALTITUDE survival study. *Circulation* 2010;122(23):2359–2367.

72. Adamson PB, Ginn G, Anker SD, et al. Remote haemodynamic-guided care for patients with chronic heart failure: a meta-analysis of completed trials. *Eur J Heart Fail* 2017;19(3):426–433.

73. Safadi A, Etzioni T, Fliss D, et al. The effect of the transition to home monitoring for the diagnosis of OSAS on test availability, waiting time, patients' satisfaction, and outcome in a large health provider system. *Sleep Disord* 2014;418246.

74. Chew EY, Clemons TE, Harrington M, et al. Effectiveness of different monitoring modalities in the detection of neovascular age-related macular degeneration: the home study, report number 3. *Retina* 2016;36(8):1542–1547.

75. Liu L, Stroulia E, Nikolaidis I, et al. Smart homes and home health monitoring technologies for older adults: a systematic review. *Int J Med Inform* 2016;91:44–59.

Rehabilitation

Trevor G. Russell, BPhty, PhD and
Deborah G. Theodoros, BSp Thy (Hons), PhD

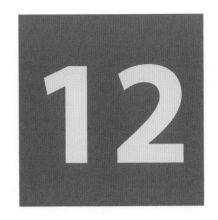

Living in a small country town, John, a 49-year-old owner of a hardware store, found that his capacity to return to his everyday life was significantly restricted following his stroke. John's aphasia and difficulties with walking, balance, and the use of his right arm and hand made it impossible for him to manage his hardware business unassisted. Access to the in-person rehabilitation services at the tertiary hospital where he was managed when he had his stroke was difficult due to distance, his physical and communication difficulties, and his need to continue to work. However, on discharge from the center-based rehabilitation unit, John transitioned to the hospital's home-based telerehabilitation program that enabled him to continue to access physical therapy, speech pathology, occupational therapy, psychology, and social work services. Using specialty telerehabilitation software on his iPad, John's rehabilitation team could assess his progress, provide interventions to maximize his function and independence, modify and progress his physical and speech exercise regimen, and provide education and support from a distance. These services were critical for John to remain in his community and support his family.

Telerehabilitation, "the delivery of rehabilitation services by information and communication technologies"[1] at a distance, offers a plausible alternative or supplement to center-based rehabilitation services. For patients with conditions associated with stroke, head and spinal injury, progressive neurological disorders, musculoskeletal disorders, and respiratory and cardiac disease, long-term rehabilitation is often required to restore function, regain everyday skills, and maintain an acceptable quality of life. The ease of access and timely intervention facilitated by telerehabilitation promotes a client-centered approach along a continuum of care.

Although "telerehabilitation" is the umbrella term adopted to denote technology-enabled rehabilitation and is used by some professional groups,[2] there is diversity in terminology across disciplines. For example, the broader term of "telepractice" is used by speech-language pathologists,[3,4] "telehealth" is used by the American Physical Therapy Association,[5] and other terms have been used to denote a specific discipline such as "telepsychology."[6]

NATURE OF TELEREHABILITATION

Telerehabilitation is distinctly different from conventional telemedicine consultations with respect to the range of health professionals involved, the frequency and type of interactions that occur with a single patient, the service settings, and the variety and utility of technologies that may be used across the continuum of care. A broad range of health professionals, including physical therapists, occupational therapists, speech-language pathologists, psychologists, audiologists, teachers, rehabilitation engineers, dieticians, rehabilitation physicians, and nurses, can be involved in telerehabilitation.[1] The services that can be provided via telerehabilitation are extensive and include education to the patient and family, counseling, assessment, intervention, ongoing monitoring, and offline self-management programs.[1] Interdisciplinary rehabilitation can also be supported by telerehabilitation through multipoint real-time videoconferencing.

The types of interactions between the client and health professional in telerehabilitation consist of a variety of intervention schedules and different types of exchanges, activities, and technologies. These include intensive and distributed intervention scheduling, individual and group therapy, the use of measurement software to quantify client function, and the use of both synchronous and asynchronous technologies to provide real-time interaction and enable client self-management in the home. It is possible for a patient undergoing rehabilitation to engage in different modes of telerehabilitation at varying times throughout their continuum of care.

A major advantage of telerehabilitation is that it can be implemented within the individual's own environment (eg, home, community, workplace) consistent with the World Health Organization recommendation to consider the contextual factors in rehabilitation.[7] Telerehabilitation models of care fall into four main categories: center-based hub and spoke, in-home real-time rehabilitation services, remote telemonitoring of patient performance, and in-home therapy activities that are supported or supervised remotely by a clinician.[8] The latter three models focus on rehabilitation within the person's own home. The hub and spoke model involves a rehabilitation service being delivered from a specialist center to a patient (and a health professional) at another center underserved by similar care.[9] Real-time rehabilitation services can be provided into the home or place of primary residence (eg, residential aged care facility) by various health professionals.[10,11] Remote telemonitoring of patient performance involves the use of technologies that provide physiological information to the clinician to enable assessment and adjustment of the rehabilitation program.[12] Asynchronous technologies can be used to enable patients to engage in a self-managed program of rehabilitation within the home while being monitored and directed by the clinician remotely.[13–16]

The delivery of services into the home via technology has become the preferred model of care in keeping with rehabilitation research evidence and social and demographic trends worldwide. Research suggests that rehabilitation for people with chronic conditions is optimized when conducted in the home. Skills taught during rehabilitation are more likely to be retained and transferred to everyday activities if taught in the environment in which they will be used.[17] Benefits of home-based rehabilitation following stroke have been identified as reduced costs and hospital length of stay, improved client decision making and outcomes,[18] and reduced carer strain.[19] A systematic review of randomized controlled trials of home-based vs. center-based stroke rehabilitation found that home-based rehabilitation was significantly more effective in improving functional independence than center-based care up to six months poststroke.[20] When provided with options for stroke rehabilitation services, patients have expressed a preference for home-based services due to the convenience and the opportunity for more meaningful engagement with carers.[21]

Social and demographic trends indicate that the aging population wants to remain independent as long as possible, preferably in their own homes.[22,23] Together with an inevitable reduction in the capacity to drive or use public transport[24] and the physical difficulties experienced by people with chronic disabilities in accessing center-based services, the demand for rehabilitation services in the home will increase. To date, there have been numerous studies of home-based telerehabilitation reported in the literature that support the validity and viability of services via this mode.[10,11,25,26]

Although telerehabilitation improves access to services and is a valid mode of service delivery, the value of this mode of service delivery in complementing and enhancing the quality of rehabilitation services is often underestimated. Telerehabilitation may be used exclusively as a mode of service delivery or as complementary to existing in-person services. Either way this mode of service delivery in all its formats provides clinicians with a mechanism by which they can optimize the rehabilitation process for their patients. Winters and Winters[8] postulated that telerehabilitation can optimize the timing, intensity, and duration of the rehabilitation program and facilitate self-efficacy and compliance with home programs.

Contemporary neurorehabilitation of people with brain impairment requires frequent access to services based on evidence-based intensive treatment protocols. For example, LSVT LOUD, the evidence-based treatment for the speech disorder in Parkinson disease (PD) involves a commitment of one hour per day, four days per week for four weeks. This level of attendance at a center-based treatment facility is problematic and often impossible for people with a movement disorder and their families. A recent study has demonstrated the validity of this intensive speech treatment when delivered online into the home.[27] Similarly, for people with progressive disorders such as PD, the timing of intervention is crucial in ensuring maintenance of function and safety within the home. Online assessment of physical[28,29] and swallowing[30] function in people with PD allows for regular monitoring of changes and the initiation of intervention from physical therapists, occupational therapists, and speech pathologists as required.

TELEREHABILITATION TECHNOLOGIES

The technologies used to deliver telerehabilitation can vary widely depending on the clinical discipline, the nature of the consultation (eg, initial appointment vs. review appointment, assessment vs. treatment), and the complexity of the rehabilitation tasks that are being undertaken. Some clinical interactions require minimal technology and minimal interaction between the clinician and the client. For example, a dietitian may request that a client log their food intake through a website on a daily basis to monitor their diet quality and their fruit, vegetable, and dietary sodium intake.[31] This interaction can occur through any web-enabled device at a time and location that suits the client. Other telerehabilitation consultations may require real-time interaction between the clinician and client to achieve the objectives of the session. A cognitive behavioral therapy (CBT) session for a patient with anxiety is an example of an interaction where two-way video communication is required for the consultation to be effective.[32] Other interactions required more complex technologies still. Consider the case where an occupational therapist wishes to conduct a home safety assessment which requires measurements of the physical environment, where a speech pathologist wishes to perform a remote swallowing assessment, or where a physical therapist wishes to measure up a child for a

wheelchair or provide upper limb rehabilitation after a stroke. In these cases, more complex technologies may be required to equip the clinician with the tools that they require to achieve the objectives of the session.

The complexity of the technology required for many rehabilitation interactions is thought to be one of the reasons for the late adoption of this service delivery model by the rehabilitation professions. Rehabilitation practice often relies heavily on objective measurement and standardized testing procedures to drive the diagnostic process and monitor the outcomes of therapeutic intervention. Early technologies did not provide a means for clinicians to obtain these measurements, requiring a trained assistant at the remote end of the consultation. Perhaps more significant a barrier is the conceptual difficulty that many clinicians have of imagining how to adopt what is traditionally "hands-on" therapy into a virtual medium. Practitioners often rely on touch and feel to perform client assessment and physical contact to provide resistance, guidance, facilitation, and cueing and to ensure that the patient is safe while receiving treatment. Hands-on manual therapy, manual facilitation, and tactile stimulus are examples of traditional approaches that cannot be replicated in the telerehabilitation context, and new and inventive ways of providing these services remotely need to be adopted. In addition to these challenges, patients who require rehabilitation often have physical impairments that affect their ability to interact with technology at the remote end of the consultation. For this reason Pramuka and van Roosmalen[33] recommend careful consideration of the accessibility and usability of technology that will be used at the patient end of the consultation, especially where the client will have an active role in the use of the equipment.

The last 10 to 15 years have seen a dramatic increase in the complexity and availability of technologies that can be used to deliver rehabilitation at a distance. It would have been inconceivable 10 years ago that many readers of this chapter would be wearing simple low-cost devices on their wrist that can monitor and tabulate movement and wirelessly sync these data to the cloud. These technology advances have seen an increase in the number of sustainable and effective telerehabilitation programs. The technologies that are used to delivered telerehabilitation interventions can largely be divided into three different classes: image-based technologies such as videoconferencing, technology to create virtual environments for rehabilitation, and sensors and asynchronous technologies.[27,34]

Image-Based Technologies

Within the field of telerehabilitation, the use of real-time image-based technologies such as videoconferencing dominates the literature. Of the 146 articles included in their review of telerehabilitation technologies, Rogante et al.[34] report that over 70% of papers involving patient treatment use image-based technologies to deliver care. Videoconferencing was also used in the first telerehabilitation paper in the early 1990s where Delaplain et al.[35] describes a service (including physical therapy) provided via a satellite-based videoconferencing system.

Videoconferencing involves the two-way transmission of video and audio data between the remote parties over a communication network. Videoconferencing end points were traditionally dedicated pieces of hardware that captured, encoded, and transmitted the visual and auditory information. The development of low-cost and computationally powerful consumer-grade devices such as laptop computers, tablets, and smart phones have provided an alternative low-cost method of videoconferencing communication that can be used for rehabilitation consultations (Figure 12-1). Videoconferencing using these devices is often referred to as software-based videoconferencing, as a specific software application usually is installed onto these devices that performs the required encoding and decoding of information. The networks used to transmit videoconferencing data have also changed over time. Dedicated (and expensive) point-to-point connections such as Integrated Services Digital Network (ISDN) telephone lines have gradually been replaced with Internet Protocol (IP) connections, which uses the ubiquitous (and relatively low-cost) infrastructure of the Internet to communicate the videoconferencing data. The domination of IP networks for video and audio communication has led to some major carriers discontinuing their support of ISDN networks as early as the end of 2017.[36]

The rise of software-based videoconferencing options has had a major impact on telerehabilitation services as the flexibility of the software environment opens the possibility of including additional features and functions into the videoconferencing experience. For example, some advanced software-based videoconferencing systems now include the ability to perform objective measurement of the patient at the remote end of the consultation and advanced media tools for the demonstration and recording of video clips during a videoconference.[37,38] These systems are removing some of the real and perceived barriers for the adoption of telerehabilitation services. Software-based videoconferencing clients can be thought of in two categories: general videoconferencing software such as Skype and Face Time, which are widely available and provide basic videoconferencing functionality, and specialized videoconferencing software for rehabilitation consultations, such as eHAB (NeoRehab, Brisbane) which combine high-quality and secure videoconferencing with advanced measurements and multimedia tools to facilitate the provision of rehabilitation via the Internet. Some of the broad features of each of these different videoconferencing systems are provided in Table 12-1.

Videoconferencing technologies are primarily appropriate when real-time interaction between the client and the therapist is required to facilitate the clinical interaction. Research using this technology is extensive, but for illustrative purposes, clinical trials have used videoconferencing technology to provide service to children with autism[39] and to adults with stroke,[10,40]

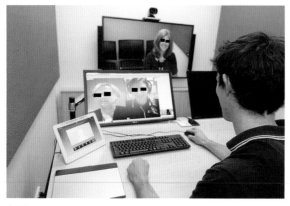

▲ **Figure 12-1.** Using both hardware (wall mounted) and software (computer monitor) videoconferencing systems to interact with remote clients.

Table 12-1. Comparative Features of Different Videoconferencing Options for Rehabilitation Consultations

Type	Quality	Standards based	Security	Multipoint support	Portability	Cost
Dedicated Hardware	Very High	Yes	Yes	Yes	No	Very High
Generic Software Based (eg, Skype)	Variable	No	Variable	Yes	Yes	Free
Specialized Software for rehab	High	Variable	Yes	Yes	Yes	Variable

PD,[38] traumatic brain injury,[41] multiple sclerosis,[42] and orthopedics.[37,43,44]

Virtual Environments

A virtual environment or virtual world is a computer-generated environment in which a user can move and interact in such a way that they feel part of the scene. There are many different types of virtual environments, each relying on different technologies and infrastructure to immerse the user in the virtual world. These range from fully immersive "goggle-and-gloves" environments, where goggle-like head mount displays are fixed over the eyes of the user to immersive them fully in a virtual three-dimensional world and instrumented gloves, which allow the world to be manipulated in real-time; to desktop virtual environments, where two-dimensional environments are presented to the user on computer monitors. In a rehabilitation sense, virtual environments provide the opportunity for various sensory information (such as vision, hearing, or touch) to be manipulated such that a desired response (such as a motor, cognitive, social, or emotional response) is elicited from the user. Keshner[45] describes the opportunity of virtual environments for rehabilitation and notes that a virtual environment "provides the opportunity for ecological validity, stimulus control and consistency, real-time performance feedback, independent practice, stimulus and response modifications that are contingent on a user's physical abilities, a safe testing and training environment, the opportunity for graduated exposure to stimuli, the ability to distract or augment the performer's attention, and perhaps most important to therapeutic intervention, motivation for the performer."[45]

Virtual environments can provide a functional, purposeful, and motivating context to rehabilitation and have been extensively researched in client groups such as stroke where early intervention, task-oriented training, and dose intensity are critical elements. Research has demonstrated the potential of this technology to restore upper and lower extremity motor control,[46–49] hand and finger function,[50] gait,[47,51] balance,[52] wheelchair use,[53] cognition,[54,55] and spatial neglect,[56] among others.

The use of virtual environments for rehabilitation is likely to receive a significant boost from the consumer gaming market in which virtual reality (VR) headsets have seen a meteoric rise in popularity in 2016. These headsets vary from extremely low cost, cardboard viewers such as the Google VR (available for $15 USD) which use a smart phone to render the video element, to expensive offerings from Sony (PlayStation VR, $549.95 USD), Oculus (Oculus Rift, $599.00 USD), and HTC (HTC Vive, $799.00 USD). The VR gaming industry is now a $5 billion a year industry with a global audience of over 55 million users,[57] and the momentum generated from this will likely result in a greater diversity, availability, and complexity of rehabilitation applications.

Sensors and Asynchronous Technologies

The use of sensor technology to remotely monitor movement and physiological parameters of a client at a distance has always been attractive to providers of telerehabilitation services. These sensors can be sophisticated and specialized movement sensors, such as those designed to measure tremor, dyskinesia, and mobility in people with PD,[58] or simple low-cost and ubiquitous activity monitors such as the Fitbit (San Francisco, California). Sensors can provide great insight into the physiological and movement status of a remote client, which assists in their management via telerehabilitation.

The physiological, movement, or speech-related information that can be gathered from sensors can be used in several ways, depending on the nature of the service. For example, Theodoros et al.[38] describe a noninferiority randomized controlled trial in which the voice disorder associated with PD was managed via telerehabilitation. In this project, the telerehabilitation system was able to gather and relay sound pressure level information during a real-time telerehabilitation intervention in the home. The use of sensors to relay this information both informs the assessment process for these clients and enables the monitoring of the progress of clients during the telerehabilitation session.

Other applications have used the information provided by sensors in a more asynchronous manner. For example, De San Miguel et al.[59] conducted a randomized controlled trial to compare the outcomes of a telehealth monitoring group with a control group that received information only. This trial used sensors to collect and display vital sign information (blood pressure, weight, temperature, pulse, and oxygen saturation levels) and required participants to answer questions relating to their general state of health on a daily basis. This study demonstrated that sensor information, even when used outside of a clinical consultation context, was able to improve a participant's self-management and control over their condition.

The ubiquitous rise of the smart phone and tablets in the community has provided another avenue for the development of applications for rehabilitation. Mobile health applications, or m-health apps, experienced a growth of 57% in 2015, bringing the total number of health apps in the marketplace to over 250,000 globally available to the consumer.[60] In the rehabilitation sector these apps provide both diagnostic and intervention functions. For example, both the UHear (Unitron Hearing Limited, Kitchener, Canada) and Mimi Hearing Test (Mimi Hearing Technologies, Berlin, Germany) apps for iPhone provide the user with a self-directed hearing test. Others, such as the Wellpepper app (Wellpepper, Seattle, WA), enable rehabilitation clinicians to record and specify home exercise programs using a tablet computer. These exercises are displayed to the client as high-resolution video clips, and the app is able to monitor parameters such as pain and compliance with the exercise program and display this information back to the clinician through a client dashboard.

SELECTING TECHNOLOGIES

With a wide range of technology options available, it can be confusing when it comes to selecting the best technology for a new telerehabilitation service or intervention. The authors advocate the use of a four-step process to select an appropriate technology, which is based upon the specific tasks that are to be undertaken within the telerehabilitation session, the type of interaction between the client and the therapist (eg, real time or asynchronous), the stimulus material that may be required during the session and the desired responses that are required from the client (Figure 12-2). It is advisable to consider all the possible tasks over the course of an intervention, and this may be easier to do if well-defined treatment protocols are developed prior to selecting the telerehabilitation technology. Predefining the treatment protocol will ensure that the needs and requirements of the service drive the technology selection rather than the other way around. When considering the interaction with the client, it is important to be as widely inclusive as possible. For example, consider what will happen not only during the telerehabilitation session, but also consider how the technology may be used to support the client *between* telerehabilitation sessions.

An example of a telerehabilitation intervention is provided next to illustrate the four-step process. The telerehabilitation intervention is a home-based telerehabilitation service for clients who have undergone total

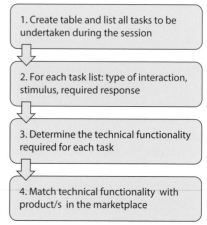

▲ **Figure 12-2.** Four-step task analysis process for selecting telerehabilitation technology.

Table 12-2. Task Analysis Table Outlining the Requirements of a Telerehabilitation Service for Clients Who Have Undergone Total Knee Arthroplasty

Task	Interaction	Stimuli	Client response	Technical function
Increase range of motion	Real-time	Instructions provided to patient via VC, video demonstration	Active movement, passive stretching	VC, media display, measurement (angles and linear distance)
Muscle strengthening	Real-time	Instructions provided to patient via VC, video demonstration of exercises	Performance of exercise	VC, media display, measurement
Management of swelling	Real-time	Instructions provided to patient via VC, video demonstration, education	Active movement, participation in discussion	VC, media display, measurement (linear distance), white board
Management of pain	Real-time	Education, media demonstrations	Participation in discussion	VC, media display, white board
Gait re-education	Real-time	Instructions provided to patient via VC, video demonstration of exercises	Walking perpendicular and parallel to camera	VC, media display, measurement (linear distance), white board
Home exercise Program	Asynchronous	Video demonstration of home-based exercises to complete between telerehabilitation sessions	Performance of exercises	Media display, diary of completed exercises, pain response to exercises

VC, videoconferencing.

knee arthroplasty. Following an acute postoperative period in hospital, clients return home and access rehabilitation care through telerehabilitation, with the aim of improving physical outcomes (such as knee range of motion and muscle strength) and functional outcomes (such as their ability to mobilize in the community and return to their day-to-day activities). Table 12-2 provides a list of all the tasks to be addressed with the clients via the telerehabilitation service. For this service, it is desirable that many of the tasks be completed in real time with the clients to enable the progression of exercises and the development of a specific treatment plan, which is customized to the needs of the client. However, it is also noted that there is a need for the client to independently complete a home exercise program between telerehabilitation sessions, and this is listed as a specific task in the table.

The stimulus column details the resources that are required for the consultation. For example, being able to provide instructions in real time via videoconferencing and the ability to show high-quality video clips to the patient during the consultation are both required to teach exercises to the patient and to demonstrate manual therapy techniques. The client response column

outlines the various responses that are expected from the client in response to the stimulus. In the majority of cases in this example, this involves the client performing manual therapy techniques on themselves or completing exercises. Finally, the technical function column outlines the functionality that would be required from a telerehabilitation platform to facilitate the performance of the task. For instance, real-time videoconferencing is highly desirable for many of the tasks in this example, along with the ability to play high-quality video clips and perform various measurements (such as the range of motion of the client's knee). Once these technical requirements are understood, an appropriate technology can be sourced from the market that best meets the needs of the service.

TELEREHABILITATION RESEARCH

Telerehabilitation is a relatively new discipline, with the first papers in the field emerging within the last 20 years. Similar to the development of literature in the broader field of telemedicine, the first few years of publication were characterized by studies with small sample sizes and low methodological rigor, resulting in the studies having low generalizability.[27] The quantity of research in the field of telerehabilitaiton has experienced a dramatic increase over the past 6 to 7 years with the number of papers rising over 500% between 2009 and 2016 (see Figure 12-3). This increase has been accompanied by a rise in the methodological quality of publications in the field. A PubMed search using the keyword "telerehabilitation" reveals a total of 483 papers published between 1998 and 2017. Figure 12-4 presents an overview of these papers categorized according to study type.

Early studies were primarily focused on the technical aspects of the field and opinions or discussions on the potential direction of the field. Prior to 2004 these papers represented approximately 70% of all published papers in the field. From 2004, the number of these papers has gradually reduced and now accounts for approximately 30% of the annual number of telerehabilitation papers. A reduction in the number of these papers has been associated with an increase in the number of higher-quality studies such as validity studies, cohort studies, and randomized controlled trials. In 2016, these papers represented 5%, 2.5%, and 14.5% of all papers, respectively. Since 2010, there has also been a dramatic rise in the number of systematic reviews and meta-analyses. In 2013–2015 there were an equal number of systematic reviews and randomized controlled trials published. Increases are also evident in studies primarily focused on the economics and sustainability of telerehabilitation and as telerehabilitation services

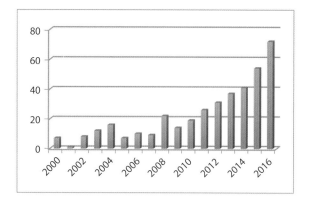

▲ **Figure 12-3.** Telerehabilitation publication count by year.

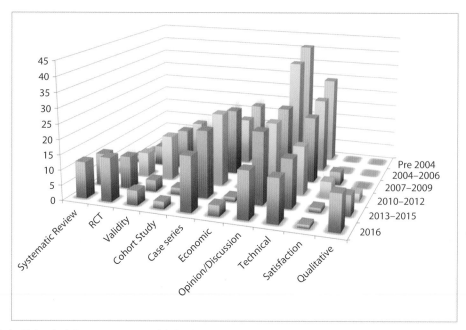

▲ **Figure 12-4.** Telerehabilitation papers published between 1998 and 2016 according to study type. Bars represent the percentage of papers in each category grouped by year.

emerge in the mainstream, qualitative studies investigating the client and clinician experience with telerehabilitation are becoming more prevalent. In 2016, these papers accounted for 12% of all published papers in the field. Interestingly, although many studies report elements of client satisfaction, there have generally been very few studies with this as the primary focus.

A total of 21 systematic reviews have been published covering many topics, including the telerehabilitation management of patients with stroke,[61,62] spinal cord injury,[63] low vision,[64] multiple sclerosis,[42,65] acquired brain injury,[66] aphasia,[67] autism,[39] neurological conditions,[68] cardiopulmonary disease,[69-71] and various orthopedic,[72] musculoskeletal,[73,74] and speech disorders.[11] In addition to these, systematic reviews that are more general in nature have been published focused on long-term conditions,[75] routine care,[76] recovery of motor function,[77] and postoperative care.[78] A summary of these studies, including the number and type of papers reviewed and the main outcomes and conclusions, is presented in Table 12-3.

Although many of these systematic reviews acknowledge a low to moderate level of evidence in the quality of the literature available, most conclude that telerehabilitation interventions produce clinical outcomes that are at least similar to usual care or control conditions. This appears to be true across the broad range of clinical conditions covered by the reviews. These results are overwhelmingly positive, as the goal of telerehabilitation applications is often to present a viable alternative for those where conventional in-person services are not available. Interestingly, a few of the systematic reviews, including some where large meta-analyses have been performed, have found that telerehabilitation can produce clinical outcomes that are in fact superior to conventional in-person services.

Of these 21 systematic reviews, 6 combined data from multiple studies to perform a meta-analysis on at least one outcomes measure. Chan et al.[69] combined the results of eight studies (782 participants) and analyzed aggregate data on peak oxygen consumption, peak workload, exercise test duration, and 6-minute walk test distance. This study concludes with a high level of confidence that no difference exists in exercise outcomes between usual care and telerehabilitation groups. They did, however, conclude that telerehabilitation exercise testing takes a statistically significantly longer duration to complete when compared to usual care.

Four of the systematic reviews completed to date have performed meta-analysis on the physical and functional outcomes achieved when using telerehabilitation to rehabilitate patients after total knee arthroplasty surgery. Two of these trials, Shukla et al.[79] and Cottrell et al.,[73] who reviewed three and four trials, respectively, found that pain, physical outcomes measures such as knee flexion, knee extension, quads strength, and satisfactions were equivalent between the telerehabilitation and control arms of the trials. These conclusions contrast with those of Jiang et al.[72] and Agostini et al.,[77] who reviewed four and three studies, respectively, and reported superior physical outcomes, including quadriceps strength, knee extension range of motion, and functional outcomes, on the Western Ontario and McMaster Universities Osteoarthritis Index favoring the telerehabilitation intervention.

Another meta-analysis that found results favoring the telerehabilitation intervention was reported in a study by Lundell et al.[71] This study investigated the effect of "telehealthcare" on physical activity levels, physical capacity, and dyspnea in clients with chronic obstructive pulmonary disease. "Telehealthcare" included management given via phone calls, websites or mobile platforms. Including only randomized controlled trails, a meta-analysis on the results of nine trials (982 patients) found a significant effect favoring telehealthcare over control group comparators on the outcome measures related to physical activity level. In addition, this paper found equivalent outcomes in physical capacity and dyspnea between the trial groups.

Although these systematic reviews support the efficacy of telerehabilitation interventions across a broad range of clinic settings, they must be interpreted with some caution. Rogante et al.[80] performed a quality assessment of 10 systematic reviews focused on telerehabilitation trials. They rated all papers according to the 11-item AMSTAR—Assessment of Multiple Systematic Reviews—checklist, which is designed to differentiate good-quality from poor-quality reviews. The median AMSTAR scores across the trials was 7 (interquartile range 4.5–8) with only 50% of systematic reviews achieving a score great than 8 indicating a high-quality review.

Table 12-3. Summary of Systematic Reviews Investigating the Efficacy of Telerehabilitation Interventions

Author (year)	Population	No. papers (participants)	Study types	Meta-analysis	Conclusions
Boisvert (2010)	Autism	8 (46)	7 Case study 1 Quasi-exp	No	low quality evidence † primary outcomes
Hailey (2011)	Routine care	61 (?)	–	No	71% studies successful 18% unsuccessful 51% clinically sig.
Johansson (2011)	Stroke	9 (724)	4 RCT 4 Obs 1 Qual	No	low quality evidence † motor function ✓ satisfaction ✓ QoL ✓ anxiety
Steel (2011)	Chronic conditions	35 (2684)	8 RCT 27 service eval, pilot, case studies	No	✓ psychological outcomes ✓ physical outcomes ✓ satisfaction ✓ therapeutic alliance
Dorstyn (2013)	Managing mental health following spinal cord injury	7 (272)	Quasi-exp	No	✓ pain and sleep ✓ QoL at 12 Mo ✓ time efficiency ✓ satisfaction
Hall (2013)	Aphasia	10 (153)	6 Single case 2 Crossover 1 RCT 1 Obs	No	† assessment outcomes † treatment outcomes
Laver (2013)	Stroke	10 (933)	RCT	No	insufficient evidence ✓ ADL ✓ UL function
Steins (2014)	Neurological populations	12 (522)	Validation	No	† type, quantity, quality measure of functional activities † discriminate nonhealthy/healthy
Agostini (2015)	Motor function recovery (neuro, ortho, cardiac)	12 (1047)	RCT	Yes	✓ neurological studies ✓✓ cardiac studies ✓✓ ortho studies
Amatya (2015) (Same study as Khan with extra papers)	Multiple sclerosis	12 (564)	10 RCT 2 Obs	No	low to mod evidence ✓ short-term disability ✓ fatigue ✓ functional activities ✓ symptoms ✓ QoL
Bittner (2015)	Low-vision	0	RCT CCT	No	Nil
Coleman (2015)	Acquired brain injury	10 (272)	Quasi-exp	No	† assessment outcomes † treatment outcomes
Hwang (2015)	Cardiopulmonary disease	11 (908)	RCT	No	✓ 6-min walk test ✓ peak 02 consumption QoL ✓ adherence

Table 12-3. Summary of Systematic Reviews Investigating the Efficacy of Telerehabilitation Interventions (*continued*)

Author (year)	Population	No. papers (participants)	Study types	Meta-analysis	Conclusions
Khan (2015)	Multiple sclerosis	9 (469)	RCT CCT	No	low quality evidence ✓ short-term disability ✓ fatigue ✓ functional activities ✓ participation
Lundell (2015)	Chronic obstructive pulmonary disease	9 (982)	RCT	Yes	✓✓ physical activity ✓ physical capacity ✓ dyspnea
Molini-Avejonas (2015)	Speech, language, and hearing science	103 (?)	-	No	† satisfaction
Chan (2016)	Cardiac and pulmonary rehabilitation	9 (782)	CCT	Yes	*Cardiac Rehab* ✓ peak oxygen ✓ peak workload ✓ 6-min walk test X test duration *Pulmonary Rehab* ✓ 6-min walk test
Cottrell (2016)	Musculoskeletal disorders	13 (1520)	RCT CCT	Yes	✓✓ physical function ✓ pain
Jiang (2016)	Total knee arthroplasty	4 (220)	RCT	Yes	✓ pain ✓ physical function ✓✓ WOMAC ✓✓ knee extension ✓✓ Quads strength
Mani (2016)	Musculoskeletal disorders	11 (?)	11 Validity	No	† concurrent validity † reliability (inter, intra) X lumbar spine posture X ortho special tests X neuro tests X scar mobilization
Shukla (2016)	Total knee arthroplasty	6 (408)	4 RCT 1 CCT 1 single arm	Yes	✓ satisfaction ✓ knee flexion ✓ knee extension ✓ physical ✓ functional
Van der Meij (2016)	Postoperative care	33 (3510)	22 RCT CCT	No	✓ physical function ✓ psychological outcomes ✓ general outcomes ✓ pain ✓ complications ✓ QoL ✓✓ satisfaction ✓✓ length of recovery

X Favors control; ✓ Telerehab equivalent; ✓✓ Favors telerehab; † Positive result (no comparison)

ADL, activities of daily living; CCT, clinical controlled trial; Eval, evaluation; Exp, experimental; Mo, month; O2, oxygen; Obs, observation; Ortho, orthopedic; Quads, quadriceps; Qual., quality; QoL, quality of life; RCT, randomized controlled trial; Sig, significant; UL, upper limb; WOMAC, Western Ontario and McMaster Universities Osteoarthritis Index.

PRACTICAL CONSIDERATIONS FOR THE IMPLEMENTATION OF A TELEREHABILITATION SERVICE

For clinicians considering the inclusion of telerehabilitation in their practice, numerous resources can be consulted to guide the development of a robust and sustainable service. The professional organizations that represent the members of each of the rehabilitation professions are an important place to start, as many have published position statements and guidelines on telerehabilitation practice. These position statements have been crafted to best address the needs of each discipline. Organizations including the American Physical Therapy Association,[5] the American Occupational Therapy Association,[81] the American Speech-Language-Hearing Association,[3] the American Psychological Association,[6] the Australian Physiotherapy Association,[2] and Speech Pathology Australia,[4] among others, have all released position papers with important professional and regional information. Where discipline-specific guidelines are not available, several general guidelines can be referred to which outline the various elements that must be considered when establishing a telerehabilitation service. These included the "blueprint for telerehabilitation guidelines" prepared by the American Telemedicine Association Special Interest Group for Telerehabilitation[1] and a policy digest provided by the Centre for Research Excellence in Telehealth.[82] These guidelines include elements such as licensure, security, privacy, reimbursement, and the appropriate selection of technology, among other topics. Such elements can have a major impact on the quality and sustainability of a telerehabilitation service and have many legal and practical implications. Table 12-4 provides a list of the most common core standards and guidelines which are addressed in position and policy statements from many discipline-specific organizations.

In addition to the resources listed earlier, the interested reader is directed to the Telerehabilitation Special Interest Group (SIG) of the American Telemedicine Association.[83] As the largest special interest group in telerehabilitation, this group aims to enhance access to rehabilitation services through the use of telehealth technologies. The special interest group includes occupational therapists, physical therapists, speech-language pathologists, rehabilitation engineers,

Table 12-4. Core Standards and Guidelines in Telerehabilitation

Core Standard and Guideline	Description
Adherence to professional code of ethics and scope of practice	Applicable to each discipline
Adherence to institutional, state, federal, and international country laws	• Licensure • Security • Privacy • Reimbursement
Selection of appropriate technologies "fit for purpose" and of high quality	• Hardware • Software • Peripheral devices • Connectivity • Technical support
Client selection	• Based on clinical reasoning • Consideration of physical and sensory, cognitive, behavioral, communication characteristics, and motivation • Client supports
Client safety	Necessary supports at client end to ensure safety during telepractice session
Clinician education and professional development in telepractice	Achieve competency in telepractice
Telepractice underpinned by evidence-based practice	At least equivalent to standard care
Modification to assessment and treatment materials	Identify and create adaptations to materials for delivery via telepractice
Environment for telepractice	• Must be conducive to telepractice • Clinician and client end • Room location, lighting, etc.
Stakeholder support	• Need to enlist support of all stakeholders • Knowledge translation process

assistive technologists, rehabilitation physicians, audiologists, educators, rehabilitation nurses, neuropsychologists, disability specialists, policy experts, and telehealth agencies. The SIG includes three subcommittees devoted to research and education, policy and coding, and outreach and is an excellent resource for finding out more information and seeking advice when establishing a telerehabilitation service.

REFERENCES

1. Brennan DM, Tindall L, Theodoros D, et al. A blueprint for telerehabilitation guidelines. *Telemed J E Health* 2011;17(8):662–665.

2. APA. *Telerehabilitation Position Statement*. 2009; https://www.physiotherapy.asn.au/DocumentsFolder/Advocacy_Position_Telerehabilitation_2009.pdf. Accessed March 2017.

3. ASHA. *Speech-Language Pathologists Providing Clinical Services via Telepractice: Position Statement*. 2005. www.asha.org/policy. Accessed March 2017.

4. SPA. *Telepractice in Speech Pathology Position Statement*. 2014. http://www.speechpathologyaustralia.org.au/spaweb/Document_Management/Public/Position_Statements.aspx. Accessed March 2017.

5. APTA. *Telehealth*. 2012. http://www.apta.org/uploadedFiles/APTAorg/About_Us/Policies/Practice/TelehealthDefinitionsGuidelines.pdf. Accessed March 2017.

6. APA. *Guidelines for the Practice of Telepsychology*. 2013. http://www.apapracticecentral.org/ce/guidelines/telepsychology-guidelines.pdf. Accessed March 2017.

7. WHO. *International Classification of Functioning, Disability and Health (ICF)*. 2001. http://www.who.int/classifications/icf/en/. Accessed March 2017.

8. Winters JM, Winters JM. A telehomecare model for optimizing rehabilitation outcomes. *Telemed J E Health* 2004;10(2):200–212.

9. Burns CL, Ward EC, Hill AJ, et al. A pilot trial of a speech pathology telehealth service for head and neck cancer patients. *J Telemed Telecare* 2012;18(8):443–446.

10. Chen J, Jin W, Zhang XX, et al. Telerehabilitation approaches for stroke patients: systematic review and meta-analysis of randomized controlled trials. *J Stroke Cerebrovasc Dis* 2015;24(12):2660–2668.

11. Molini-Avejonas DR, Rondon-Melo S, Amato CA, Samelli AG. A systematic review of the use of telehealth in speech, language and hearing sciences. *J Telemed Telecare* 2015;21(7):367–376.

12. Kraal JJ, Peek N, van den Akker-Van Marle ME, Kemps HM. Effects and costs of home-based training with tele-monitoring guidance in low to moderate risk patients entering cardiac rehabilitation: the FIT@Home study. *BMC Cardiovasc Disord* 2013;13:82.

13. Anton D, Nelson M, Russell T, et al. Validation of a Kinect-based telerehabilitation system with total hip replacement patients. *J Telemed Telecare*. 2016;22(3):192–197.

14. Fink RB, Brecher A, Sobel P, Schwartz MF. Computer-assisted treatment of word retrieval deficits in aphasia. *Aphasiology* 2005;19:943–954.

15. Laganaro M, Di Pietro M, Schnider A. Computerised treatment of anomia in acute aphasia: treatment intensity and training size. *Neuropsychol Rehabil* 2006;16(6):630–640.

16. Mortley J, Wade L, Enderby P. Superhighway to promoting a client-therapist partnership? Using the internet to deliver word-retrieval computer therapy, monitored remotely with minimal speech and language therapy input. *Aphasiology* 2004;18:193–211.

17. McCue M, Fairman A, Pramuka M. Enhancing quality of life through telerehabilitation. *Phys Med Rehabil Clin N Am* 2010;21(1):195–205.

18. Geddes JM, Chamberlain MA. Home-based rehabilitation for people with stroke: a comparative study of six community services providing co-ordinated, multidisciplinary treatment. *Clin Rehabil* 2001;15(6):589–599.

19. Anderson C, Mhurchu CN, Rubenach S, et al. Home or hospital for stroke rehabilitation? Results of a randomized controlled trial: II: cost minimization analysis at 6 months. *Stroke* 2000;31(5):1032–1037.

20. Hillier S, Inglis-Jassiem G. Rehabilitation for community-dwelling people with stroke: home or centre based? A systematic review. *Int J Stroke* 2010;5(3):178–186.

21. Weiss Z, Snir D, Zohar R, Klein N, et al. Allocation and preference of patient for domiciliary or institutional rehabilitation after stroke. *Int J Rehabil Res* 2004;27(2):155–158.

22. Kahana E, Kahana B. Baby boomers' expectations of health and medicine. *Virtual Mentor* 2014;16(5):380–384.

23. Morris J, Mueller J, Jones M. Tomorrow's elders with disabilities: what the wireless industry needs to know. *J Eng Design* 2010;21:131–146.

24. Liddle J, Gustafsson L, Bartlett H, McKenna K. Time use, role participation and life satisfaction of older people: impact of driving status. *Aust Occup Ther J* 2012;59(5):384–392.

25. Hoaas H, Andreassen HK, Lien LA, et al. Adherence and factors affecting satisfaction in long-term telerehabilitation for patients with chronic obstructive pulmonary disease: a mixed methods study. *BMC Med Inform Decis Mak* 2016;16:26.

26. Levy CE, Silverman E, Jia H, et al. Effects of physical therapy delivery via home video telerehabilitation on functional and health-related quality of life outcomes. *J Rehabil Res Dev* 2015;52(3):361–370.

27. Theodoros D, Russell T. Telerehabilitation: current perspectives. *Stud Health Technol Inform* 2008;131:191–209.

28. Hoffmann T, Russell T, Thompson L, et al. Using the Internet to assess activities of daily living and hand function in people with Parkinson's disease. *NeuroRehabilitation* 2008;23(3):253–261.

29. Russell TG, Hoffmann TC, Nelson M, et al. Internet-based physical assessment of people with Parkinson disease is accurate and reliable: a pilot study. *J Rehabil Res Dev* 2013;50(5):643–650.

30. Ward EC, Sharma S, Burns C, et al. Validity of conducting clinical dysphagia assessments for patients with normal to mild cognitive impairment via telerehabilitation. *Dysphagia* 2012;27(4):460–472.

31. Kelly JT, Reidlinger DP, Hoffmann TC, Campbell KL. Telehealth methods to deliver dietary interventions in adults with chronic disease: a systematic review and meta-analysis. *Am J Clin Nutr* 2016;104(6):1693–1702.

32. Stubbings DR, Rees CS, Roberts LD, Kane RT. Comparing in-person to videoconference-based cognitive behavioral therapy for mood and anxiety disorders: randomized controlled trial. *J Med Internet Res* 2013;15(11):e258.

33. Pramuka M, van Roosmalen L. Telerehabilitation technologies: accessibility and usability. *Int J Telerehabil* 2009;1(1):85–98.

34. Rogante M, Grigioni M, Cordella D, Giacomozzi C. Ten years of telerehabilitation: a literature overview of technologies and clinical applications. *NeuroRehabilitation* 2010;27(4):287–304.

35. Delaplain CB, Lindborg CE, Norton SA, Hastings JE (1993). Tripler pioneers telemedicine across the Pacific. *Hawaii Medical Journal* 1993; 52(12), 338–339.

36. Sunrise. *Information about the Discontinuation of ISDN Calling by the 31.12.2017.* 2017. https://www.sunrise.ch/content/dam/sunrise/business/telefonie/abschaltung-isdn-und-analog-telefonie/information-sheet-iscontinuation-isdn-calling.pdf. Accessed March 2017.

37. Russell TG, Buttrum P, Wootton R, Jull GA. Internet-based outpatient telerehabilitation for patients following total knee arthroplasty: a randomized controlled trial. *J Bone Joint Surg Am* 2011;93(2):113–120.

38. Theodoros DG, Hill AJ, Russell TG. Clinical and quality of life outcomes of speech treatment for Parkinson's disease delivered to the home via telerehabilitation: a noninferiority randomized controlled trial. *Am J Speech Lang Pathol* 2016;25(2):214–232.

39. Boisvert M, Lang R, Andrianopoulos M, Boscardin ML. Telepractice in the assessment and treatment of individuals with autism spectrum disorders: a systematic review. *Dev Neurorehabil* 2010;13(6):423–432.

40. Huijgen BC, Vollenbroek-Hutten MM, Zampolini M. Feasibility of a home-based telerehabilitation system compared to usual care: arm/hand function in patients with stroke, traumatic brain injury and multiple sclerosis. *J Telemed Telecare* 2008;14(5):249–256.

41. Ng EM, Polatajko HJ, Marziali E, et al. Telerehabilitation for addressing executive dysfunction after traumatic brain injury. *Brain Inj* 2013;27(5):548–564.

42. Khan F, Amatya B, Kesselring J, Galea M. Telerehabilitation for persons with multiple sclerosis. *Cochrane Database Syst Rev* 2015;4:CD010508.

43. Eriksson L, Lindstrom B, Gard G, Lysholm J. Physiotherapy at a distance: a controlled study of rehabilitation at home after a shoulder joint operation. *J Telemed Telecare* 2009;15(5):215–220.

44. Moffet H, Tousignant M, Nadeau S, et al. In-home telerehabilitation compared with face-to-face rehabilitation after total knee arthroplasty: a noninferiority randomized controlled trial. *J Bone Joint Surg Am* 2015;97(14):1129–1141.

45. Keshner EA. Virtual reality and physical rehabilitation: a new toy or a new research and rehabilitation tool? *J Neuroeng Rehabil* 2004;1(1):8.

46. Lucca LF. Virtual reality and motor rehabilitation of the upper limb after stroke: a generation of progress? *J Rehabil Med* 2009;41(12):1003–1100.

47. Mirelman A, Patritti BL, Bonato P, Deutsch JE. Effects of virtual reality training on gait biomechanics of individuals post-stroke. *Gait Posture* 2010;31(4):433–437.

48. Piron L, Turolla A, Agostini M, et al. Exercises for paretic upper limb after stroke: a combined virtual-reality and telemedicine approach. *J Rehabil Med* 2009;41(12):1016–1102.

49. Turolla A, Dam M, Ventura L, et al. Virtual reality for the rehabilitation of the upper limb motor function after stroke: a prospective controlled trial. *J Neuroeng Rehabil* 2013;10:85.

50. Merians AS, Tunik E, Adamovich SV. Virtual reality to maximize function for hand and arm rehabilitation: exploration of neural mechanisms. *Stud Health Technol Inform* 2009;145:109–125.

51. Baram Y, Aharon-Peretz J, Lenger R. Virtual reality feedback for gait improvement in patients with idiopathic senile gait disorders and patients with history of stroke. *J Am Geriatr Soc* 2010;58(1):191–192.

52. In T, Lee K, Song C. Virtual reality reflection therapy improves balance and gait in patients with chronic stroke: randomized controlled trials. *Med Sci Monit* 2016;22:4046–4053.

53. Buxbaum LJ, Palermo MA, Mastrogiovanni D, et al. Assessment of spatial attention and neglect with a virtual wheelchair navigation task. *J Clin Exp Neuropsychol* 2008;30(6):650–660.

54. Kang YJ, Ku J, Han K, et al. Development and clinical trial of virtual reality-based cognitive assessment in people with stroke: preliminary study. *Cyberpsychol Behav* 2008;11(3):329–339.

55. Kim BR, Chun MH, Kim LS, Park JY. Effect of virtual reality on cognition in stroke patients. *Ann Rehabil Med* 2011;35(4):450–459.

56. Ogourtsova T, Souza Silva W, Archambault PS, Lamontagne A. Virtual reality treatment and assessments for post-stroke unilateral spatial neglect: a

systematic literature review. *Neuropsychol Rehabil* 2017;27(3):409–454.

57. Fortune. *Virtual Reality Video Games Industry to Generate $5.1 Billion in 2016*. 2016. http://fortune.com/2016/01/05/virtual-reality-game-industry-to-generate-billions/. Accessed March 2017.

58. Great Lakes Neurotechnologies. *Kinesia 360*. 2017. http://glneurotech.com/kinesia/products/kinesia-360/. Accessed March 2017.

59. De San Miguel K, Smith J, Lewin G. Telehealth remote monitoring for community-dwelling older adults with chronic obstructive pulmonary disease. *Telemed J E Health* 2013;19(9):652–657.

60. Research 2 Guidance. *mHealth App Developer Economics 2016*. 2016. http://research2guidance.com/product/mhealth-app-developer-economics-2016/. Accessed March 2017.

61. Johansson T, Wild C. Telerehabilitation in stroke care: -a systematic review. *J Telemed Telecare* 2011;17(1):1–6.

62. Laver KE, Schoene D, Crotty M, et al. Telerehabilitation services for stroke. *Cochrane Database Syst Rev* 2013;12:CD010255. doi: 10.1002/14651858.CD010255.pub2

63. Dorstyn D, Mathias J, Denson L. Applications of telecounselling in spinal cord injury rehabilitation: a systematic review with effect sizes. *Clin Rehabil.* 2013;27(12):1072–1083.

64. Bittner AK, Wykstra SL, Yoshinaga PD, Li T. Telerehabilitation for people with low vision. *Cochrane Database Syst Rev* 2015;8:CD011019.

65. Amatya B, Galea MP, Kesselring J, Khan F. Effectiveness of telerehabilitation interventions in persons with multiple sclerosis: a systematic review. *Mult Scler Relat Disord* 2015;4(4):358–369.

66. Coleman JJ, Frymark T, Franceschini NM, Theodoros DG. Assessment and treatment of cognition and communication skills in adults with acquired brain injury via telepractice: a systematic review. *Am J Speech Lang Pathol* 2015;24(2):295–315.

67. Hall N, Boisvert M, Steele R. Telepractice in the assessment and treatment of individuals with aphasia: a systematic review. *Int J Telerehabil* 2013;5(1):27–38.

68. Steins D, Dawes H, Esser P, Collett J. Wearable accelerometry-based technology capable of assessing functional activities in neurological populations in community settings: a systematic review. *J Neuroeng Rehabil* 2014;11:36.

69. Chan C, Yamabayashi C, Syed N, et al. Exercise telemonitoring and telerehabilitation compared with traditional cardiac and pulmonary rehabilitation: a systematic review and meta-analysis. *Physiother Can* 2016; 68(3):242–251.

70. Hwang R, Bruning J, Morris N, et al. A systematic review of the effects of telerehabilitation in patients with cardiopulmonary diseases. *J Cardiopulm Rehabil Prev* 2015;35(6):380–389.

71. Lundell S, Holmner A, Rehn B, et al. Telehealthcare in COPD: A systematic review and meta-analysis on physical outcomes and dyspnea. *Respir Med* 2015;109(1):11–26.

72. Jiang S, Xiang J, Gao X, Guo K, Liu B. The comparison of telerehabilitation and face-to-face rehabilitation after total knee arthroplasty: a systematic review and meta-analysis. *J Telemed Telecare*. 2016 Jan 1:1357633X16686748. doi: 10.1177/1357633X16686748. [Epub ahead of print].

73. Cottrell MA, Galea OA, O'Leary SP, et al. Real-time telerehabilitation for the treatment of musculoskeletal conditions is effective and comparable to standard practice: a systematic review and meta-analysis. *Clin Rehabil* 2017;31(5):625–638.

74. Mani S, Sharma S, Omar B, et al. Validity and reliability of Internet-based physiotherapy assessment for musculoskeletal disorders: a systematic review. *J Telemed Telecare* 2017;23(3):379–391.

75. Steel K, Cox D, Garry H. Therapeutic videoconferencing interventions for the treatment of long-term conditions. *J Telemed Telecare* 2011;17(3):109–117.

76. Hailey D, Roine R, Ohinmaa A, Dennett L. Evidence of benefit from telerehabilitation in routine care: a systematic review. *J Telemed Telecare* 2011;17(6):281–287.

77. Agostini M, Moja L, Banzi R, et al. Telerehabilitation and recovery of motor function: a systematic review and meta-analysis. *J Telemed Telecare* 2015;21(4):202–213.

78. van der Meij E, Anema JR, Otten RH, et al. The effect of perioperative e-health interventions on the postoperative course: a systematic review of randomised and non-randomised controlled trials. *PLoS One* 2016;11(7):e0158612.

79. Shukla H, Nair SR, Thakker D. Role of telerehabilitation in patients following total knee arthroplasty: evidence from a systematic literature review and meta-analysis. *J Telemed Telecare* 2017;23(2):339–346.

80. Rogante M, Kairy D, Giacomozzi C, Grigioni M. A quality assessment of systematic reviews on telerehabilitation: what does the evidence tell us? *Ann Ist Super Sanita* 2015;51(1):11–18.

81. AOTA. Telerehabilitation. *Am J Occup Ther* 2010; 64:S92–S102.

82. CRE Telehealth. Policy Digest. 2016. http://www.cretelehealth.org.au/policy-digest. Accessed March 2017.

83. ATA TR SIG. *Telerehabilitation SIG*. 2017. http://www.americantelemed.org/main/membership/ata-members/ata-sigs/telerehabilitation-sig. Accessed March 2017.

Clinical Services—Pediatric

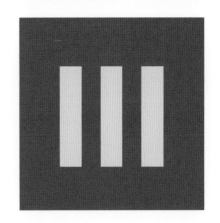

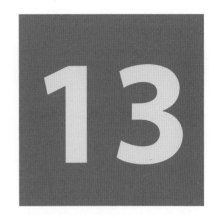

Pediatric Emergency and Critical Care Telehealth

Alison L. Curfman, MD and
James P. Marcin, MD, MPH

CASE STUDY 1

A 7-year-old boy is found unresponsive at the bottom of a swimming pool. Cardiopulmonary resuscitation is initiated by first responders, and the child is rushed to the closest hospital. The internal medicine physician covering the emergency department (ED) at this critical access hospital has limited experience with critically ill children. Upon arrival, the staff continues resuscitation and immediately activates a pediatric tele-emergency consultation. Within a minute, a pediatric emergency medicine physician from the regional pediatric quaternary care center is connected to the bedside with telemedicine, with high-quality audiovisual communications, ready to assist the team. With the expert guidance and teamwork, the resuscitation is successful, and the child is transported to the regional pediatric hospital for definitive care.

CASE STUDY 2

A 4-year-old girl with a history of asthma presents to a community hospital ED in respiratory distress. The physician administers IV steroids and initiates breathing treatments, but it becomes clear that the patient needs hospital admission and close observation. Previously, a child on continuous albuterol would need to be transported several hours to the closest pediatric intensive care unit (ICU), but with a remote monitoring program in place, the child is
admitted to the local community hospital with 24/7 monitoring by a pediatric critical care physician. With this collaborative treatment between the bedside team of respiratory therapists, nurses and physicians, and the telemedicine team, the child improves and after 3 days is able to go home. An expensive, risky interfacility transfer was avoided, and the patient received high-quality pediatric care in her home town, which provided good outcomes and patient-and-family-centered care.

CASE STUDY 3

A 6-month-old with a diffuse rash presents to a small rural ED. The general emergency medicine physician has seen many rashes, but never one like this. The child is otherwise well appearing, but the physician does not feel comfortable making a diagnosis. Previously, he would have transferred the child 4 hours to the closest pediatric referral center, but with their telemedicine program, she is able to activate a consultation with a pediatric emergency medicine physician. The remote physician takes a full history and performs a physical exam and is able to efficiently diagnose and treat the child without the patient ever leaving their hometown.

INTRODUCTION

Each of these scenarios illustrates how the use of telemedicine by pediatric emergency and critical care clinicians can address disparities in timely access to care, improve clinical outcomes, and reduce health care costs, all while improving the quality of care delivered to children.

According to the 2010 Census, rural areas of the United States are home to nearly 20% of the population. As a result, many children face significant access barriers to important pediatric health services.[1,2] These barriers include geographic challenges for families living in rural communities, a relative shortage and maldistribution of general pediatricians and pediatric subspecialists, and social and economic barriers that make it difficult to travel to locations where pediatric health services are provided. Primary care pediatricians working in rural communities also report greater barriers in accessing subspecialty care compared to other providers.[3] These barriers and differential access to pediatric care are at least partly to blame for disparities in health outcomes, particularly for children with special health care needs living in underserved, rural communities.[4] Children with suboptimal access to care have been shown to more frequently forgo visits to pediatric subspecialists and to rely more heavily on the ED for care.[5,6]

For critically ill children where access to expertise is urgent, these health care disparities can mean the difference between life and death. The care provided in the ICU is increasingly complex and requires state-of-the-art facilities, the most modern technologies, and a comprehensive team of specially trained multidisciplinary providers and ancillary personnel. As a result, care of ICU patients has become more complicated, and patients are increasingly exposed to failures in the care delivery that result in mistakes, complications, and even death. In fact, it is estimated that on average, every patient admitted to an average U.S. ICU experiences 1.7 potentially life-threatening errors each day, and each year some 50,000 patients die from preventable deaths.[7]

In the past two decades, two major health system factors have been identified that maximize the chances of high-quality care and minimize risks of mistakes and complications in the ICU. The first factor is the regionalization of specialty ICU services. ICU regionalization is a means of concentrating medical expertise and increasing patient volumes at designated referral and tertiary care hospitals. Higher patient volumes often result in increased care efficiency and improved patient outcomes. Well-known examples include the regionalization of trauma, specialty surgical procedures, adult critical care, and neonatal and pediatric intensive care.[8–14]

The second factor shown to improve outcomes and quality of care in the ICU is to ensure that all patients are actively cared for by critical care physicians. In both adult and pediatric ICUs, research demonstrates that critically ill patients have a lower risk of death, shorter ICU and hospital length of stay, and receive higher-quality care when critical care physicians are involved in their management.[15–18] In fact, researchers estimate that ICU mortality is reduced by some 10% to 25% when critical care physicians direct patient care compared to ICUs, where critical care physicians have little to no involvement in patient care.[15,18]

Unfortunately, not all critically ill patients are cared for in regionalized ICUs, nor are they uniformly treated by critical care physicians. Although regionalization improves patient care, by its design it also creates disparities in access. For example, Figure 13-1 shows a map of the United States with the geographical region surrounding the children's hospitals registered with the Children's Hospital Association; those living in the shaded area are within a one-hour drive of a regionalized children's hospital, and those living outside the shaded area live more than one hour from a regionalized children's hospital. Using census data from 2016 and an estimated total U.S. population of 322,431,073, the total pediatric population (age less than 18 years) that live within the shaded area is 57,244,788, or 77.3% of the total pediatric population, and the total pediatric population living outside the shaded area (and residing more than 60 minutes from a children's hospital) is 16,810,409, or 22.7% of the total pediatric population.

Acutely ill patients living in nonurban areas are by necessity treated and cared for in hospitals that lack full pediatric ICU (PICU) services and critical care expertise,[19] resulting in risk of both delays in care and inappropriate care.[20,21] Magnifying this problem is the continued shortages of critical care physicians for both adult and PICUs, which is expected to worsen in future years.[22,23]

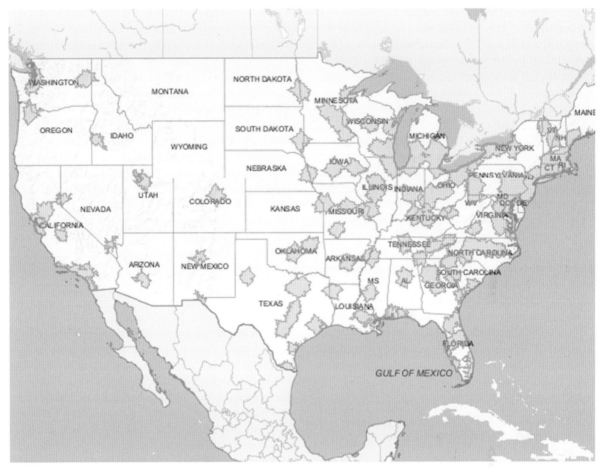

▲ **Figure 13-1.** A map of the United States with the geographic region surrounding the children's hospitals registered with the Children's Hospital Association. Those living in the shaded area are within a one-hour drive of a regionalized children's hospital, and those living outside the shaded area live more than one hour from a regionalized children's hospital.

TELEMEDICINE AS A SOLUTION

Telemedicine is defined as the provision of health care over a distance using telecommunications technologies. It can be used to supplement efforts to both maintain the regionalization of ICU services and help specially trained critical care physicians participate in the care of critically ill patients in other locations. Telemedicine technologies can be used to more efficiently increase access to specialty care services, including critical care physicians, to patients living in underserved and remote communities and in community hospitals where the full spectrum of ICU and critical care services are not available.[24,25] By importing specialty expertise using telemedicine, EDs, inpatient wards, and intensive care units are given the means to increase their capacity to provide a higher quality of care to critically ill patients. Critical care physicians can also increase their efficiency with these technologies so that their expertise can be shared with more patients at more than one ICU or hospital at a time. In addition, telemedicine use can potentially reduce patient transfers of less severely ill and injured children to referral centers, thus reserving limited ICU beds to those most in need of care at a regionalized center.[26,27] For these reasons, use of telemedicine in pediatric emergency and critical care is increasing and is expected to become a technology that most centers will use in future practice.

Although telemedicine can be part of the solution to disparities in access to critical care physicians and specialized care, it is not meant to obviate the transfer of critically ill patients in need of services at a regional ICU, nor is it meant to replace an onsite critical care physician. Instead, as numerous clinical programs across the country have demonstrated, critical care providers can use telemedicine and remote monitoring technologies to immediately share their expertise in a variety of clinical scenarios.

In this chapter, we review how telemedicine can be used by pediatric emergency and critical care physicians. Specifically, we review how telemedicine can be used in remote hospital EDs during the transport of critically ill children, in hospital inpatient wards, and in remote ICUs where pediatric critical care specialists are not immediately available.

MODELS OF USE

▶ Telemedicine for Critically Ill Children Presenting to Remote Hospitals

It is well documented that critically ill children presenting to EDs without pediatric expertise receive a lower quality of care compared with those receiving care provided in EDs with that expertise.[20,28–31] Many of these EDs are at times inadequately equipped to care for pediatric emergencies.[28,31–37] In addition, the staff working in smaller, general EDs—including physicians, nurses, pharmacists, and support staff—are often less experienced in caring for critically ill children and may do so infrequently. The combined inherent stresses of caring for a critically ill child with this lack of equipment, infrastructure, and experienced personnel can result in delayed or incorrect diagnoses, suboptimal therapies, and imperfect medical management.[17,20,38,39] As a consequence, acutely ill or injured children often receive a lower quality of care than children presenting to EDs in regionalized children's hospitals.[20,40–43] This is succinctly reflected in the aphorism that children are not just little adults.

The use of telemedicine technologies for disaster victims[44] or in remote or underserved EDs can be a means of obtaining subspecialty expert consultation.[45–51] Telemedicine has also been shown to be a feasible method of providing specialty expertise from the United States internationally, namely to augment the care of children with congenital heart disease.[52,53] The benefit of using this technology as opposed to using the telephone (the current standard of care) is that the consultant (ie, the pediatric critical care physician) has the ability to have a virtual presence at the patient's bedside. The consultant has full control of the remote camera, including movement about the room and high-resolution zoom, allowing access to high-definition video views of the patient, the treating providers, and the family, as well as monitors and other medical equipment.

▶ Telemedicine During Transport of Critically Ill Pediatric Patients

The use of telemedicine by physicians to assist in the care of critically ill patients during transport has the potential to improve processes of care at several levels. For example, telemedicine allows physicians to be an immediate part of the monitoring, identification, and management of changes in the patient's status that occur during transport. With more immediate physician supervision using telemedicine, medical decisions, including new medication orders, have the potential to occur more rapidly and efficiently than without direct physician supervision.

At present, mobile telephone technologies are used to transmit two-way audio as well as data, including electrocardiogram data. However, to create a model of care that uses telemedicine during transport, much more robust mobile broadband telecommunications are needed. Only a few transport programs in the United States use these technologies because high-quality broadband mobile telecommunication is expensive and not always or easily available,[54] particularly if continuous video transmission or large amounts of data streaming is desired. Common methods of transmitting video include the use of high-fidelity cell phone services (sometimes combining several cell phone lines) and the use of the Internet, which can be available with citywide WiFi or satellite services.[55,56] Although satellite technologies can be used to provide mobile telemedicine connections, this technology is most often prohibitively expensive.

There have been anecdotal reports documenting the feasibility of cell phone and WiFi transmitted telemedicine consultations during transport. In one study, the outcomes of adult patients with simulated trauma were compared among scenarios that used telemedicine and scenarios that used telephone communications during transport.[57] Use of telemedicine resulted in a reduction in adverse clinical events, including fewer episodes of desaturation and hypotension and less tachycardia, compared with identical simulated patients without telemedicine use. In addition, recognition rates for key physiologic signs and the need for critical interventions were higher in the transport simulations that used telemedicine.[57] These data are encouraging and support the possibility that telemedicine can be used during patient transport. However, until more reliable and affordable mobile telecommunications are available to implement telemedicine during transport and until more research is conducted on the impact that telemedicine has during transport and on workflow, the effectiveness and benefit of this technology remain undetermined.

▶ Critical Care Telemedicine Consultations for Hospitalized Children

Pediatric critical care services are more regionalized and less available than adult critical care services. Therefore children living in nonurban communities who may need critical care services are often transported to a pediatric ICU, exposing them to the inherent risks and costs. At times, pediatric patients who are not critically ill are overtriaged and transferred to the regional center, because there may be a need for the specialty services provided by the pediatric ICU.[58] Adding to this inefficiency, regionalized quaternary pediatric ICUs frequently run at full capacity. The transfer of some pediatric patients to a quaternary pediatric referral center is often not necessary if there is a closer hospital with adequate pediatric capabilities, such as a level II or community pediatric ICU, an intermediate or step-down pediatric care unit, or a general ICU with pediatric expertise.[59]

Admitting some of the less ill children to hospitals other than regional quaternary referral centers can result in a high quality of care provided with shorter length of stays, less resource use, and lower costs.[60–62] It is therefore logical that some mildly or moderately ill children (eg, children with asthma who require continuous albuterol or children with known diabetes and mild diabetic ketoacidosis) can be cared for in level II or community pediatric ICUs or other non-children's hospital ICUs under the care of pediatric nurses and physicians with supervision from a regional children's hospital pediatric critical care team using telemedicine and remote monitoring.[63]

Telemedicine can be used by pediatric critical care clinicians using a broad range of applications to assist in the care of hospitalized children in a variety of clinical scenarios.[64] Physician consultations, nurse and physician monitoring, and medical oversight can range from a simple model of intermittent, need-based consultations (*reactive model*) to a model that integrates continuous oversight via monitoring and proactive medical decision making (*continuous model*).[65] In a reactive model, a pediatric critical care physician can provide bedside telemedicine consultations to patients in remote EDs, inpatient wards, high-acuity units, or ICUs. Such consultations could prompt a variety of clinical interventions, including recommendations on diagnostic studies, medications, or other therapies. The consultation may also conclude the need to transport the patient to the regional pediatric ICU. This type of model could result in a range of interventions from a one-time consultation to multiple videoconferencing interactions during the course of the day or hospital stay.[66,67]

In the continuous model, oversight by critical care physicians and nurses is provided by telemedicine in combination with comprehensive electronic remote monitoring. In such a model, a remote team of physicians and nurses is able to monitor many patient beds, often covering several ICUs. This continuous oversight model of telemedicine is more proactive with medical interventions and often involves nontelemedicine guidelines such as the implementation of evidence-based protocols. This electronic ICU is created by centralizing electronic health records, ICU monitoring technologies, and nurse/physician video oversight. Tele-ICUs can be created internally by large health systems or can be contracted out to third-party technology and physician organizations that specialize in remote ICU monitoring services.

There is a trend within pediatric critical care toward 24-hour in-house attending-level coverage, but many pediatric ICUs continue to use a system of overnight coverage by trainees at the bedside, with attending backup from home. Another novel use of telemedicine allows at-home pediatric ICU physicians to connect to the ICU at night to assist the onsite team in a reactive mode.[68] This method has been shown to be feasible, although it has not been rigorously assessed with regard to quality. The reactive telemedicine model has also been reported by other pediatric specialists to provide inpatient consultations, including cardiology consultations and ethics consultations.[69,70]

TECHNOLOGIES

Telemedicine ICU consultations involve real-time, interactive, high-definition video and audio communication between the specialist at the regional children's hospital and health care provider at the remote hospital. Therefore, in developing a telemedicine program that originates from a children's hospital, there are many technical challenges to address, considering the goal is to provide 24/7 immediate assistance to critically ill infants and children. It is a requirement to have on-call systems for both clinicians and the technical personnel at both the remote and regional ED and ICU.

Telecommunication lines need to be reliable and have adequate bandwidth to maintain quality of service. In the past, this required the use of dedicated telecommunication lines, such as complete or fractionated T1 lines, Integrated Services Digital Network (ISDN), or some other private networking telecommunication systems. Currently, however, the Internet is more often used, as the connection speeds and audio-video quality have become more reliable. Further, modifications to allow encryption need to be made so that the communications are compliant with the Health Insurance Portability and Accountability Act (HIPAA). A common solution to this is built-in videoconferencing unit encryption, the use of private networks, and/or establishing a virtual private network (VPN) tunnel. Careful consideration of the telemedicine imaging equipment is also needed. Remotely controlled videoconferencing devices offer a range of quality and can be ceiling mounted, wall mounted, pole mounted, or even mounted on mobile robotic platforms. Peripheral devices, such as high-resolution exam cameras, stethoscopes, otoscopes, and ophthalmoscopes, are available; however, it may be easier to have the remote physician or nurse describe physical findings, such as pupillary responses, than to have a remote operator use the camera. In the continuous oversight telemedicine models, the connections for live cardiorespiratory and pressure monitors are needed, as well as the option for live monitoring of ventilators or other devices. In some cases where these monitoring systems are not used, as in the consultative model, a remotely controlled video camera can be directed for close-up, real-time monitor visualization and other equipment with interpretations similar to physical bedside interpretations.

SUMMARY OF EVIDENCE

Previous studies have shown that the use of telemedicine in the ED to deliver consultations is similar to in-person consultations in terms of diagnostic accuracy, treatment plans, and plans for disposition.[46,63,71–74] The use of telemedicine to urgently obtain a consultation from a neurologist in the ED to treat a patient with an acute stroke is now common practice.[71,74–76] Similarly, telemedicine is used to provide emergency medicine consultations to critical access hospitals, which are staffed by physician assistants.[77] Both of these examples have been shown to result in high-quality, cost-effective care.[77–79]

There is increasing evidence and acceptance that providing pediatric emergency and critical care consultations to remote EDs for critically ill children can improve the quality of care and increase provider, patient, and parent/guardian satisfaction.[72,80] Three studies have described how pediatric critical care physicians use telemedicine to provide consultations to critically ill children presenting to several rural EDs.[63,72,80] Heath and colleagues[72] at the University of Vermont concluded that use of telemedicine was associated with improved patient care and was superior to telephone consultations.[81] A study by Dharmar and colleagues[82] showed that patients receiving telemedicine consultations in remote EDs received higher overall care quality compared with similar patients receiving telephone consultations.[80] Both of these programs also reported that referring ED physicians more frequently changed their diagnoses and/or therapeutic interventions than when consultations were provided by telephone. In addition, the use of telemedicine to provide critical care consultations has been shown to result in significantly higher parent/guardian satisfaction and perceived quality compared with telephone consultations.[80]

Published data from a consultative telemedicine program show excellent clinical outcomes for the reactive consultative model described earlier, including mortality and length of stay, similar to severity-adjusted benchmark data from a set of national pediatric ICUs.[66,67] Programs have reported a high degree of satisfaction among remote providers and parents/guardians and allowed patients to remain in their local communities, thereby lessening the burden on family members. In addition, implementation of this consultative telemedicine model resulted in an overall reduction in health care costs because of more appropriate transport use and decreased use of the more costly regional pediatric ICU.[83] Moreover, the use of telemedicine to assist with cardiopulmonary resuscitation has been reported.[84]

REIMBURSEMENT/LEGAL/REGULATORY/LICENSING RELATED ISSUES

Success factors for current programs for pediatric emergency and critical care telemedicine in a recent survey included identifying spoke hospitals based on receptivity and cultivating clinical champions at the spoke facilities.[85] Several barriers were also identified, including credentialing, workflow integration at both sites because telemedicine consults require more time compared to telephone consults, usability of the technology, lack of physician buy-in, and misaligned incentives between the sites. Uneven reimbursement was also mentioned, but was not perceived as a major issue because many programs operate independently of reimbursement.

Most of the hub sites are academic institutions that may have motivations other than reimbursement. Overall, although more research is needed, there is mounting evidence that pediatric critical care consultations to rural and underserved EDs using telemedicine can be used to help address disparities in access to specialists and, in doing so, improve the overall quality of care. It is also likely that because of better care and

the reduction in unnecessary transports, telemedicine consultations to rural and underserved EDs can be provided in a cost-efficient manner that reduces the health care costs that would otherwise be incurred if telemedicine were not used.[83]

QUALITY IMPROVEMENT/CARE IMPROVEMENT/ETHICS/PITFALLS

Pediatric telehealth, particularly in times of emergency or critical care consultation, should be held to the same standard of quality as in-person care. The necessary equipment and connections described earlier must be available, and telemedicine must operate on a sustainable infrastructure in order to provide quality care for children. It is essential that providers use all the same diagnostic tools necessary to assess and treat children. Many refer to this as an "in-person equivalent." Even if the telehealth providers cannot physically be at the bedside to examine the child, they need to collaborate with the bedside team using appropriate equipment to virtually emulate the exam that they would perform in person.

Improvements in technology, including connection speeds, radiology image transfer, and integrated electronic medical records systems, will all be essential in improving care of children through telemedicine. Quality care should also reflect the "medical home model of quality pediatric care: care that is patient-centered, comprehensive, team-based, coordinated, accessible, and focused on quality and safety."[86]

GUIDELINES

In 2015, the American Academy of Pediatrics (AAP) Section on Telehealth Care published a technical report on the use of telemedicine in pediatrics.[87] This report chronicled the use of telemedicine by pediatricians and pediatric medical and surgical specialists to deliver inpatient and outpatient care. It also provided a report on the use of telemedicine in response to emergencies and disasters and the use of telemedicine to provide subspecialty consultations to remote and underserved populations.

The AAP Committee on Pediatric Workforce also released a policy statement in 2015 about the use of telemedicine to address access and physician workforce shortages.[86] A key point of this guideline is that telemedicine should be used in the context of the medical home. Telemedicine should improve access to care while also preventing further fragmentation of care.

The American Telemedicine Association released a set of guidelines regarding tele-ICU care in 2014.[88] The purpose of these guidelines was to assist administrators, practitioners, and information technology specialists in establishing safe and effective models of care using telemedicine. This document established core guidelines for tele-ICU operations, including administrative guidelines, guidelines for the clinical application for the practice of tele-ICU, and technical guidelines.

CONCLUSION

The use of telemedicine in pediatric emergency and critical care is expanding, as there is increasing evidence that it can improve access, timeliness, quality of care, and cost of care for critically ill pediatric patients. Telemedicine can help provide children with subspecialist care in their moment of need while also reducing unnecessary testing and transfers. Studies in pediatric emergency medicine and critical care telemedicine have shown promising results. By continuing to operate in a manner to support the pediatric medical home, telehealth can continue to make a positive impact on pediatric emergency and critical care.

REFERENCES

1. Randolph GD, Pathman DE. Trends in the rural-urban distribution of general pediatricians. *Pediatrics* 2001;107(2):E18.

2. Basco WT, Rimsza ME, Committee on Pediatric Workforce, American Academy of Pediatrics. Pediatrician workforce policy statement. *Pediatrics* 2013;132(2):390–397.

3. Pletcher BA, Rimsza ME, Cull WL, et al. Primary care pediatricians' satisfaction with subspecialty care, perceived supply, and barriers to care. *J Pediatr* 2010; 156(6):1011–1015, 1015.e1.

4. Skinner AC, Slifkin RT. Rural/urban differences in barriers to and burden of care for children with special health care needs. *J Rural Health* 2007;23(2):150–157.

5. Johnson WG, Rimsza ME. The effects of access to pediatric care and insurance coverage on emergency department utilization. *Pediatrics* 2004;113(3 Pt 1):483–487.

6. Ray KN, Bogen DL, Bertolet M, Forrest CB, Mehrotra A. Supply and utilization of pediatric subspecialists in the United States. *Pediatrics* 2014;133(6):1061–1069.

7. Donchin Y, Gopher D, Olin M, et al. A look into the nature and causes of human errors in the intensive care unit. *Crit Care Med* 1995;23(2):294–300.

8. Birkmeyer JD, Finlayson EV, Birkmeyer CM. Volume standards for high-risk surgical procedures: potential benefits of the Leapfrog initiative. *Surgery* 2001;130(3):415–422.

9. Phibbs CS, Bronstein JM, Buxton E, Phibbs RH. The effects of patient volume and level of care at the hospital of birth on neonatal mortality. *JAMA* 1996;276(13): 1054–1059.

10. Tilford JM, Simpson PM, Green JW, Lensing S, Fiser DH. Volume-outcome relationships in pediatric intensive care units. *Pediatrics* 2000;106(2 Pt 1):289–294.

11. Marcin JP, Li Z, Kravitz RL, et al. The CABG surgery volume-outcome relationship: temporal trends and selection effects in California, 1998-2004. *Health Serv Res* 2008;43(1 Pt 1):174–192.

12. Marcin JP, Song J, Leigh JP. The impact of pediatric intensive care unit volume on mortality: a hierarchical instrumental variable analysis. *Pediatr Crit Care Med* 2005;6(2):136–141.

13. Finks JF, Osborne NH, Birkmeyer JD. Trends in hospital volume and operative mortality for high-risk surgery. *N Engl J Med* 2011;364(22):2128–2137.

14. Lorch SA, Myers S, Carr B. The regionalization of pediatric health care. *Pediatrics* 2010;126(6):1182–1190.

15. Blunt MC, Burchett KR. Out-of-hours consultant cover and case-mix-adjusted mortality in intensive care. *Lancet* 2000;356(9231):735–736.

16. Pollack MM, Alexander SR, Clarke N, Ruttimann UE, Tesselaar HM, Bachulis AC. Improved outcomes from tertiary center pediatric intensive care: a statewide comparison of tertiary and nontertiary care facilities. *Crit Care Med* 1991;19(2):150–159.

17. Pollack MM, Cuerdon TT, Patel KM, et al. Impact of quality-of-care factors on pediatric intensive care unit mortality. *JAMA* 1994;272(12):941–946.

18. Pronovost PJ, Angus DC, Dorman T, Robinson KA, Dremsizov TT, Young TL. Physician staffing patterns and clinical outcomes in critically ill patients: a systematic review. *JAMA* 2002;288(17):2151–2162.

19. Kanter RK. Regional variation in child mortality at hospitals lacking a pediatric intensive care unit. *Crit Care Med* 2002;30(1):94–99.

20. Dharmar M, Marcin JP, Romano PS, et al. Quality of care of children in the emergency department: association with hospital setting and physician training. *J Pediatr* 2008;153(6):783–789.

21. Marcin JP, Dharmar M, Cho M, et al. Medication errors among acutely ill and injured children treated in rural emergency departments. *Ann Emerg Med* 2007;50(4):361–367, 367 e361–e362.

22. Angus DC, Kelley MA, Schmitz RJ, White A, Popovich J Jr. Caring for the critically ill patient. Current and projected workforce requirements for care of the critically ill and patients with pulmonary disease: can we meet the requirements of an aging population? *JAMA* 2000;284(21):2762–2770.

23. Committee on Pediatric Workforce. Pediatrician workforce statement. *Pediatrics* 2005;116(1):263–269.

24. Marcin J, Ellis J, Mawis R, Nagrampa E, Nesbitt T, Dimand R. Telemedicine and the medical home: providing pediatric subspecialty care to children with special health care needs in an underserved rural community. *Pediatrics* 2004 Jan;113(1 Pt 1):1–6.

25. Marcin JP, Ellis J, Mawis R, Nagrampa E, Nesbitt TS, Dimand RJ. Using telemedicine to provide pediatric subspecialty care to children with special health care needs in an underserved rural community. *Pediatrics* 2004;113(1 Pt 1):1–6.

26. Haskins PA, Ellis DG, Mayrose J. Predicted utilization of emergency medical services telemedicine in decreasing ambulance transports. *Prehosp Emerg Care* 2002;6(4):445–448.

27. Tsai SH, Kraus J, Wu HR, et al. The effectiveness of video-telemedicine for screening of patients requesting emergency air medical transport (EAMT). *J Trauma* 2007;62(2):504–511.

28. Athey J, Dean JM, Ball J, Wiebe R, Melese-d'Hospital I. Ability of hospitals to care for pediatric emergency patients. *Pediatr Emerg Care* 2001;17(3):170–174.

29. Bowman SM, Zimmerman FJ, Christakis DA, Sharar SR, Martin DP. Hospital characteristics associated with the management of pediatric splenic injuries. *JAMA* 2005;294(20):2611–2617.

30. Li J, Monuteaux MC, Bachur RG. Interfacility transfers of noncritically ill children to academic pediatric emergency departments. *Pediatrics* 2012;130(1): 83–92.

31. McGillivray D, Nijssen-Jordan C, Kramer MS, Yang H, Platt R. Critical pediatric equipment availability in Canadian hospital emergency departments. *Ann Emerg Med* 2001;37(4):371–376.

32. Burt CW, Middleton KR. Factors associated with ability to treat pediatric emergencies in US hospitals. *Pediatr Emerg Care* 2007;23(10):681–689.

33. Gausche-Hill M, Schmitz C, Lewis RJ. Pediatric preparedness of US emergency departments: a 2003 survey. *Pediatrics* 2007;120(6):1229–1237.

34. Middleton KR, Burt CW. *Availability of pediatric services and equipment in emergency departments:*United States, 2002-03. *Adv Data.* 2006(367):1–16.

35. Bourgeois FT, Shannon MW. Emergency care for children in pediatric and general emergency departments. *Pediatr Emerg Care* 2007;23(2):94–102.

36. Remick K, Kaji AH, Olson L, et al. Pediatric readiness and facility verification. *Ann Emerg Med* 2016;67(3): 320–328.

37. Gausche-Hill M, Ely M, Schmuhl P, et al. A national assessment of pediatric readiness of emergency departments. *JAMA Pediatr* 2015;169(6):527–534.

38. Keeler EB, Rubenstein LV, Kahn KL, et al. Hospital characteristics and quality of care. *JAMA* 1992;268(13): 1709–1714.

39. Tilford JM, Roberson PK, Lensing S, Fiser DH. Improvement in pediatric critical care outcomes. *Crit CareMed* 2000;28(2):601–603.

40. Durch J, Lohr KN, Institute of Medicine (U.S.). Committee on Pediatric Emergency Medical Services. *Emergency Medical Services for Children.* Washington, DC: National Academy Press; 1993.

41. Durch JS, Lohr KN. From the institute of medicine. *JAMA* 1993;270(8):929.

42. Seidel JS, Henderson DP, Ward P, et al. Pediatric prehospital care in urban and rural areas. *Pediatrics* 1991;88(4):681–690.

43. Seidel JS, Hornbein M, Yoshiyama K, et al. Emergency medical services and the pediatric patient: are the needs being met? *Pediatrics* 1984;73(6):769–772.

44. Burke RV, Berg BM, Vee P, et al. Using robotic telecommunications to triage pediatric disaster victims. *J Pediatr Surg* 2012;47(1):221–224.

45. Brennan JA, Kealy JA, Gerardi LH, et al. A randomized controlled trial of telemedicine in an emergency department. *J Telemed Telecare* 1998;4(Suppl 1):18–20.

46. Brennan JA, Kealy JA, Gerardi LH, et al. Telemedicine in the emergency department: a randomized controlled trial. *J Telemed Telecare* 1999;5(1): 18–22.

47. Hicks LL, Boles KE, Hudson ST, et al. Using telemedicine to avoid transfer of rural emergency department patients. *J Rural Health* 2001;17(3):220–228.

48. Lambrecht CJ. Emergency physicians' roles in a clinical telemedicine network. *Ann Emerg Med* 1997;30(5): 670–674.

49. Rogers FB, Ricci M, Caputo M, et al. The use of telemedicine for real-time video consultation between trauma center and community hospital in a rural setting improves early trauma care: preliminary results. *J Trauma* 2001;51(6):1037–1041.

50. Stamford P, Bickford T, Hsiao H, Mattern W. The significance of telemedicine in a rural emergency department. *IEEE Eng Med Biol Mag* 1999;18(4):45–52.

51. Latifi R, Hadeed GJ, Rhee P, et al. Initial experiences and outcomes of telepresence in the management of trauma and emergency surgical patients. *Am J Surg* 2009;198(6):905–910.

52. Munoz RA, Burbano NH, Motoa MV, et al. Telemedicine in pediatric cardiac critical care. *Telemed J E Health* 2012;18(2):132–136.

53. Alverson DC, Swinfen LR, Swinfen LP, et al. Transforming systems of care for children in the global community. *Pediatr Ann* 2009;38(10):579–585.

54. Liman TG, Winter B, Waldschmidt C, et al. Telestroke ambulances in prehospital stroke management: concept and pilot feasibility study. *Stroke* 2012;43(8):2086–2090.

55. Hsieh JC, Lin BX, Wu FR, et al. Ambulance 12-lead electrocardiography transmission via cell phone technology to cardiologists. *Telemed J E Health* 2010;16(8):910–915.

56. Qureshi A, Shih E, Fan I, et al. Improving patient care by unshackling telemedicine: adaptively aggregating wireless networks to facilitate continuous collaboration. *AMIA Annu Symp Proc* 2010;2010:662–666.

57. Charash WE, Caputo MP, Clark H, et al. Telemedicine to a moving ambulance improves outcome after trauma in simulated patients. *J Trauma* 2011;71(1):49–55.

58. Wakefield DS, Ward M, Miller T, et al. Intensive care unit utilization and interhospital transfers as potential indicators of rural hospital quality. *J Rural Health* 2004;20(4):394–400.

59. Rosenberg DI, Moss MM. Guidelines and levels of care for pediatric intensive care units. *Critical Care Med* 2004;32(10):2117–2127.

60. Gupta RS, Bewtra M, Prosser LA, Finkelstein JA. Predictors of hospital charges for children admitted with asthma. *Ambul Pediatr* 2006;6(1):15–20.

61. Merenstein D, Egleston B, Diener-West M. Lengths of stay and costs associated with children's hospitals. *Pediatrics* 2005;115(4):839–844.

62. Odetola FO, Gebremariam A, Freed GL. Patient and hospital correlates of clinical outcomes and resource utilization in severe pediatric sepsis. *Pediatrics* 2007;119(3):487–494.

63. Labarbera JM, Ellenby MS, Bouressa P, et al. The impact of telemedicine intensivist support and a pediatric hospitalist program on a community hospital. *Telemed J E Health* 2013;19(10):760–766.

64. Dharmar M, Smith AC, Armfield NR, et al. Telemedicine for children in need of intensive care. *Pediatr Ann* 2009;38(10):562–566.

65. Reynolds HN, Rogove H, Bander J, et al. A working lexicon for the tele-intensive care unit: we need to define tele-intensive care unit to grow and understand it. *Telemed J E Health* 2011;17(10):773–783.

66. Marcin JP, Nesbitt TS, Kallas HJ, et al. Use of telemedicine to provide pediatric critical care inpatient consultations to underserved rural Northern California. *J Pediatr* 2004;144(3):375–380.

67. Marcin JP, Schepps DE, Page KA, et al. The use of telemedicine to provide pediatric critical care consultations to pediatric trauma patients admitted to a remote trauma intensive care unit: a preliminary report. *Pediatr Crit Care Med* 2004;5(3):251–256.

68. Yager PH, Cummings BM, Whalen MJ, Noviski N. Nighttime telecommunication between remote staff intensivists and bedside personnel in a pediatric intensive care unit: a retrospective study. *Crit Care Med* 2012;40(9):2700–2703.

69. Huang T, Moon-Grady AJ, Traugott C, Marcin J. The availability of telecardiology consultations and transfer patterns from a remote neonatal intensive care unit. *J Telemed Telecare* 2008;14(5):244–248.

70. Kon AA, Rich B, Sadorra C, Marcin JP. Complex bioethics consultation in rural hospitals: using telemedicine to bring academic bioethicists into outlying communities. *J Telemed Telecare* 2009;15(5):264–267.

71. Demaerschalk BM, Raman R, Ernstrom K, Meyer BC. Efficacy of telemedicine for stroke: pooled analysis of the Stroke Team Remote Evaluation Using a Digital Observation Camera (STRokE DOC) and STRokE DOC Arizona telestroke trials. *Telemed J E Health* 2012;18(3):230–237.

72. Heath B, Salerno R, Hopkins A, Hertzig J, Caputo M. Pediatric critical care telemedicine in rural underserved emergency departments. *Pediatr Crit Care Med* 2009;10(5):588–591.

73. Kofos D, Pitetti R, Orr R, Thompson A. Telemedicine in pediatric transport: a feasibility study. *Pediatrics* 1998;102(5):E58.

74. Meyer BC, Raman R, Hemmen T, et al. Efficacy of site-independent telemedicine in the STRokE DOC trial: a randomised, blinded, prospective study. *Lancet Neurol* 2008;7(9):787–795.

75. Emsley H, Blacker K, Davies P, O'Donnell M. Telestroke. When location, location, location doesn't matter. *Health Service J* 2010;120(6227):24–25.

76. Pervez MA, Silva G, Masrur S, et al. Remote supervision of IV-tPA for acute ischemic stroke by telemedicine or telephone before transfer to a regional stroke center is feasible and safe. *Stroke* 2010;41(1):e18–e24.

77. Galli R, Keith JC, McKenzie K, Hall GS, Henderson K. TelEmergency: a novel system for delivering emergency care to rural hospitals. *Ann Emerg Med* 2008; 51(3):275–284.

78. Henderson K. TelEmergency: distance emergency care in rural emergency departments using nurse practitioners. *J Emerg Nurs* 2006;32(5):388–393.

79. Nelson RE, Saltzman GM, Skalabrin EJ, Demaerschalk BM, Majersik JJ. The cost-effectiveness of telestroke in the treatment of acute ischemic stroke. *Neurology* 2011;77(17):1590–1598.

80. Dharmar M, Romano PS, Kuppermann N, et al. Impact of critical care telemedicine consultations on children in rural emergency departments. *Crit Care Med* 2013;41(10):2388–2395.

81. Dharmar M, Marcin JP. A picture is worth a thousand words: critical care consultations to emergency departments using telemedicine. *Pediatr Crit Care Med* 2009;10(5):606–607.

82. Dharmar M, Marcin JP, Kuppermann N, et al. A new implicit review instrument for measuring quality of care delivered to pediatric patients in the emergency department. *BMC Emerg Med* 2007;7:13.

83. Marcin JP, Nesbitt TS, Struve S, Traugott C, Dimand RJ. Financial benefits of a pediatric intensive care unit-based telemedicine program to a rural adult intensive care unit: impact of keeping acutely ill and injured children in their local community. *Telemed J E Health* 2004;10(suppl 2):S-1–5.

84. Kon AA, Marcin JP. Using telemedicine to improve communication during paediatric resuscitations. *J Telemed Telecare* 2005;11(5):261–264.

85. Uscher-Pines L, Kahn JM. Barriers and facilitators to pediatric emergency telemedicine in the United States. *Telemed J E Health* 2014;20(11):990–996.

86. Marcin JP, Rimsza ME, Moskowitz WB. The use of telemedicine to address access and physician workforce shortages. *Pediatrics* 2015;136(1):202–209.

87. Burke BL Jr, Hall RW. Telemedicine: pediatric applications. *Pediatrics* 2015;136(1):e293–e308.

88. Bluemke DA. Coronary computed tomographic angiography and incidental pulmonary nodules. *Circulation* 2014;130(8):634–637.

Child Telepsychiatry

Peter Yellowlees, MD, Maryann Waugh, MEd
and Jay H. Shore, MD, MPH

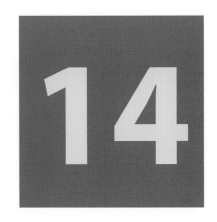

Zac, a 12-year-old Native American child living on an isolated reservation, was referred for a telepsychiatry consultation by his primary care physician for a diagnostic opinion as to whether he had attention deficit hyperactivity disorder (ADHD). He had a colorful history of recurrent aggression, fighting, truancy and school suspensions going back several years, and had already been diagnosed by a pediatrician visiting the community as having an oppositional disorder and possible ADHD, with the suggestion that a trial of stimulants would be worthwhile. Zac had likely suffered from fetal alcohol syndrome at birth, and his polysubstance-abusing mother died when he was 2. He lived with his father, an ex-alcoholic who had been sober since then, and who came to the consultation with him. During the consultation Zac was observed sitting quietly and politely next to his father, who gave most of the history and confirmed on questioning that there was minimal evidence supporting ADHD and that Zac could be well behaved, calm, and loving when he wanted to be, but also had significant tantrums and poor behavior if he felt threatened. His behavior was generally reported to be much worse at school than at home, and Zac openly admitted that he liked being suspended as he had more "freedom." When seen alone Zac admitted to taking marijuana quite regularly and expressed concern that he found it hard to keep up with his classmates academically and knew that poor behavior led to exclusion which, for him, solved this problem. During feedback to

his primary care physician (PCP), the telepsychiatrist confirmed that Zac did not have ADHD and that stimulants were not required. Instead changes to his Individual Educational Plan to help support him academically were recommended, as well as commencing a urine monitoring program, with rewards for negative screens, and a similar positive behavioral program across school and home. Zac's father and PCP were both pleased with these recommendations, as neither had felt he had ADHD, but they had been put in a difficult position by the pediatrician's recommendations.

INTRODUCTION

Technological advances and changing demands from health care consumers and payors have led to significant changes in psychiatric service delivery models.[1] There is a particular dearth of child and adolescent psychiatrists in the United States, with recent estimates of need exceeding 15 million children and adolescents and a current workforce of 6,800 child and adolescent psychiatrists.[2] This makes it even more critical that care systems maximize psychiatric expertise to serve a large population of youth in need.

Like adult psychiatry, youth psychiatry is not dependent upon peripheral devices or instruments for patient assessment or treatment and is well suited for virtual treatment modalities. In addition, youth populations are particularly amenable to virtual treatment options. Members of the millennial generation, born after the 1989 debut of the Internet, are described as "digital natives," having never experienced life without the ubiquitous presence of laptops, smart phones, tablets, and other e-devices. In 2015, the average two-year-old child had an online presence estimated to include over a thousand posted photos, and the average three-year old was quite familiar with the use of a smart phone. For digital natives, physical travel for services that can easily be accessed virtually may be considered outdated and wasteful, and concerns about digital personal health information (PHI) are negligible compared to prior generations—if those concerns exist at all.[1,3,4] As members of the millennial generation become parents and their digital-native children receive treatment, child telepsychiatry services will be increasingly in demand. This chapter is designed to describe the treatment modalities and models that are used to support telepsychiatry services for children; summarize the evidence for virtual treatment efficacy; and provide an overview of the reimbursement, licensing, and legal and ethical considerations related specifically to telepsychiatry implementation for child populations—while not duplicating the adult telepsychiatry content of Chapter 10.

MODALITIES/MODELS

Child and adolescent telepsychiatry leverages the same two primary modalities as adult telepsychiatry. Synchronous modalities allow a child/adolescent; or a child/adolescent, a pediatrician, or other provider; and/or parent/guardian to virtually interact in real time using audio and/or video technology.[5] Asynchronous applications will likely expand future opportunities for cost savings and efficiency and may allow, for example, a pediatrician or other general practice professional to collect semi-structured interview data and store-and-forward this information via email or another web application for later review by a psychiatric provider.[6–9] The asynchronous modality may be particularly helpful for youth and adolescent patients, but there are few clinical trials with youth populations, in contrast to more ample research with adults.

Asynchronous youth applications are receiving some attention as feasible intervention modalities for youth in supervised situations. Emerging research is promising, and a variety of online interventions are associated with reduced symptoms for depressed and anxious youth and adolescents. These seem to work best with mild disorder symptoms and as part of a care plan that also involves in-person treatment time. A noted advantage of asynchronous interventions is fidelity of treatment implementation.[10]

Child and adolescent psychiatry typically goes beyond diagnoses and medication management and includes parent and teacher education and training. Home-based telepsychiatry can help to more accurately portray actual parent–child interactions for psychiatrist review and help refine parental education, training, and support.[11]

CONTINUUM OF MODELS

Like adult telepsychiatry, child telepsychiatry can be implemented using a variety of models that range from traditional behavioral health outpatient models to integrated primary care models. Some of those models are described in Chapter 10. Other common child-specific models include school-based and juvenile justice–based telepsychiatry.

School-based models are gaining increasing attention as a way to increase mental health access to youth, particularly those unlikely to access mental health services otherwise, reduce the stigma associated with mental health treatment, provide opportunities for mental health promotion and not just treatment, and substantially increase typical rates of care plan follow-up.[12] Given the shortage of child and adolescent psychiatrists, many school-based models incorporate the psychiatrist as a consultant for medication management support into a multidisciplinary treatment team that may include parents, teachers, nurses, occupational therapists, and school-based mental health professionals such as school psychologists. School-based health clinics are a natural fit for telepsychiatry as they establish primary and integrated care settings within the school. Less frequently, psychiatrists provide direct, virtual patient care in the school setting. In instances of direct patient care, the virtual modality decreases the need for travel for both the psychiatrist and the patient and limits missed appointments as patients are already in the school setting.[12]

Although more research is still needed, school-based telepsychiatry appears an effective and acceptable model. Both consultative and direct care applications have advantages for patients and families such as reduced scheduling demands, the opportunity for parents to participate in virtual sessions from their own work or homes, the support and engagement in school personnel in implementing and monitoring the patients' progress on the care plan, and the potential increase in comfort level for parents who already trust the school's personnel.

A disadvantage for some patients/families is the reduced privacy that comes from having a multidisciplinary school team involved in student mental health care. Other disadvantages from the psychiatric provider perspective include the potential for limited parent engagement in the care plan and the additional challenge presented by practicing psychiatry not just virtually, but within the unfamiliar culture of a school and a multidisciplinary school team. Some providers have recommended a hybrid model of in-person and virtual care for the most effective, culturally competent school-based telepsychiatry.[12]

Juvenile justice populations have particularly high rates of psychopathology, barriers to care access, and particularly high care costs. As such, juvenile justice–based telepsychiatry models are increasingly being implemented in settings from community-based probation to secure commitment facilities to increase care access and decrease costs.[13] Similar to school-based models, juvenile justice–based models typically require the psychiatrist to work with a team of professionals and not just the parent and child, as in a typical outpatient application. In addition, juvenile justice settings must maintain a safety and security priority—which may affect the traditional patient–provider alliance and privacy assurances, as well as the ability of patients, parents, and/or correctional staff to implement care plans as designed. Other challenges may include treatment-resistant youth and/or parents/staff and particular difficulty accessing patient medical histories. Overall, however, there is growing evidence of feasibility across juvenile justice settings, and psychiatrists willing to work within the challenging environment have an opportunity to work at the top of their clinical scope and affect a population in severe need.[13,14]

TECHNOLOGY

Early videoconferencing applications demanded rare audio-video connections and bulky hardware and were expensive to implement. Now, most laptops, cell phones, and tablets enable patients and providers to use wireless Internet access to stream secure, integrated health care information using high-resolution cameras and display screens, audio input and output, and other data applications.[1,15] Millennials and younger generations are best situated to benefit from continuing technological advances, as some are more comfortable with virtual than in-person interactions with psychiatrists and other providers. Their high levels of comfort with various forms of virtual interaction, including avatars, creates more opportunity for youth to access more cost-effective services in settings that reduce any stigma and discomfort, relative to their adult counterparts.[1]

SUMMARY EVIDENCE/LITERATURE

Telepsychiatry has been well established as a feasible modality for psychiatric diagnosis, assessment, and treatment for children and adolescents.[16,17] Virtual psychiatry is associated with increased care access and quality[18] across a variety of care settings from more traditional community mental health outpatient settings, to primary care and pediatric settings, as well as schools, daycare centers, juvenile justice, and child welfare settings.[17–19] Telepsychiatry has been associated with measures of feasibility, efficacy, and acceptability across a variety of minority youth groups in the United States, including youth from Black, Hispanic, Hawaiian, Native American, and Alaskan Native populations.[17] It has been used to diagnose and treat a variety of disorders in children and adolescents, including depression, ADHD, obsessive compulsive disorder, oppositional defiant disorder, and others.[11]

Although more randomized controlled trials will help to inform situations in which virtual and in-person care is optimal in terms of patient outcomes and cost, telepsychiatry is increasingly practiced in diverse youth care settings. In many ways, these child and adolescent applications are similar to adult telepsychiatry applications. There are, however, important distinctions. Some are specific to the virtual modality, and others involve child-specific adaptations of traditional clinical practice to virtual settings.

In a recent and comprehensive review of current and evidence-based telemental and telepsychiatry practices for youth, Glof and colleagues[11] note that Schedule

II stimulants are frequently prescribed to youth and adolescents for behavioral health treatment and that these stimulants fall under specific rules that regulate online prescription. Further, youth behavioral health diagnoses typically require the evaluation/rule-out of a variety of developmental and cognitive disorders. The originating and provider sites must have the capacity to meet the criteria for both situations. Additionally, most youth care plans require the family and other important caregivers to be engaged in effective implementation. In some virtual care settings, including integrated and collaborative care models, the psychiatrist may have little to no direct contact with parents or other caregivers and must flexibly operate within alternative care models for the telepsychiatry to pragmatically work.[11]

REIMBURSEMENT/ LEGAL/REGULATORY/ LICENSING RELATED ISSUES

Reimbursement and legal/regulatory issues are essentially the same for youth and adult patients, with payor-directed constraints on reimbursable activities and locations representing the primary obstacle to developing and sustaining youth telepsychiatry programs.[20] Please see Chapter 10 for more detail about reimbursement and legal/regulatory issues related to telepsychiatry. The one regulatory exception where there is a child-specific legal requirement is consent. Telepsychiatrists must get informed consent to treat via telehealth from guardians, rather than directly from their minor patients, although the specifications for how this consent is obtained (ie, verbal or written format) falls under state jurisdiction and varies from state to state.[21] In what is described as the first attempt to develop practice guidelines and parameters for child and adolescent telepsychiatry, researchers Myers and Cain[22] note that child-specific originating sites such as schools, child welfare, or correctional facilities will likely complicate regulatory issues related to confidentiality, records management, and ethical standards. Whereas traditional medical clinics like hospital-based clinics and primary care clinics will be well versed in patient health records and Health Insurance Portability and Accountability Act (HIPAA) regulations, nonmedical originating sites will need support in maintaining secure medical information according to HIPAA

rules, as well as other regulating policies such as Family Educational Rights and Privacy Act (FERPA).[22]

ETHICS AND POTENTIAL PITFALLS

Similarly, the same ethical issues and potential pitfalls in a telepsychiatry environment apply to youth and adult populations. An important consideration in high-quality, ethical psychiatric care, whether in-person or virtual, however, is ensuring that diagnoses and treatment plans are made in the context of the patient's cultural identity and environment. For child and adolescent patients, these cultural considerations must extend equally to the patient's parents or caregivers. Savin and colleagues[17] note that clinicians must be familiar with parents' childrearing practices, ideas about normal child behavior, and beliefs about mental illness etiology and effective treatment. This process of clinical ethnography is equally relevant to in-person and virtual treatment; however, the virtual medium may bring a psychiatrist into contact with increasingly diverse patient populations and make the ethnographic investigation more challenging. Whereas youth populations are increasingly comfortable with all forms of technology, parents and older caregivers may resist tele-interactions or may alter behavior during virtual sessions because of discomfort with the medium. Current guidelines recommend allowing time for parents and caregivers to ask questions and get used to the tele-interactions through casual conversation before initiating the first clinical session.[17]

Despite reimbursement challenges from the majority of health care payors, home-based telepsychiatry is starting to expand, and this expansion presents the opportunity for new ethical concerns and potential clinical pitfalls. Child and adolescent psychiatrists must be aware of home-based safety concerns due to lack of onsite staff, privacy and technology concerns inherent in diverse individual home situations, and the increased risk for youth who are distracted to more easily leave a home telesession than they can an office visit.[11] It is important for providers to think through various home-based pitfalls and develop back-up plans collaboratively with patients (ie, continue visit via phone if Internet connection is unstable, parent diversion for siblings if they are home and distracting, and/ or ways to encourage youth patients to successfully

Table 14-1. Suggestions for Youth Providers

Considerations Prior to Implementing Telepsychiatry with Youth Populations

1. Check for state- and payor-specific reimbursement restrictions related to originating site, provider licensing, malpractice insurance, etc.
2. Identify any potential privacy complications related to nonclinical originating sites (ie, FERPA for school-based clinics).
3. Establish a clear process for obtaining parent/guardian consent and youth assent prior to starting service delivery.
4. Conduct practice sessions with clinical staff prior to use with patients to ensure adequate bandwidth and connectivity, as well as audiovisual quality.
5. Establish back up plans (ie, phone) for technology glitches.
6. Establish emergency procedures aligned with the resources of the originating site.
7. Describe the scope of the telepsychiatry service to families in advance; for example, describe the scope of service, how prescriptions will be managed, and how communication and follow-up will occur.
8. Practice cultural humility with the understanding that the virtual environment may further accentuate communication differences.
9. Ensure that the patient setting has appropriate space to observe child behavior and family interactions, and on a related note, ensure that the angle of the camera allows the psychiatrist a good view.
10. Allow adequate time for patients and families to get used to the virtual medium and build rapport with the psychiatrist.
11. Leverage onsite staff to facilitate some one-on-one or smaller group time during clinical sessions.

complete sessions), as well as establish safety planning in the event of expressed and immediate suicide ideation or other emergencies (Table 14-1).

STANDARDS/GUIDELINES

Children usually respond positively to videoconferencing and find it a natural and easy environment within which to interact. In general, videoconference-based youth assessments are similar to in-person consultation. Typically, parents are the primary respondents during a youth assessment. The child and possibly other family members initially listen and are invited to contribute later in the session, if they wish. This style of interviewing gives the telepsychiatrist the opportunity to both take a history and observe the parent–child interaction. Teleclinicians have noted that children are actually more natural in interactions with their parents over videoconferencing, as they are not as aware of being observed as they are when in a physical office. Therefore from a clinical perspective, some have argued that for certain clinical situations, the use of telepsychiatry with children should be the new standard of practice.[23–24]

It is very important that parents, family members, and/or legal guardians provide informed consent and be involved as clinically appropriate. The recent guidelines from the American Academy of Child Psychiatry[2] note that ideally the room at the patient's end should be large enough for children to move around and play separately from their parents so that the virtual psychiatrist can assess motor skills and other important abilities and issues. Just as in the clinic setting, children may be asked to wait outside the room with a caregiver during parts of the interview, and parents or other family members may be asked to wait outside during other parts. This allows issues to be discussed privately with individuals as necessary, rather than with a whole family group. A separate table, paper, crayons, and age-appropriate toys should be available for children to use, and the formal child psychiatry assessments should follow the guidelines from the American Academy of Child and Adolescent Psychiatry.[16]

The telepsychiatry parameters developed specifically for child and adolescent populations note that the inclusion of an onsite clinical "presenter" can help ease any technology issues, help manage agitated or uncooperative children, and help succinctly present clinical concerns to maximize the time of the virtual psychiatrist. This presenter is often a nurse or psychologist who may be responsible for diverse duties such as obtaining vital signs, providing patient/family education, and coordinating care. In some models they may provide more onsite assessment and treatment—roles that may be relegated to the psychiatric provider in other models. As with adult implementations, the guidelines recommend written telepsychiatry protocols to specify which professional performs what function across intake, evaluation, and treatment to clarify roles and address process issues quickly.[22] The American Telemedicine Association has a special interest group that is in the process of developing telehealth guidelines specifically for pediatric patients. Some of their specific goals include promoting sound state and federal policies to improve access to care for children in both rural and in urban areas; encouraging a research agenda specific to pediatric applications of telehealth; and engaging the American Academy of Pediatrics, the Society for Pediatric Research, the Pediatric Academic Societies, and the American Association of Family Practice in collaborative work regarding pediatric telehealth service.[25]

SUMMARY AND CONCLUSIONS

Telepsychiatry is expanding as a care modality that can leverage technology to maximize a limited supply of child and adolescent specialists. As a patient population, youth are particularly well suited for technology-based care delivery, typically regarding virtual treatment as not only acceptable, but preferable, to in-person care that includes long wait times and unnecessary physical travel. The youth telepsychiatry research is currently focused on synchronous models, with outcomes that include increased care access and quality across a variety of models and settings, as well as diverse youth populations. Youth-specific settings with a growing evidence base include school and juvenile justice, and there are also documented applications in daycare and child welfare agencies. There is less research regarding asynchronous applications with youth populations. As the adult telepsychiatry literature identifies expanding cost savings and efficiencies associated with this store-and-forward model, however, it is likely to receive more research attention as a promising model in pediatric and other youth settings.

The majority of youth-specific telepsychiatry considerations mirror in-person care considerations and include obtaining informed consent from parents/guardians in addition to obtaining youth consent and identifying appropriate strategies to solicit youth and parent/guardian input, both separately and in group settings. A potential benefit associated with the virtual medium is the ability to observe youths' natural interactions with other family members via camera, which clinicians report, is more easily forgotten by young patients than the in-person presence of the psychiatry specialist. A challenge specifically associated with the virtual medium includes online prescribing limitations associated with common prescriptions for childhood behavioral challenges. With the evidence base for telepsychiatry continually growing and policy decisions providing increasing support for virtual care applications, child and adolescent telepsychiatry currently faces payment and reimbursement issues as its predominant obstacles. As research increases for home-based applications and practices and payors develop and pilot new and innovative payment models, it is likely that models and applications of child and adolescent telepsychiatry will continue to expand opportunities for increased care access, quality, and efficiency.

REFERENCES

1. Chan S, Parish M, Yellowlees P. Telepsychiatry today. *Curr Psychiat Rep* 2015;17(11):89.
2. American Academy of Child and Adolescent Psychiatry (AACAP). 2016. http://www.aacap.org/aacap/resources_for_primary_care/Workforce_Issues.aspx. Accessed June 20, 2016.
3. Yellowlees P, Chan S, Parish M. The hybrid doctor-patient relationship in the age of technology - Telepsychiatry consultations and the use of virtual space. *Int Rev Psychiatr* 2015;27(6):476–489.
4. Yellowlees P, Nafiz N. The psychiatrist-patient relationship of the future: anytime, anywhere? *Harvard Rev Psychiatr* 2010;18(2):96–102.
5. Malhotra S, Chakrabarti S, Shah R. Telepsychiatry: promise, potential, and challenges. *Indian J Psychiatr* 2013;55(1):3–11.
6. Odor A, Yellowlees P, Hilty D, et al. Psych VACS: a system for asynchronous telepsychiatry. *Telemed J E Health* 2011;17(4):299–303.
7. Yellowlees P, Odor A, Patrice K, et al. Disruptive innovation: the future of healthcare? *Telemed J E Health* 2011;17(3):231–234.
8. Butler TN, Yellowlees P. Cost analysis of store-and-forward telepsychiatry as a consultation model for primary care. *Telemed J E Health* 2012;8(1):74–77.
9. Yellowlees PM, Odor A, Parish MB. Cross-lingual asynchronous telepsychiatry: disruptive innovation? *Psychiatr Serv* 2012;63(9):945.
10. Myers K, Comer JS. The case for telemental health for improving the asccessibility and quality of children's mental health services. *J Child Adol Psychop* 2016;26(3):186–189.
11. Gloff NE, LeNoue DR, Novins DK, et al. Telemental health for children and adolescents. *Int Rev Psychiatr* 2015;27(6):513–524.
12. Stepaan S, Lever N, Bernstein L, et al. Telemental health in schools. *J Child Adol Psychop* 2016;26(3):266–272.

13. Kaliebe K., Heneghan J, Kim TJ. Telepsychiatry in juvenile justice settings. *Child Adol Psych Cl* 2011;20: 113–123.

14. Myers K, Valentine J, Morganthaler R, et al. Telepsychiatry with incarcerated youth. *J Adolescent Health* 2006;38:643–648.

15. Chan S, Torous J, Hinton L, et al. Towards a framework for evaluating mobile mental health apps. *Telemed J E Health* 2015;21(12):1038–1041.

16. Myers KM, Valentine JM, Melzer SM. Feasibility, acceptability, and sustainability of telepsychiatry for children and adolescents. *Psychiatr Serv* 2007;58(11):1493–1496.

17. Savin D, Glueck DA, Chardavoyne J, et al. Bridging cultures: child psychiatry via videoconferencing. *Child Adol Psych Cl* 2011;20:125–134.

18. Hilty DM, Ferrer DC, Parish MB, et al. The effectiveness of telemental health: a 2013 review. *Telemed J E Health* 2013;19(6): 444–454.

19. Keilman P. Telepsychiatry with child welfare families referred to a family service agency. *Telemed J E Health* 2005;11(1):98–101.

20. Lambert D, Gale J, Hartley D, et al. Understanding the business case for telemental health in rural communities. *J Behav Health Ser R* 2016;43(3):366–379.

21. Thomas L, Capistrant G. State telemedicine gaps analysis. American Telemedicine Association. http://www.americantelemed.org/main/policy-page/state-telemedicine-gaps-reports. Accessed September 12, 2016.

22. Myers K, Cain S. Practice parameters for telepsychiatry with children and adolescents. *Child and Adol Psychiatr* 2008;47(12):1468–1483.

23. Hilty DM, Yellowlees PM, Parrish MB, et al. Telepsychiatry: effective, evidence-based and at a tipping point in health care delivery? *J Psychiatr Clin North Am* 2015;38(3):559–592.

24. Pakyurek M, Yellowlees PM, Hilty D. The child and adolescent telepsychiatry consultation: can it be a more effective clinical process for certain patients than conventional practice? *Telemed J E Health* 2010;16(3):289–292.

25. American Telemedicine Association. Pediatric Telehealth SIG. http://www.americantelemed.org/main/membership/ata-members/ata-sigs/pediatric-telehealth-sig. Accessed November 15, 2016.

School and Childcare Center Telehealth

Neil E. Herendeen, MD, MS

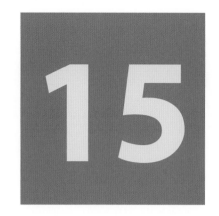

CASE STUDY

Jackie is a working mother of five children who works as a teacher's aide and cooks for the childcare center that her youngest two children attend. Three of her kids have asthma, and her youngest has recurrent otitis, which added together have required 15 medical visits (pediatrician, pulmonologist, emergency department) in a three-month period. As with many low-paying service jobs, Jackie does not get paid if she is not at work and feels caught in a no-win situation. She either feels guilty for being a bad mom if she doesn't take her children in for their medical appointments or lets her family down by not getting paid when she takes off work but then doesn't have enough money at the end of the month to pay her bills. Her childcare center director appreciates her dilemma and is excited to tell her about a new telemedicine service that will allow her children to see their primary care medical home without having to leave school or the childcare center. Jackie can now stay at work and have her kids get the medical attention they deserve. She still has to come to the hospital for her specialist visits and well-child visits but is able to schedule those for later in the afternoon after her breakfast and lunchtime duties at the childcare center are completed. So far, her youngest has avoided getting pressure equalization tubes with careful management by her primary care provider, and her older children with asthma have improved their attendance at school with better asthma control and an earlier response to exacerbations.

Children younger than 18 years of age in the United States made 127.5 million office visits in 2012 for problem-focused concerns.[1] These visits account for 75% of all office visits for children and represent the leading cause of parents having to miss time from work.[1,2] Fewer than 50% of working women in the United States believe that they can avoid conflict between family and work responsibilities the next time one of their children is sick.[2] Clearly, the social and economic burden associated with caring for ill children is substantial, but there may be opportunities to rethink how and when children receive medical care. Telemedicine offers new options for evaluating and treating children with both acute and chronic illnesses with potential efficiencies for patients, parents, providers, and payors.[3]

Telemedicine models for schools and childcare centers have evolved as the technology and connectivity have improved in the new millennium. State regulations and insurance company expectations have tried to keep up with the growing direct-to-consumer telemedicine applications, and terms like "face to face" have been replaced with "real-time video interaction" to distinguish virtual connections from in-person physical interactions. The idea of telemedicine providing an "in-office equivalent" visit allows providers to choose a telemedicine platform that allows them to conduct a history and physical that is the same as what they would conduct in person. For acute illness visits, that might include peripherals to look in the child's ears, eyes, and throat; an electronic stethoscope for listening to the child's lungs; and a general camera for observing the child's behavior or looking at a rash. For behavioral health follow-up visits, the provider may be satisfied with a simple webcam to provide two-way video communication for counseling and education. Telemedicine units may be fixed in the school nurse's office or may be mobile with laptop computers and a suitcase of attachments traveling with a telepresenter from one school to another as the need arises.

Pediatric researchers have contributed to the scientific evidence base establishing that telemedicine visits for children can be conducted safely, effectively, conveniently, and economically. In one of the few head-to-head comparisons of pediatric telemedicine versus in-person examination for common acute childhood illnesses, there was 86% agreement in diagnosis and treatment between the telemedicine and in-person providers compared to a 92% agreement for duplicate in-person examinations.[4] Ninety-six percent of school- and childcare-based telemedicine visits were able to be completed in a model using telepresenters connecting to primary care pediatric offices and diagnostic capabilities of otoscope, stethoscope, videoconference, and point-of-care testing (rapid strep tests).[5]

Satisfaction surveys of patients and providers rank telemedicine high for convenience, quality of interaction, clarity of images, and confidentiality of information being discussed. After just one telemedicine encounter, 98% of parents of preschoolers would choose a childcare center that offered telemedicine if given a choice over a similar center without telemedicine services.[6] Absence due to illness from childcare in Rochester, New York, was decreased by 63% during an 18-month period after telemedicine was implemented in five inner-city childcare centers.[6] On average, parents report a savings of 4.5 work hours that would have otherwise been lost if telemedicine had not been available to their ill child.[6]

Evaluation and management of children with chronic conditions can also be enhanced with school-based telemedicine. Children with type 1 diabetes ages 5 to 14 years receiving remote diabetes care management via telemedicine at school were able to lower their hemoglobin A1c levels and experience fewer hospital and emergency department visits during the school year.[7] Other programs in Kansas and Georgia have shown the effectiveness of using school-based telemedicine to enhance psychiatry services to treat attention deficit hyperactivity disorder (ADHD), depression, and autism spectrum disorders.[8,9]

Utilization studies show a slight increase in overall use of health services when telemedicine access is made available in elementary schools and childcare centers during the day.[10] This may represent an increase in nonessential convenience-driven visits, or more likely, fulfillment of a previously unmet need (ie, underutilization of health care in a vulnerable population). The cost associated with this slight increase in primary care visits was more than offset by a 22% reduction in costly emergency room visits for children.[10]

Reimbursement for telemedicine services for children in school and childcare varies greatly from state to state. In the best case, school-based telemedicine visits are reimbursed at the same rate as an in-person office visit plus a small fee for the originating site to help cover the infrastructure cost of equipment and personnel at the school. Many states have passed legislation for "parity" bills that require insurers to cover a telemedicine visit if that service would be otherwise eligible for payment if conducted in person in the office. Some states have different rules for commercial insurers and Managed Medicaid programs. Pediatricians are finding that parity of coverage does not equal parity in reimbursement rates, with insurers gladly reimbursing for telemedicine services but at only half the local rate of an office visit. In the worst case are states that adopt the Centers for Medicare and Medicaid (CMS) guidelines for Medicare and apply them to services for children. These guidelines restrict the geographic location of the originating site, require licensed providers to act as telepresenters, and define the type and location of the telemedicine provider, essentially eliminating any chance of setting up a school-based telemedicine program. Quality metrics for asthma and ADHD have shifted the focus from patient adherence to population management, with providers having a greater incentive to deliver timely, high-quality care. As pay-for-performance metrics become a larger part of primary care reimbursement, some providers are using telemedicine visits in the school to help meet or exceed goals for chronic care management, especially in urban practices with notoriously high no-show rates.

As is the case in all pediatric care, good communication is at the core of any telemedicine encounter. Policies and procedures must specifically address the need for secure, private communication with both the child and his or her guardian. Consideration must be given to the educational laws called Family Educational Rights and Privacy Act (FERPA) in addition to health system Health Insurance Portability and Accountability Act (HIPAA) regulations. Confidential adolescent care is another challenge for telemedicine providers to know the specific rules of their state and sometimes of their school district when it comes to obtaining consent for evaluation and treatment for mental health, substance abuse, or reproductive health issues. Contingency plans should be developed in the event of technologic failures or medical emergencies that require immediate intervention at the originating site.

Operating procedures and guidelines are being developed to address the unique aspects of delivering pediatric telemedicine care. The American Telemedicine Association has published multiple guidelines to help establish a safe and effective telemedicine program. They have also helped define the core terms used to describe and differentiate the spectrum of services that can be delivered under the heading of telemedicine. Pediatric providers and program managers are encouraged to check with their regional telemedicine resource center and professional organizations to keep abreast of any changes that may affect your ability to perform telemedicine services. The following websites will help:

http://www.americantelemed.org/main/policy-page/state-policy-resource-center

http://hub.americantelemed.org/resources/telemedicine-practice-guidelines

https://www.aap.org/en-us/about-the-aap/Committees-Councils-Sections/sotc/Pages/External-Resources.aspx

REFERENCES

1. Uddin SG, O'Connor KS, Ashman JJ. Physician office visits by children for well and problem-focused care: United States, 2012. *NCHS Data Brief* 2016;(248):1–8.

2. Ranji U, Salganicoff A. *Women's Health Care Chart Book*. Kaiserfamilydoundation.files.wordpress.com/2013/01/8164.pdf. Accessed December 28, 2013.

3. Herendeen N, Deshpande P. Telemedicine and the patient-centered medical home. *Pediatr Ann* 43(2):2014;e28–e32.

4. McConnochie KM, Conners GP, Brayer AF, et al. Differences in diagnosis and treatment using telemedicine versus in-person evaluation of acute illness. *Ambul Pediatr* 2006;6(4):187–195; discussion 196–197.

5. McConnochie KM, Conners GP, Brayer AF, et al. Effectiveness of telemedicine in replacing in-person evaluation for acute childhood illness in office settings. *Telemed J E Health* 12(3):2006;308–316.

6. McConnochie KM, Wood NE, Kitzman HJ, et al. Telemedicine reduces absence resulting from illness in urban child care: evaluation of an innovation. *Pediatrics* 2005;115(5):1273–1282.

7. Daniels SR. School-centered telemedicine for type 1 diabetes mellitus. *Pediatrics* 2009;155(3):A2.

8. Spaulding RJ, Cook DJ, Doolittle GC. School-based telemedicine in Kansas: parent perceptions of health and economic benefits. In: Yfantopoulos JN, Papanikos GT, Boutsioli Z, eds. *Health Care Issues: An International Perspective*. Athens Institute for Education and Research;2006: 371–386.

9. Knopf A. School-based telehealth brings psychiatry to rural Georgia. *Behav Healthc* 2013;33(1):47–48.

10. McConnochie KM, Tan J, Wood NE. Acute illness utilization patterns before and after telemedicine in childcare for inner-city children: a cohort study. *Telemed J E Health* 2007;13(4):381–390.

Telehealth in Pediatric Cardiology

Craig Sable, MD

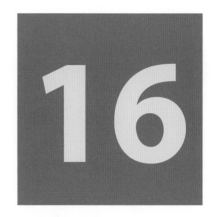

CASE STUDY

The first-time parents of a healthy two-day-old baby are anxiously awaiting discharge from a community hospital in the upper peninsula of Michigan so they can start their new life. The nurse explains to the parents that the baby must "pass" a few routine tests prior to discharge. This includes a pulse oximetry screening test to rule out critical congenital heart disease. Unexpectedly, the baby's oxygen level is 93%, lower than the acceptable value for discharge. A family practitioner meets with the family and tells them that after following the recommended algorithm, he is not comfortable sending the baby home without a more definitive test to rule out a life-threatening heart problem. The baby needs to have an echocardiogram (ultrasound of heart) performed. The hospital does offer this test in babies, but the cardiologists in the hospital are only qualified to interpret studies in adults. The nearest pediatric cardiologist is 300 miles away and only visits the region one time per month. If this had happened two years ago, the baby would have needed to be transferred via helicopter to a children's hospital hundreds of miles away.

Fortunately, the hospital has an established telemedicine link with a children's hospital. A local sonographer performs the echocardiogram and transmits it immediately to a cloud server. Within 30 minutes of completing the test, a pediatric cardiologist meets the family via live videoconference consultation and tells them their baby's heart is normal and there is

nothing to worry about. Had something abnormal been detected, the pediatric cardiologist could have watched the echocardiogram as it was being performed; instructed the sonographer to obtain additional images; made management recommendations to the local physician; and counseled the family about the diagnosis, treatment, and prognosis.

This scenario plays out hundreds of times a day across the United States; congenital heart defects occur in 1% of all children and one-quarter of them are critical. Many additional newborns have findings concerning for a heart defect; as a result echocardiography is requested in approximately 40/1,000 newborns prior to hospital discharge.[1] Many of these infants are born at hospitals that have adult cardiology programs that include echocardiography but don't have immediate access to onsite pediatric cardiology. Over the last 20 years telemedicine has become the standard of care in this setting, allowing for initiation of lifesaving treatment and urgent transport for babies with critical heart disease and obviating the need for unnecessary transport in cases where congenital heart disease can be excluded.

Telemedicine has changed the practice of pediatric cardiology. Pediatric cardiology is one of the largest users of telemedicine, with multiple modalities, clinical models, and technology (Tables 16-1 and 16-2). In this chapter we will provide an overview of how tele-echocardiography and other modalities of telemedicine are used in pediatric cardiology, with focus on shifting

Table 16-1. Modalities and Clinical Use Cases for Telecardiology

Modality	Indication	Setting	Patient location	Provider location	Population	Telemedicine goals
Echocardiography	Suspected congenital/acquired heart disease	Clinical Academic	Hospital Outpatient	Hospital Clinic Home	Fetal Newborns Older children	Test interpretation Sonographer training Clinical consultation Family counseling Second opinion Research
Electrophysiology	Rhythm assessment	Clinical	Hospital Home	Hospital Clinic Home	All	Inpatient monitor review Longitudinal rhythm assessment
Intensive care (telemedicine cart)	Pre/postoperative management	Clinical	Hospital	Hospital Home	Newborns Older children	Direct patient care Clinical consultation
Remote monitoring	Home interstage (single ventricle) monitoring	Clinical	Home	Hospital	Infants	Direct patient care Triage for escalation of care
Direct to consumer	Preventive cardiology Follow-up outpatient visits (syncope, chest pain, heart failure)	Clinical	Home	Hospital Clinic	Older children	Direct patient care Family counseling
Global health	Case review conferences Image interpretation	Clinical Conference Academic Education	Hospital Outpatient	Hospital Clinic Home	All	Direct patient care Second opinion Program building Research
Multimodality conferencing	Patient care conferences	Conference Education	Hospital	Anywhere	All	Multidisciplinary patient review Clinical decision making Cardiac surgery planning Second opinion

Table 16-2. Technology for Telecardiology

Technology	Endpoints	Connectivity	Examples
Live videoconferencing	Room systems: CODEC Carts/peripheral devices (camera, stethoscope, ultrasound machine) Personal computers Tablets Smart phones	Standard Internet 3G/4G/LTE Historic (ISDN, T1/3)	Echocardiography Intensive care Multimodality conferencing Global health
Store and forward	Medical devices PACs systems Personal computer (thick client or URL based)	SFTP VPN Cloud server Standard Internet 3G/4G/LTE	Echocardiography Electrophysiology Remote monitoring Auscultation Global health
Collaboration (includes direct to consumer and standard commercial products; eg, Skype, Webex)	Personal computers Tablets Smart phones	Standard Internet 3G/4G/LTE	Direct to consumer Multimodality conferencing

technology and expanding clinical use cases. We will also provide a brief discussion of how the pediatric cardiology literature can be leveraged for regulatory advocacy. For a more detailed review of telemedicine use in pediatric cardiology, the reader is referred to the recent scientific statement from the American Heart Association, *Telemedicine in Pediatric Cardiology.*[2]

ECHOCARDIOGRAPHY

Telemedicine has become the standard of care in pediatric echocardiography. Pediatric tele-echocardiography can be carried out in real time via live videoconference or store-and-forward of images to be viewed remotely. Initial telemedicine studies utilized point-to-point Integrated Services Digital Network (ISDN) and Terrestrial-1 (T1) connections for live telemedicine with good image quality and acceptable temporal resolution (frame rates of 23–30/second).[1,3–8] Rapid progression of technology over the last five years has made this ISDN and T1 connectivity technology obsolete. Today, Internet Protocol (IP) allows for multipoint network connectivity that enables use of codecs or videoconferencing software from anywhere on any device. These include room systems, desktop or laptop computers, tablets, and smart phones.

Modern technology with high-speed connections greatly enhances store-and-forward

telemedicine as well. As a result, the field of pediatric tele-echocardiography has evolved to primarily be dependent on store-and-forward solutions that, in many cases, are extensions of existing echocardiography Picture Archiving and Communication System (PACS) systems with special considerations for data transfer. Direct point-to-point study transmission options include secure File Transfer Protocol (FTP) and Virtual Private Network (VPN). Cloud servers enable transmission of and access to echocardiograms from anywhere in the world with subsequent download into local PACS servers.[9,10] Many physicians access echocardiograms via remote connection to PACS networks through client or web-based programs. In our hospital we have a mix of all of these technologies, but prefer studies being transferred into our PACS system for uniform interpretation and reporting. However, some partner hospitals insist on us reporting in their local PACS and electronic medical records. Diligent attention to security, licensure and credentialing requirements, and compliance issues, as well as a need for 24/7 technical support staff, are critical for maintenance of a tele-echocardiography network.

We reported on our technology transition experience of over 10,000 telemedicine transmissions from 24 sites in seven states and territories between 1998 and 2014.[11] Figures 16-1, 16-2, and 16-3 show how we transitioned our program over this period. A significant

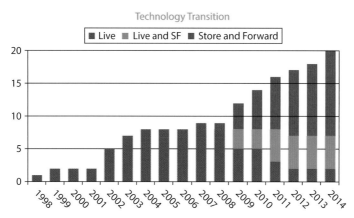

▲ **Figure 16-1.** Transition of our program (by sites) from live to store-and-forward telemedicine. (From Krishnan A, Fuska M, Dixon R, et al. The evolution of pediatric tele-echocardiography: 15-year experience of over 10,000 transmissions. *Telemed J E Health* 2014;20(8):681–686.)

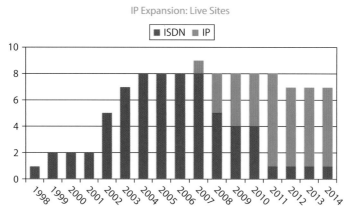

▲ **Figure 16-2.** Transition of live telemedicine in our program (by sites) from ISDN to Internet Protocol. (From Krishnan A, Fuska M, Dixon R, et al. The evolution of pediatric tele-echocardiography: 15-year experience of over 10,000 transmissions. *Telemed J E Health* 2014;20(8):681–686.)

increase in telecardiology utilization took place after IP expansion without detrimental effects on efficiency or diagnostic accuracy. This occurred in parallel to a change from a predominance of real-time telemedicine to store-and-forward transmissions. Over 150 patients were transported for surgical, catheter-based, or medical intervention, and critical heart disease was ruled out in over 75 patients, preventing unnecessary transport. Medical management and/or outpatient follow-up was recommended in approximately half of the studies for minor heart defects.

Multiple studies have found neonatal tele-echocardiography to be accurate and cost effective, to have a positive impact on patient care, to prevent unnecessary transports, and to improve sonographer proficiency.[4,5,7,12–17] In older children, tele-echocardiography is equally feasible from the technical standpoint, but most clinical scenarios dictate that the best practice is to have a pediatric cardiologist evaluate the patient prior to ordering an echocardiogram. Fetal telecardiology is also possible; it has shown to be accurate and can improve sonographer proficiency.[18,19] A multicenter

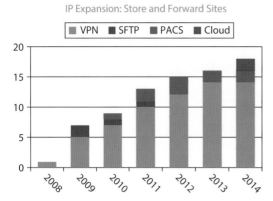

IP Expansion: Store and Forward Sites

▲ **Figure 16-3.** Utilization of different store-and-forward telemedicine protocols in our program (by sites). (From Krishnan A, Fuska M, Dixon R, et al. The evolution of pediatric tele-echocardiography: 15-year experience of over 10,000 transmissions. *Telemed J E Health* 2014;20(8):681–686.)

study from nine centers assessed the impact of telemedicine on infants with no or minor heart disease. Three hundred thirty-eight pairs of infants with and without access to telemedicine were matched for study indication, diagnosis, gestational age, birth weight, and gender.[20] Access to telemedicine resulted in statistically significant reductions in rate of transfer to a tertiary care hospital (10% vs. 5%), total and intensive care unit length of stay, and inappropriate use of inotropic support and indomethacin. Table 16-3 provides a summary of other pediatric tele-echocardiography studies reported in the literature (modified from an American Heart Association [AHA] scientific statement).[2]

Pulse oximetry screening for critical congenital heart disease is mandated in almost every state and is a driver for the establishment of telemedicine links between community hospitals and tertiary care pediatric cardiac centers.[21-23] If a positive screen is obtained, telemedicine can provide timely access to pediatric subspecialists in cardiology and neonatology for assessment and treatment recommendations. There is a theoretical concern that false-positive pulse oximetry screens would dramatically increase the number of tele-echocardiograms, pushing up costs and overburdening pediatric cardiologists providing interpretation. However, a recent study shows that the additional increase in echocardiograms from pulse oximetry screening is negligible when

compared to the number of false-positive echocardiograms generated by heart murmurs.[24]

ELECTROPHYSIOLOGY

Telemedicine has been used for several years for simple transmission of electrophysiological data through transtelephonic event recorders and pacemaker evaluations. Remote monitoring of rhythm data from bedside monitors is also commonplace. Leveraging applications for smart phones and tablets for rhythm analysis makes monitoring of cardiac electrical activity for detection of arrhythmias and myocardial infarction feasible. The SEARCH-AF trial from Australia evaluated nearly 1,000 patients with a single-lead electrocardiogram (ECG) device built into an iPhone case. The technology was accurate and cost effective and has the potential to prevent stroke.[25,26] A modification of the existing single-lead device was used in a recent study for assessment of ST elevation myocardial infarction (STEMI). There was agreement in six patients (four with STEMI and two with non-STEMI) when comparing the smart phone tracing to 12-lead ECG.[27] This technology can generate tracings of diagnostic quality in children, with positive user satisfaction and could be used to manage children with supraventricular tachycardia and atrial fibrillation.[28]

INTENSIVE CARE UNIT

Telemedicine has many applications in the pediatric intensive care unit (PICU)[29-34] and in the emergency department,[35-37] using a broad range of applications to assist in the care of hospitalized children in a variety of clinical scenarios.[38,39] Telemedicine can be used in a reactive or continuous model for support of critical care patients. In the reactive model, physician consultations, nurse and physician monitoring, and medical oversight are provided on an intermittent, as-needed basis. In a reactive model, a pediatric cardiologist or intensivist can evaluate and provide recommendations on diagnostic studies, medications, or other therapies.[29,32,33] The other end of the spectrum integrates continuous oversight via monitoring and proactive medical decision making.[40] All models require compliance with best critical care practices and maintenance of training, including advanced life support certifications and participation in quality assurance programs.

Table 16-3. Pediatric Tele-echocardiography Publications*

Location	Year(s)	Key findings
Nova Scotia[12,74,75]	1989, 97, 2004	Real time over POTS, cost savings, tele-education
Kentucky[13]	1993	Store-and-forward over POTS
Chicago[3,4]	1996	Real time over single ISDN line
Ireland[16,76–78]	1996, 1998, 2008	Real time over low-bandwidth connection
North Carolina[79–81]	1997, 1998	Outcomes and reduced length of stay
Glasgow[5]	1999	100% accuracy requires 3 ISDN lines
Minnesota[82]	1999	Accuracy, management over T1
New Orleans[7]	1999	Accuracy, proficiency, cost savings over 3 ISDN lines
Iowa[15,83]	1999, 2001	Minimal difference: cardiologist vs. pediatrician ordering echo in children less than one year of age.
Washington, DC[1]	2002	500 studies/3 ISDN lines/Impact on practice
Switzerland[84]	2003	Real time over 3 ISDN lines/feasibility and accuracy
Hawaii[85]	2004	Live and store-and-forward between Hawaii and Guam
Portland[86]	2004	Remote real-time image control and optimization
Washington, DC[8]	2004	"Forward-and-store" tele-echocardiography
Portugal[87]	2005	1761 consultations over 5 years/mostly elective
Seattle[14]	2006	769 studies/3 ISDN lines/99% accurate
South Dakota[17]	2006	Neonatal tele-echocardiography triage
India[88]	2007	Real time/small aperture satellite bandwidth
London[89]	2007	Belgrade to London conference over single ISDN line
Portugal[90]	2010	Fetal, neonatal, and pediatric consultations in real time
Arizona[91]	2012	Real-time telemed more accurate than recorded echos
Canada[92]	2013	Videoconferencing for ACHD management

Abbreviations *ACHD*: adult with congenital heart disease, *ISDN*: integrated services digital network, *POTS*: plain old telephone systems, *T1*: Terrestrial 1.
*Modified from Satou GM, Rheuban K, Alverson D, et al. Telemedicine in pediatric cardiology: a scientific statement from the American Heart Association. *Circulation* 2017;135(11):e648-e678.

Patients in critical care settings with access to telemedicine can be more quickly evaluated, stabilized, and triaged to determine the need for transport and more advanced treatment.[41] Case reviews, education, and quality improvement between referral and tertiary care sites can utilize the same technology to complement clinical telemedicine.[42] Use of telemedicine in a variety of critical care programs around the globe results in improvements in clinical outcomes, including length of stay and mortality.[29,32,33,43,44] These studies also report high levels of satisfaction among providers at both ends of the telemedicine encounter, as well as patients and parents. Reductions in health care costs occur due to more appropriate transport utilization and decreased utilization of the more costly regional ICU.[34,38,45–47] Munoz et al. reported on a telemedicine-supported cardiac intensive care unit collaboration between Pittsburgh and Bogota, Columbia.[32,33,48] This program included a web interface of physiological monitors and videoconferencing via a mobile telemedicine cart. Face-to-face videoconferencing, sharing of medical images, and review of rhythm disturbances resulted in 71 recommendations in 53 patients, including management of arrhythmias and surgical and catheterization planning.

REMOTE MONITORING

Home monitoring incorporates automated telemedicine technology[49] for a wide variety of diseases in adults, including diabetes,[50] chronic respiratory disease,[51] congestive heart failure,[52] and hypertension,[49] as well as children with asthma.[53] These devices are usually tablet sized and connect to a variety of peripheral devices (hard wired or wireless, usually Bluetooth), including scales, heart rate and pulse oximeter monitors, blood pressure devices, glucometers, and peak flow meters. Many vendors are now integrating directly with commercially available tablets and smart phones. These devices can combine standardized management with patient and parent education modules. Data can also be manually entered. These devices then transmit data (cellular network or wired or wireless Internet connection) can be reviewed with software that allows for serial comparisons and red flags for outlying or missing data.

Home telemedicine models for adult patients with heart disease could be translatable to children. Home telemonitoring programs for adults with congestive heart failure using automated daily capture of weight, blood pressure, heart rate, and oxygen saturation transmitted to a nurse practitioner resulted in fewer admissions, shorter lengths of stay during admissions, lower health care costs, and improved quality of life.[54] A meta-analysis of home telemedicine monitoring of patients with congestive heart failure showed reduced mortality, decreased number of hospitalizations and the use of other health services, and improved quality of life.[52]

The National Pediatric Cardiology Quality Improvement Collaborative (NPC-QIC) has focused on reduction of interstage morbidity and mortality for single ventricle patients after stage I palliation.[55-59] This program includes home surveillance of pulse oximetry, weight, nutritional intake, and warning signs of deterioration.[60-62] One of the consistent findings from the NPC-QIC is the importance of weight gain on positive outcomes. Cross et al. reported utilization of a telemedicine solution for interstage single ventricle care that incorporated automated transmission of pulse oximetry, weight, and formula intake, along with answering questions about the status of the infant.[63] This solution included a website with automated warning alerts and a patient dashboard for easy access to subtle changes over time. The weight for age percentile for patients with access to home telemedicine was more likely to increase than in those patients without access to home telemedicine (Figure 16-4).

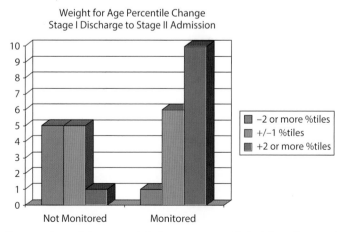

▲ **Figure 16-4.** Impact of home telemedicine on weight for age percentile in infants between stage 1 and stage 2 single ventricle palliation. (From Cross R, Steury R, Randall A, et al. Single-ventricle palliation for high-risk neonates: examining the feasibility of an automated home monitoring system after stage I palliation. *Future Cardiol* 2012;8(2):227–235.)

DIRECT TO CONSUMER TELEMEDICINE

The marketing of and demand for "direct to consumer" medical care in the home via web-based applications that include tablet and smart phone applications are growing rapidly.[64] Many insurance providers and large employee health plans are adopting this technology as a way to provide lower-cost care for common problems that might otherwise result in an emergency room visit.[65] Direct to consumer telemedicine primarily relies on video and audio connections between a physician (or other health care provider) and patient. The tablet, smart phone, or computer-based application may include additional features that allow for scheduling, billing, and sharing of still-frame images and documentation. In some models, peripherals may be available such as smart phone–compatible heart rhythm detection devices[27] and otoscopes.[66] In our program, we are utilizing our own physicians to provide this service for follow-up visits for syncope, preventive cardiology (obesity and hypercholesterolemia), and neurodevelopmental assessment. We are in the process of adding this service for our transplant and chronic heart failure population as well.

The most common model for direct to consumer telemedicine is a turnkey service that includes access to technology and a physician group provided through the same vendor that provides the technology. This could, in theory, create a threat to the delivery of high-quality care, especially for complex pediatric patients. Additionally, as the use of these devices grows, careful attention must be paid to patient safety and privacy. In response to this concern, the American Telemedicine Association has implemented an accreditation program for consumer-directed telehealth services provision.[67]

GLOBAL TELEMEDICINE

Less than 10% of the world's population has access to lifesaving surgical and catheter-based interventions to treat even low-risk congenital heart defects,[68] and rheumatic heart disease remains endemic across most of the globe.[69] Collaboration between cardiology and cardiac surgery experts in high-income countries and programs in low-income and lower middle–income countries is essential to closing the gap in care. Telemedicine can be a powerful tool to facilitate care and disease prevention in low-income and middle-income countries.[70] Educational web conferences can

have a significant impact on improving outcomes for congenital heart surgery in resource-poor countries.[71] Live patient care conferences and sharing of images via the cloud can advance research collaboration for congenital and rheumatic heart disease.[72] We recently reported on using telemedicine to facilitate screening of over 4,000 Brazilian children for rheumatic heart disease.[73] Echocardiograms performed in schools in Brazil were uploaded to the cloud and interpreted jointly by physicians in Belo Horizonte Brazil and Washington, DC. However, there are several challenges to successful implementation of global telemedicine. These include differences in time zone, language, culture, local government regulations, Internet security, maintenance of equipment, and lack of access to affordable broadband connectivity, especially in more remote regions.

PATIENT CARE CONFERENCES

Although most of the published telemedicine data is on clinical applications, the most prevalent use case may be multimodality videoconferencing. We conduct multiple patient care and educational conferences each week that includes physicians within our practice, referring physicians, and trainees who connect via telemedicine. ECGs, echocardiograms, angiograms, magnetic resonance images (MRIs), and computed tomography (CT) scans are shared along with relevant patient data for clinical decision making with input from a multidisciplinary team, many of whom are not available to attend these meetings in person. Secure login and encryption are utilized to protect patient confidentiality. Participants who connect remotely can do so from telemedicine rooms that have been set up at remote sites, as well as personal computers, tablets, and smart phones with installed videoconferencing programs and applications. Additional technology enables a connection between the videoconference and collaboration tools so that those without direct access to the videoconferencing program can connect via a secure website.

REIMBURSEMENT/LICENSING/ CREDENTIALING/REGULATORY ISSUES

Regulatory issues surrounding reimbursement, licensing, and credentialing for telemedicine remain significant obstacles for widespread adoption of telemedicine for pediatric cardiology. A detailed discussion of these issues is provided elsewhere in this book. However, the large amount of data from pediatric cardiology, especially surrounding newborns with suspected heart defects, can be leveraged to make a strong case for a more favorable health care environment that supports broader acceptance of telemedicine. The priorities of cost containment, quality and outcomes, patient-centered care, and optimal use of technology are best served by increased utilization of telemedicine. In order to realize this potential, the following guiding principles must be adopted: 1) legislation and policies that will allow for reimbursement for telemedicine to be equal to traditional health care must be enacted at state and federal levels, 2) state medical boards must work together to enable the practice of telemedicine across state lines, and 3) medical staff of hospitals must lobby for and accept universal credentialing by proxy procedures.

SUMMARY

Pediatric cardiology is one of the most prevalent applications of telemedicine. Multiple publications support that tele-echocardiography is accurate and diagnostic, improves care of the sickest children, appropriately triages patients—preventing unnecessary transports, is cost effective, and improves sonographer proficiency and physician efficiency. Evolving technology allows for seamless integration of tele-echocardiography into routine practice, making it a standard of care in 2017. Near-universal adoption of newborn pulse oximetry screening for critical congenital heart disease mandates a renewed focus on telemedicine for many delivery hospitals in the United States. Telemedicine also affects many other areas of pediatric cardiology with innovative solutions for electrophysiology, intensive care unit, home monitoring, direct to consumer telemedicine, global health, and patient care and education conferences. Removal of reimbursement, licensure, and credentialing obstacles is needed to realize the full benefit that telemedicine can have for our pediatric cardiology patients and on our health care system in general.

REFERENCES

1. Sable CA, Cummings SD, Pearson GD, et al. Impact of telemedicine on the practice of pediatric cardiology in community hospitals. *Pediatrics* 2002;109(1):E3.

2. Satou GM, Rheuban K, Alverson D, et al. Telemedicine in pediatric cardiology: A scientific statement from the American Heart Association. *Circulation* 2017;135(11): e648-e678.

3. Alboliras ET, Berdusis K, Fisher J, et al. Transmission of full-length echocardiographic images over ISDN for diagnosing congenital heart disease. *Telemed J* 1996;2(4):251–258.

4. Fisher JB, Alboliras ET, Berdusis K, et al. Rapid identification of congenital heart disease by transmission of echocardiograms. *Am HeartJ* 1996;131(6):1225–1227.

5. Houston A, McLeod K, Richens T, et al. Assessment of the quality of neonatal echocardiographic images transmitted by ISDN telephone lines. *Heart* 1999;82(2):222–225.

6. Sable C. Digital echocardiography and telemedicine applications in pediatric cardiology. *Pediatric Cardiol* 2002;23(3):358–369.

7. Sable C, Roca T, Gold J, et al. Live transmission of neonatal echocardiograms from underserved areas: accuracy, patient care, and cost. *Telemed J* 1999;5(4):339–347.

8. Woodson KE, Sable CA, Cross RR, et al. Forward and store telemedicine using Motion Pictures Expert Group: a novel approach to pediatric tele-echocardiography. *J Am Soc Echocardiogr* 2004;17(11):1197–1200.

9. Singh S, Bansal M, Maheshwari P, et al. American Society of Echocardiography: Remote Echocardiography with Web-Based Assessments for Referrals at a Distance (ASE-REWARD) Study. *J Am Soc Echocardiogr* 2013;26(3):221–233.

10. Hsieh JC, Li AH, Yang CC. Mobile, cloud, and big data computing: contributions, challenges, and new directions in telecardiology. *Int J Environ Res Public Health* 10(11):6131–6153, 2013.

11. Krishnan A, Fuska M, Dixon R, et al. The evolution of pediatric tele-echocardiography: 15-year experience of over 10,000 transmissions. *Telemed J E Health* 2014;20(8):681–686.

12. Finley JP, Sharratt GP, Nanton MA, et al. Paediatric echocardiography by telemedicine – nine years' experience. *J Telemed Telecare* 1997;3(4):200–204.

13. Sobczyk WL, Solinger RE, Rees AH, et al. Transtelephonic echocardiography: successful use in a tertiary pediatric referral center. *J Pediatr* 1993;122(6):S84–S88.

14. Lewin M, Xu C, Jordan M, et al. Accuracy of paediatric echocardiographic transmission via telemedicine. *J Telemed Telecare* 2006;12(8):416–421.

15. Scholz TD, Kienzle MG. Optimizing utilization of pediatric echocardiography and implications for telemedicine. *Am J Cardiol* 1999;83(12):1645–1648.

16. McCrossan BA, Grant B, Morgan GJ, et al. Diagnosis of congenital heart disease in neonates by

videoconferencing: an eight-year experience. *J Telemed Telecare* 2008;14(3):137–140.

17. Awadallah S, Halaweish I, Kutayli F. Tele-echocardiography in neonates: utility and benefits in South Dakota primary care hospitals. *S D Med* 2006;59(3):97–100.

18. McCrossan BA, Sands AJ, Kileen T, et al. A fetal telecardiology service: patient preference and socio-economic factors. *Prenat Diag* 2012;32(9):883–887.

19. Sharma S, Parness IA, Kamenir SA, et al. Screening fetal echocardiography by telemedicine: efficacy and community acceptance. *J Am Soc Echocardiogr* 2003;16(3):202–208.

20. Webb CL, Waugh CL, Grigsby J, et al. Impact of telemedicine on hospital transport, length of stay, and medical outcomes in infants with suspected heart disease: a multicenter study. *J Am Soc Echocardiogr* 2013;26(9):1090–1098.

21. Mahle WT, Newburger JW, Matherne GP, et al. Role of pulse oximetry in examining newborns for congenital heart disease: a scientific statement from the American Heart Association and American Academy of Pediatrics. *Circulation* 2009;120(5):447–458.

22. Kemper AR, Mahle WT, Martin GR, et al. Strategies for implementing screening for critical congenital heart disease. *Pediatrics* 2011;128(5):e1259–e1267.

23. Mahle WT, Martin GR, Beekman RH 3rd, et al. Endorsement of Health and Human Services recommendation for pulse oximetry screening for critical congenital heart disease. *Pediatrics* 2012;129(1):190–192.

24. Singh A, Rasiah SV, Ewer AK. The impact of routine pre-discharge pulse oximetry screening in a regional neonatal unit. *Arch Dis Child Fetal Neonatal Ed* 2014;99(4): F297–F302.

25. Lowres N, Freedman SB, Redfern J, et al. Screening education and recognition in community pharmacies of atrial fibrillation to prevent stroke in an ambulant population aged >=65 years (SEARCH-AF stroke prevention study): a cross-sectional study protocol. *BMJ Open* 2012;2(3).pii: e001355.

26. Lowres N, Neubeck L, Salkeld G, et al. Feasibility and cost-effectiveness of stroke prevention through community screening for atrial fibrillation using iPhone ECG in pharmacies. The SEARCH-AF study. *Throm Haemost* 2014;111(6):1167–1176.

27. Muhlestein JB, Le V, Albert D, et al. Smartphone ECG for evaluation of STEMI: Results of the ST LEUIS Pilot Study. *J Electrocardiol* 2015;48(2):249–259.

28. Nguyen HH, Van Hare GF, Rudokas M, et al. SPEAR Trial: Smartphone Pediatric ElectrocARdiogram Trial. *PLoS One* 2015;10(8):e0136256.

29. Lopez-Magallon AJ, Otero AV, Welchering N, et al. Patient outcomes of an international telepediatric cardiac critical care program. *Telemed J E Health* 2015;21(8):601–610.

30. Lilly CM, Cody S, Zhao H, et al. Hospital mortality, length of stay, and preventable complications among critically ill patients before and after tele-ICU reengineering of critical care processes. *JAMA* 2011;305(21):2175–2183.

31. Morrison JL, Cai Q, Davis N, et al. Clinical and economic outcomes of the electronic intensive care unit: results from two community hospitals. *Crit Care Med* 2010;38(1):2–8.

32. Otero AV, Lopez-Magallon AJ, Jaimes D, et al. International telemedicine in pediatric cardiac critical care: a multicenter experience. *Telemed J E Health* 2014;20(7):619–625.

33. Munoz RA, Burbano NH, Motoa MV, et al. Telemedicine in pediatric cardiac critical care. *Telemed J E Health* 2012;18(2):132–136.

34. Marcin JP, Nesbitt TS, Kallas HJ, et al. Use of telemedicine to provide pediatric critical care inpatient consultations to underserved rural Northern California. *J Pediatr* 2004;144(3):375–380.

35. Dharmar M, Kuppermann N, Romano PS, et al. Telemedicine consultations and medication errors in rural emergency departments. *Pediatrics* 2013;132(6):1090–1097.

36. Dharmar M, Marcin JP. A picture is worth a thousand words: critical care consultations to emergency departments using telemedicine. *Pediatr Crit Care Med* 2009;10(5):606–607.

37. Dharmar M, Romano PS, Kuppermann N, et al. Impact of critical care telemedicine consultations on children in rural emergency departments. *Crit Care Med* 2013;41(10):2388–2395.

38. Dharmar M, Smith AC, Armfield NR, et al. Telemedicine for children in need of intensive care. *Pediatr Ann* 2009;38(10):562–566.

39. Marcin JP. Telemedicine in the pediatric intensive care unit. *Pediatr Clin North Am* 2013;60(3):581–592.

40. Reynolds HN, Rogove H, Bander J, et al. A working lexicon for the tele-intensive care unit: We need to define tele-intensive care unit to grow and understand it. *Telemed J E Health* 2011;17(10):773–783.

41. Huang T, Moon-Grady AJ, Traugott C, et al. The availability of telecardiology consultations and transfer patterns from a remote neonatal intensive care unit. *J Telemed Telecare* 2008;14(5):244–248.

42. Backman W, Bendel D, Rakhit R. The telecardiology revolution: improving the management of cardiac disease in primary care. *J R Society Med* 2010;103(11):442–446.

43. Alverson DC, Swinfen LR, Swinfen LP, et al. Transforming systems of care for children in the global community. *Pediat Ann* 2009;38:579–585.

44. Lorch SA, Myers S, Carr B. The regionalization of pediatric health care. *Pediatrics* 2010;126(6):1182–1190.

45. Marcin JP, Nesbitt TS, Struve S, et al. Financial benefits of a pediatric intensive care unit-based telemedicine program to a rural adult intensive care unit: impact of keeping acutely ill and injured children in their local community. *Telemed J E Health* 2004;10(Suppl 2):1–5.

46. Kon AA, Marcin JP. Using telemedicine to improve communication during paediatric resuscitations. *J Telemed Telecare* 2005;11(5):261–264.

47. Heath B, Salerno R, Hopkins A, et al. Pediatric critical care telemedicine in rural underserved emergency departments. *Pediatr Crit Care Med* 2009;10(5):588–591.

48. Lopez-Magallon AJ, Otero AV, Welchering N, et al. Patient outcomes of an international telepediatric cardiac critical care program. *Telemed J E Health* 2015;21(8):601–610.

49. Pare G, Moqadem K, Pineau G, et al. Clinical effects of home telemonitoring in the context of diabetes, asthma, heart failure and hypertension: a systematic review. *J Med Internet Res* 2010;12(2):e21.

50. Jia H, Feng H, Wang X, et al. A longitudinal study of health service utilization for diabetes patients in a care coordination home-telehealth programme. *J Telemed Telecare* 2011;17(3):123–126.

51. Polisena J, Tran K, Cimon K, et al. Home telehealth for chronic obstructive pulmonary disease: a systematic review and meta-analysis. *J Telemed Telecare* 2010;16(3):120–127.

52. Polisena J, Tran K, Cimon K, et al. Home telemonitoring for congestive heart failure: a systematic review and meta-analysis. *J Telemed Telecare* 2010;16(2):68–76.

53. Chan DS, Callahan CW, Hatch-Pigott VB, et al. Internet-based home monitoring and education of children with asthma is comparable to ideal office-based care: results of a 1-year asthma in-home monitoring trial. *Pediatrics* 2007;119(3):569–578.

54. Benatar D, Bondmass M, Ghitelman J, et al. Outcomes of chronic heart failure. *Arch Intern Med* 2003;163(3):347–352.

55. Anderson JB, Beekman RH 3rd, Kugler JD, et al. Improvement in interstage survival in a national pediatric cardiology learning network. *Circ Cardiovasc Qual Outcomes* 2015;8(4):428–436.

56. Anderson JB, Beekman RH 3rd, Kugler JD, et al. Use of a learning network to improve variation in interstage weight gain after the Norwood operation. *Congenit Heart Dis* 2014;9(6):512–520.

57. Bradshaw EA, Cuzzi S, Kiernan SC, et al. Feasibility of implementing pulse oximetry screening for congenital heart disease in a community hospital. *J Perinatol* 2012;32(9):710–715.

58. Cross RR, Harahsheh AS, McCarter R, et al. Identified mortality risk factors associated with presentation, initial hospitalisation, and interstage period for the Norwood operation in a multi-centre registry: a report from the national pediatric cardiology-quality improvement collaborative. *Cardiol Young* 2014;24(2):253–262.

59. Schidlow DN, Anderson JB, Klitzner TS, et al. Variation in interstage outpatient care after the Norwood procedure: a report from the Joint Council on Congenital Heart Disease National Quality Improvement Collaborative. *Congenit Heart Dis* 2011;6(2):98–107.

60. Ghanayem NS, Hoffman GM, Mussatto KA, et al. Home surveillance program prevents interstage mortality after the Norwood procedure. *J Thorac Cardiovasc Surg* 2003;126(5):1367–1377.

61. Petit CJ, Fraser CD, Mattamal R, et al. The impact of a dedicated single-ventricle home-monitoring program on interstage somatic growth, interstage attrition, and 1-year survival. *J Thorac Cardiovasc Surg* 2011;142(6):1358–1366.

62. Dobrolet NC, Nieves JA, Welch EM, et al. New approach to interstage care for palliated high-risk patients with congenital heart disease. *J Thorac Cardiovasc Surg* 2011;142(4):855–860.

63. Cross R, Steury R, Randall A, et al. Single-ventricle palliation for high-risk neonates: examining the feasibility of an automated home monitoring system after stage I palliation. *Future Cardiol* 2012;8(2):227–235.

64. Uscher-Pines L, Mulcahy A, Cowling D, et al. Access and quality of care in direct-to-consumer telemedicine. *Telemed J E Health*. 2016;22(4):282–287.

65. UnitedHealthcare. UnitedHealthcare Covers Virtual Care Physician Visits, Expanding Consumers' Access to Affordable Health Care Options. http://www.unitedhealthgroup.com/newsroom/articles/feed/unitedhealthcare/2015/0430virtualcarephysicians.aspx.

66. The iPhone Otoscope. https://www.cellscope.com/clinicians. Accessed March 3, 2017.

67. American Telemedicine Association. *Direct to Consumer Accreditation*. http://www.americantelemed.org/accreditation/online-patient-consultations/program-home-.VyZiWD_tmKI. Accessed March 3, 2017.

68. Hoffman J. The global burden of congenital heart disease. *Cardiovasc J Afr* 2013;24(4):141–145.

69. Zuhlke LJ, Steer AC. Estimates of the global burden of rheumatic heart disease. *Glob Heart* 2013;8(3):189–195.

70. Vedanthan R, Choi BG, Baber U, et al. Bioimaging and subclinical cardiovascular disease in low- and middle-income countries. *J Cardiovasc Transl Res* 2014;7(8):701–710.

71. Jenkins KJ, Castaneda AR, Cherian KM, et al. Reducing mortality and infections after congenital heart surgery in the developing world. *Pediatrics* 2014;134(5):e1422–e1430.

72. Ploutz M, Lu JC, Scheel J, et al. Handheld echocardiographic screening for rheumatic heart disease by non-experts. *Heart* 2016;102(1):35–39.

73. Lopes EL, Beaton AZ, Nascimento BR, et al. Telehealth solutions to enable global collaboration in rheumatic heart disease screening. *J Telemed Telecare* November 4, 2016. pii: 1357633X16677902. [Epub ahead of print.]

74. Finley JP, Human DG, Nanton MA, et al. Echocardiography by telephone – evaluation of pediatric heart disease at a distance. *Am J Cardiol* 1989;63(20):1475–1477.

75. Cloutier A, Finley J. Telepediatric cardiology practice in Canada. *Telemed J E Health* 2004;10(1):33–37.

76. Casey F, Brown D, Craig BG, et al. Diagnosis of neonatal congenital heart defects by remote consultation using a low-cost telemedicine link. *J Telemed Telecare* 1996;2(3):165–169.

77. Casey F, Brown D, Corrigan N, et al. Value of a low-cost telemedicine link in the remote echocardiographic diagnosis of congenital heart defects. *J Telemed Telecare* 1998;4(suppl 1):46–48.

78. Mulholland HC, Casey F, Brown D, et al. Application of a low-cost telemedicine link to the diagnosis of neonatal congenital heart defects by remote consultation. *Heart* 1999;82(2):217–221.

79. Rendina MC, Long WA, deBliek R. Effect size and experimental power analysis in a paediatric cardiology telemedicine system. *J Telemed Telecare* 1997;3(suppl 1):56–57.

80. Rendina MC, Downs SM, Carasco N, et al. Effect of telemedicine on health outcomes in 87 infants requiring neonatal intensive care. *Telemed J* 1998;4(4):345–351.

81. Rendina MC. The effect of telemedicine on neonatal intensive care unit length of stay in very low birthweight infants. *Proceedings/AMIA Annual Symposium AMIA Symposium* 1998:111–115.

82. Randolph GR, Hagler DJ, Khandheria BK, et al. Remote telemedical interpretation of neonatal echocardiograms: impact on clinical management in a primary care setting. *J Am Coll Cardiol* 1999;34(1):241–245.

83. Mehta AR, Wakefield DS, Kienzle MG, et al. Pediatric tele-echocardiography: evaluation of transmission modalities. *Telemed J E Health* 2001;7(1):17–25.

84. Widmer S, Ghisla R, Ramelli GP, et al. Tele-echocardiography in paediatrics. *Eur J Pediatr* 2003;162(4):271–275.

85. Munir JA, Soh EK, Hoffmann TN, et al. A novel approach to tele-echocardiography across the Pacific. *Hawaii Med J* 2004;63(10):310–313.

86. Sahn DJ, Catallo L, Puntel R. Remote optimization of image and diagnostic quality during real time telemedicine echo screening of neonates at risk for cardiac disease: a new capability developed in support of our DOD PRMRP-funded study. Paper presented at the PRMRP Investigators Meeting, Puerto Rico, 2004.

87. Castela E, Ramalheiro G, Pires A, et al. Five years of tele-consultation: experience of the Cardiology Department of Coimbra Pediatric Hospital. *Rev Port Cardiol* 2005;24(6):835–840.

88. Sekar P, Vilvanathan V. Telecardiology: effective means of delivering cardiac care to rural children. *Asian Cardiovasc Thorac Ann* 2007;15(4):320–323.

89. Kosutic J, Rigby ML, Mijin D, et al. Low-bandwidth tele-consultations for patients with complex congenital heart diseases. *J Telemed Telecare* 2007;13(3):113–118.

90. Gomes R, Rossi R, Lima S, et al. Pediatric cardiology and telemedicine: seven years' experience of cooperation with remote hospitals. *Rev Port Cardiol* 2010;29(2):181–191.

91. Haley JE, Klewer SE, Barber BJ, et al. Remote diagnosis of congenital heart disease in southern Arizona: comparison between tele-echocardiography and videotapes. *Telemed J E Health* 2012;18(10):736–742.

92. Dehghani P, Atallah J, Rebeyka I, et al. Management of adults with congenital heart disease using videoconferencing across Western Canada: a 3-year experience. *Can J Cardiol* 2013;29(7):873–878.

Telehealth in Children with Special Needs

Kathleen A. Webster, MD, MBA, FAAP

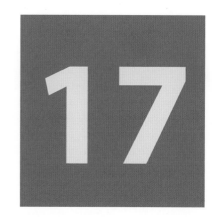

CASE STUDY

Isabella was born prematurely, with congenital heart disease and hypoplastic lungs. She underwent several surgeries, including a tracheostomy and feeding tube placement. After many months in the hospital she was able to be discharged home on a home ventilator. Her care team includes a pulmonologist, cardiologist, gastroenterologist, and the complex care team. In the year since her discharge, she has done well and now only requires a ventilator at night. During that year, however, she developed respiratory viral infections. Each illness required a trip to the local hospital, a long wait, and an exam by an unfamiliar provider who then transferred her by ambulance to the more distant children's hospital where her care team was located. Twice she was able to be sent home, and three times she was admitted to the intensive care unit for a longer hospital stay. Her mother was frustrated with the time and expense of these visits. She wanted to be able to keep her at home, but agreed that the team needed to be able to see Isabella frequently during her illness in order to adjust her support. A new telemedicine program was implemented, and Isabella's mother was given a tablet computer and a handheld device that allowed her to connect to the complex care team. When Isabella developed a slight fever and increased respiratory secretions, her mother called the care team. Her physician was able to connect by video and guide the mother through a physical exam with a stethoscope and
skin camera. Isabella was placed on her home ventilator for 4 days. Her physician and respiratory therapist connected with her every day to check in and repeat her exam. Isabella was able to remain at home, and her mother was very relieved to have the support of a team that knew her well.

BACKGROUND

The accompanying chapters explore the many uses of telemedicine to serve the pediatric population in any setting: inpatient, emergency departments, schools, child care, and outpatient clinics. These programs have succeeded in meeting the goals of increasing access to care, improving quality, reducing costs, and meeting the technology demands of patients and providers. Within this patient population, there exists a subset of children who require far more than the care needed by an average healthy child, or even one with an acute illness. Children with special health care needs (CSHCN) are recognized by the Maternal Child Health Bureau as those who require more care and resources on a chronic basis. Studies to quantify this need have stated that these children represent between 0.5% and 16% of the U.S. population, but require an estimated 10% to 50% of all health care dollars.[1–5] These children may have chronic physical needs such as diabetes, asthma, or congenital heart disease or perhaps developmental and/or behavioral issues that increase their need for care. There is overall a greater need for specialty care.[6]

Some of these children have multiple chronic needs and may be dependent on technology such as wheelchairs, feeding tubes, or ventilators. The most complex of these are classified as "medically fragile," or children with medical complexity (CMC). A variety of attempts have been made to more clearly define this group.[4,5] They are broadly characterized as those with multisystem chronic conditions, requiring multiple specialists and with frequent need to access both inpatient and outpatient care. As technology evolves, outcomes improve, and mortality decreases, the population of children meeting these definitions is increasing. CSCHN are recognized to have a particular benefit from coordination of the patient-centered medical home (PCMH). Increasingly, centers providing care for these children are recognizing the need to improve their care coordination and access to a multitude of specialists, primary care providers, nurses, case managers, therapists, nutritionists, and other providers.

The volume of health care visits needed may prohibit a parent from a regular work schedule or keep a child from attending school. Even in urban areas, the time, cost, and personnel required to bring these children to specialized care centers can be significant and are magnified if the child is located in a rural or medically underserved area.[6] As medical specialties evolve, providers may be in short supply and often must travel to outreach clinics, decreasing time available to care for patients. The costs and logistics of transportation may result in delays in seeking care for illnesses and often result in after-hours visits to the emergency department (ED). Provider comfort level with children with complex medical needs may result in more frequent hospitalizations.

As the case study illustrates, the use of telehealth technology can help achieve increased access and improved efficiency for CSHCN and CMC through remote patient monitoring, connection with the medical home, and multispecialty connections. Table 17-1 summarizes the types of services that may be provided to these children in various settings through the use of telehealth.

REMOTE PATIENT MONITORING

Remote patient monitoring in the home setting is becoming more widely used. The challenge is correctly interpreting the data and/or sharing it with a familiar health care provider for support and feedback. In CSHCN, a parent or caregiver may collect and share

Table 17-1. Types of Services Available to CMC via Telehealth

Originating Site	Type of Service
Home/School	Chronic Disease Management
	Scheduled Follow-Up
	Acute Care Visits
Outpatient Clinic	Provider->Provider Communication
	Subspecialty Consultation
Emergency Department	Primary Care Connection
	Subspecialty Consultation
Inpatient	Primary Care Connection
	Subspecialty Consultation
	Family-Centered Rounds

these data through a secure web portal in an asynchronous store-and-forward model. The most commonly described scenario is one in which measurements are taken daily or even more frequently and then uploaded to a secure site on a periodic basis. This not only allows the family or patient to view trends in the data, but also allows health care providers to provide feedback and detect the need for intervention.

Successful implementation of this type of program has been achieved for a variety of chronic conditions. Incorporation of telehealth technology to monitor oxygen saturation, nutritional intake, and weight gain contributed to the success of a home monitoring program for children with congenital heart disease.[7] Similarly, adolescents with diabetes benefitted from a program allowing monthly uploads of blood glucose and insulin pump therapy, resulting in improved compliance and better glycemic control.[8] In children with cystic fibrosis, monitoring of spirometry and pulse oximetry resulted in improved outcomes as well as significant cost savings.[9] In another program, children with asthma completed online symptom diaries and shared peak flow measurements. An additional component included uploading videos of inhaler technique. Not only was this found to be effective, but compared to children who presented in person for coaching, the inhaler technique was improved in the telemedicine group. Investigators attributed this to an ability to conduct more frequent assessments and to allow these at a time that fit the schedule of the patient and family.[10] Unique additions to home monitoring programs such as this demonstrate that there is no "one size fits all" monitoring package, but that through telemedicine, it is possible to design programs uniquely suited to a patient's needs.

CONNECTING CHILDREN WITH MEDICAL COMPLEXITY TO THE PATIENT-CENTERED MEDICAL HOME

The PCMH has become a vital element in the care of all pediatric patients, endorsed by the leading physician organizations. The core tenets are to create expanded access, better communication, and coordinated care and to do this in partnership with the patient and/or family.[11] Applying such a model of care to CMC leads to improved clinical outcomes and decreased financial and logistical burdens in providing care to this patient population.[3,6,12] For CMC, the medical home encompasses an entire team of providers, including primary care, specialists, therapists, case managers, and community resources.[3] The family is a critical part of this type of coordinated care because for the medically complex child, family members may find themselves taking on a medical role as they navigate a multitude of medical supplies, equipment, and technology. By definition, medically complex children require more frequent access to both routine and acute care visits.[6]

The importance of accessing a member of this team is critical for CMC. Having the ability to seek guidance from a member of their own medical team can help prevent ED visits, costly transfers, and hospital stays. It has been documented that parents are more likely to seek care at a hospital if they are unable to reach a provider who knows their child. The ability to connect a child with a member of their medical team may help to decrease the need for acute hospitalization.[13] Telehealth is increasingly being proven to be a valuable tool to achieve these goals and to connect patients and their families with the providers who know and understand their complex needs.

The need for these visits may arise in a host of settings. School-based programs using both synchronous real-time video consultations and store-and-forward images have been shown to be effective for all children, including those with special needs.[12,13,14] Such programs allow children with developmental disabilities and behavioral issues to be examined by a familiar local provider. In addition to the benefits of minimal disruption to the parent and child's day, these programs help avoid the need for costly and disruptive transport. Children with special health care needs may have emotional and/or behavioral issues, leading to fear of unfamiliar settings or providers. In a review of one school-based program, school staff described a perceived reduction in stress for the child and an increased likelihood of a successful examination.[14]

Parents or caregivers in the home setting often report difficulties managing CSHCN at home, and some have reported delays in seeking care to avoid the burdens of transport and hospital-based care.[13] Bringing assessments to the home via telehealth helps provide reassurance and guidance as to the appropriate management and may lead to better outcomes attributable to earlier intervention. One such home program connected children on home ventilator support and their caregivers with their care team. Telemedicine improved clinical decision making and increased parental confidence in the assessment and treatment recommendations.[15] This program provided real-time visual assessment of children in their homes. As technology advances with the development of devices that support the remote assessment of heart and breath sounds, temperature, otoscopic examination, blood pressure, blood glucose, and other parameters,[16] remotely located clinicians can replicate the in-person assessment of a medically complex child.

In addition to acute evaluations, routine assessments of the child in the home may be preferable to exams in an office setting. Having a child in a familiar environment provides invaluable insight, not only to physicians but also to therapists, counselors, and other members of a medically complex child's health care team. Other services that may be more effective in the home setting include palliative care and pain services. In caring for medically complex children, this is often required as complex diseases progress. Studies have shown the feasibility of providing palliative care in the home setting for pediatric patients, with a reduction in costs and need for travel.[17–19]

MULTISPECIALTY CONSULTATIONS

The concept of a multidisciplinary or multispecialty clinic is not new. In this model, patients with a particular condition travel to a clinic or hospital for coordinated visits with multiple physician specialists and nonphysician providers integral to their care and evaluation. This model has been associated with higher rates of patient satisfaction, less ancillary testing, a decreased number of clinic visits per child, improved outcomes, better provider-to-provider communication, and more coordinated care.[20-24] Cost savings are generally realized by the family in terms of both time and expense. With streamlined referrals and coordinated services, the evidence also suggests a reduction in overall health care costs.[20,24] For CMC, multidisciplinary clinics can reduce the need for ED visits and inpatient care.[25] Despite the proven benefits, however, there are limitations. These coordinated efforts often require many specialists, who themselves may be in limited supply and work at centralized urban tertiary or quaternary centers, presenting challenges for distantly located patients.[20] Low patient volumes may lead to limited scheduling opportunities and longer wait times for appointments. The financial viability of multidisciplinary clinics has been limited by current reimbursement models, facility costs, and practice overhead expenses.[24,26] On-site clinics risk exposure to other chronically ill children with potential infectious illnesses.[27] Children, particularly those with emotional or behavioral issues, may be overstimulated and stressed with multiple assessments and providers.

Many of these barriers can be avoided using telehealth to help facilitate multispecialty consultations. Telehealth technology allows clinicians to connect with a patient synchronously or asynchronously, reducing the need for travel. Visits can occur in a familiar environment such as a school[28,29] or primary care office.[30] Telehealth clinics allow for greater flexibility in scheduling, both for the patient and the provider, and have been associated with increased patient satisfaction and greater patient and provider productivity. Additionally, telehealth visits provide an opportunity for specialists to communicate directly with the school staff or primary care office, resulting in greater knowledge and better overall case management. As provider comfort with telemedicine grows and as technology evolves to include the use of peripheral devices that replicate the in-person exam, team-based care in the home setting will become an important adjunct for children with special health care needs.

BARRIERS

Although telehealth offers great promise for CSHCN and CMC, a number of barriers remain that impede broader implementation. A survey of providers for CSHCN regarding the use of telehealth identified significant barriers, including lack of information/ knowledge, technology costs, limited or unclear reimbursement models, and concerns regarding technology and privacy as impediments to widespread use.[2]

TECHNOLOGY AND SECURITY

Connectivity is essential to the success of every telehealth project. Solving connectivity issues requires attention in both the institutional and home environments. Although broadband to the home has become widely available, it is not ubiquitous. Even homes with broadband may lack sufficient connectivity to run certain telehealth applications with an acceptable of quality of service, and additional sources of connectivity may be needed.[17]

In any telehealth program, major considerations include security of patient data and images. The widespread availability of video and imaging tools requires that telehealth programs educate both providers and families as to the appropriate choice of technology and acceptable protocols for in-home teleconsults (eg, having everyone in the room identified and introduced). Although many people use interactive video for social reasons, appropriate protocols and processes must govern the use of telehealth and ensure both adequate security and proper functioning of the technology. Another important consideration is technical support for the technology selected. Troubleshooting tools and technical assistance should be available along with an emergency notification and access plan if either the technology fails or an emergency situation arises. A key factor identified in maintaining patient engagement with telehealth programs is the ability to quickly resolve any issues.[17]

CMC have multiple providers, often distributed across wide geographic regions and multiple health care systems. Although telehealth has become more ubiquitous, interoperability of devices and telehealth solutions systems remains an important issue. Additionally, access to consistent broadband Internet may be a limiting factor. Testing, collaboration with information technology support, and backup plans are an integral part of program development.

COST AND REIMBURSEMENT

Program costs must be evaluated. Although cost savings may be realized by the family, it is important to assess the cost of the program and the value added to the hosting institution. The move toward value-based care mandates more efficient care coordination, but there are still limitations with regard to provider reimbursement for telehealth services. Many medically complex children are insured through state Medicaid programs. Although the status of Medicaid regulations is improving,[31] there is still a great deal of variability among the states and regulations regarding provider reimbursement. Nearly half of all state Medicaid programs require a specific patient setting for care to be provided via telehealth, and some exclude the home or schools as eligible originating sites. Some states do not recognize nonphysician providers and may require the provider to be physically located in a specific setting when conducting the encounter. These barriers limit after-hours consults and in some states limit providers' ability to conduct multidisciplinary consults and visits. Only 18 states recognize school-based settings as originating sites. Others limit technology choices by excluding store-and-forward technology or remote patient monitoring from reimbursement.[32]

SUMMARY

The population of children with special and complex medical needs is growing. There is an increasing evidence base demonstrating the effectiveness of telehealth in meeting the needs of these children. The American Academy of Pediatrics recognizes telehealth as a tool to address the shortage of subspecialty providers and, in particular, as an important link to care within the context of the medical home.[33] Intuitively these benefits seem magnified for CSHCN and CMC. The importance of family engagement has been cited as

an important foundation for the medical home model.[6] For children with special needs, this involvement is critical to the achievement of high-quality outcomes. The use of telehealth to achieve these goals, via improved access to care, reduced patient and family stress, and an increased likelihood of complete assessments with familiar providers, is invaluable. Technology solutions enabling the medical support of children outside specialized medical centers have grown through a broad range of devices, programs, and broadband-facilitated telehealth services. In the care of children with complex medical conditions, these models can prove to be transformational.

REFERENCES

1. U.S. Department of Health and Human Services, Health Resources and Services Administration, Maternal and Child Health Bureau. *Child Health USA 2012.* Rockville, MD: U.S. Department of Health and Human Services; 2013.

2. Lucile Packard Foundation for Children's Health. *Realizing the Promise of Telehealth for Children with Special Health Care Needs.* 2015. http://www.lpfch.org/publication/realizing-promise-telehealth-children-special-health-care-needs. Accessed May 10, 2016.

3. Cady RG, Erickson M, Lunos S, et al. Meeting the needs of children with medical complexity using a telehealth advanced practice registered nurse care coordination model. *Matern Child Health J* 2015;19:1497–1506.

4. Coller RJ, Lerner CF, Eickhoff JC, et al. Medical complexity among children with special health care needs: a two-dimensional view. *Health Services Res* 2016;51(4):1644–1669.

5. Karpook J, Werner M. Five keys to success: advancing care models for children with complex medical needs. White paper. The Chartis Group. Boston 2016.

6. Hooshmand M, Yao K. Challenges facing children with special health care needs and their families: telemedicine as a bridge to care. *Telemed e-Health* 2017;23(1):1–7.

7. Harahsheh AS, Hom LA, Clauss SB, et al. The impact of a designated cardiology team involving telemedicine home monitoring on the care of children with single ventricle physiology after Norwood palliation. *Pediatr Cardiology* 2016;37:899.

8. Schiaffini R, Tagliente I, Carducci C, et al. Impact of long-term use of eHealth systems in adolescents with type 1 diabetes treated with sensor segmented pump therapy. *J Telemed Telecare* 2016;22(5):277–281.

9. Tagliente I, Trieste L, Solvoll T, et al. Telemonitoring in cystic fibrosis: a 4 year assessment and simulation for the next 6 years. *Interact J Med Res* 2016;5(2):e11.

10. Chen DS, Callahan CW, Hatch-Pigott VB, et al. Internet-based home monitoring and education of children with asthma is comparable to ideal office-based care; results of a 1 year asthma in-home monitoring trial. *Pediatrics* 2007;119(3):569–578.

11. Herendeen N, Deshpande P. Telemedicine and the patient-centered medical home. *Pediatr Ann* 2014;43(2):e28–e32.

12. McConnochie KM, Ronis SD, Wood NE, Ng PK. Effectiveness and safety of acute care telemedicine for children with regular and special health care needs. *Telemed and e-Health* 2015;21(8):611–622.

13. Nelson B, Coller RJ, Saenz AA, et al. How avoidable are hospitalizations for children with medical complexity? Understanding parent perspectives. *Acad Pediatr* 2016;16(6):579–586.

14. Langkamp DL, McManus MD, Blakemore SD. Telemedicine for children with developmental disabilities: a more effective clinical process than office-based care. *Telemed and e-Health* 2015;21(2):110–114.

15. Casavant DW, McManus ML, Parsons SK, et al. Trial of telemedicine for patients on home ventilator support: feasibility, confidence in clinical management and use in medical decision making. *J Telemedicine Telecare* 2014;20(4):441–449.

16. Beck M. New Gadgets that Could Give Telemedicine a Boost. *The Wall Street Journal* September 25, 2016. http://www.wsj.com/. Accessed Oct. 12, 2016.

17. Katalinic O, Young A, Doolan D. Case study: the interact home telehealth project. *J Telemed Telecare* 2013;19(7):418–424.

18. Bradford NK, Armfield NR, Young J, Smith AC. Pediatric palliative care by video consultation at home: a cost minimization analysis. *BMC Health Serv Res* 2014;28(14):328.

19. Bradford NK, Armfield NR, Young J, et al. Principles of a pediatric palliative care consultation can be achieved with home telemedicine. *J Telemed Telecare* 2014;20(7):360–364.

20. Tang M. Multidisciplinary teams in cancer care: pros and cons. *Cancer Forum* 2009;33(3).

21. Ali AS, Haney J, Payne L, Grischkan J. Initial experience from a multidisciplinary pediatric salivary gland disorder clinic. *International J Pediatric Otorhinolaryngology* 2015;79(9):1505–1509.

22. Abdel-Baki MS, Hanzlik E, Kieran MW. Multidisciplinary pediatric brain tumor clinics: The key to successful treatment? *CNS Oncol* 2015;4(3):147–155.

23. Al-Hazmi HH, Trbay MS, Gomha AB, et al. Uronephrological outcomes of patient with neural tube defects: Does Spina bifida clinic make a difference? *Saudi Med J* 2014;35(suppl 1):S64–S67.

24. Collaco JM, Aherrera AD, Au Yeung KJ. Interdisciplinary pediatric aerodigestive care and reduction in health care costs and burden. *JAMA Otolaryngol Head Neck Surg* 2015;141(2):101–105.

25. Casey PH, Lyle RE, Bird TM. Effect of hospital-based comprehensive care clinic on health costs for Medicaid-insured medically complex children. *Arch Ped Adolesc Med* 2011;165(5):392–398.

26. Melzer SM, Richards GE, Covington ML. Reimbursement and costs of pediatric ambulatory diabetes care by using the resource-based relative value scale: is multidisciplinary care financially viable? *Pediatric Diabetes* 2004;5(3):133–142.

27. Lebecque P, Leonard A, DeBoeck K, et al. Early referral to cystic fibrosis specialist centre impacts on respiratory outcome. *J Cystic Fibrosis* 2009;8(1):26–30.

28. Davis AM, Sampilo M, Gallagher KS, et al. Treating rural pediatric obesity through telemedicine vs. telephone: Outcomes from a cluster randomized controlled trial. *J Telemed Telecare* 2016;22(2):86–95.

29. Slusser W, Whitley M, Izadpanah N, et al. Multidisciplinary pediatric obesity clinic via telemedicine within the Los Angeles metropolitan area: lessons learned. *Clin Pediatr* 2016;55(3):251–259.

30. Wallace P, Barber J, Clayton W, et al. Virtual outreach: a randomised controlled trial and economic evaluation of joint teleconferenced medical consultations. *Health Technol Assess* 2004;8(50).

31. Thomas L, Capistrant G. *State Telemedicine Gaps Analysis: Coverage and Reimbursement*. http://www.americantelemed.org/policy-page/state-telemedicine-gaps-reports. Accessed September 27, 2016.

32. Center for Connected Health Policy. *State Telehealth Laws and Medicaid Program Policies*. 2015. http://cchpca.org/telehealth-medicaid-state-policy. Accessed September 27, 2016.

33. Committee on Pediatric Workforce. The use of telemedicine to address access and physician workforce shortages. *Pediatrics* 2015;136(1):202–209.

Other Telehealth Systems of Health

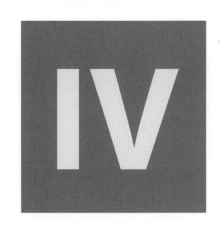

The Dawn of Direct-to-Consumer Telehealth

Ateev Mehrotra, MD, MPH,
Lori Uscher-Pines, PhD, MSc and Michelle S. Lee, BA

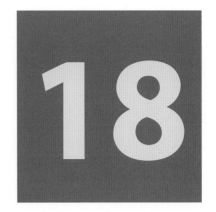

CASE STUDY

Ms. Jones lets out a groan as she wakes up. She feels the familiar pressure/burning sensation she has had with prior urinary tract infections. As someone who is prone to such infections she knows she needs a course of antibiotics. However, she worries how and when she will be able to visit her primary care physician. Although Ms. Jones has a good relationship with her physician, it usually takes a couple of days to get an appointment, and she has to budget for half a day for the drive to the physician's office and the time in the waiting room. Given her already overwhelming schedule of taking care of her children and her work responsibilities, fitting in a visit to her physician seems near impossible.

She then remembers receiving a notice from her health plan that they now cover telemedicine visits. Wondering if this may be a better alternative, Ms. Jones sets up her laptop in the kitchen; clicks her way to the telemedicine company's website; registers with her insurance card; and answers some questions about her past medical history, medications, and allergies. Ten minutes later a physician appears on her laptop's screen and asks Ms. Jones about her history and symptoms. He diagnoses Ms. Jones with a urinary tract infection and sends an antibiotic prescription to the local pharmacy.

After the visit is over, Ms. Jones marvels at the convenience and how much time it saved her. However, she cannot help but wonder whether she received high-quality care.

Both existing health systems and private companies such as Teladoc, American Well, and Doctor on Demand now offer patients around-the-clock "virtual" access to physicians for minor illnesses, rashes, or behavioral health issues. Patients can access these visits via telephone or videoconferencing on their smartphone, tablet, or laptop. On demand access to healthcare providers through personal devices represents a new type of telemedicine, direct-to consumer (DTC) telemedicine. DTC telemedicine may be the most popular form of telehealth: there were a reported 1.25 million DTC telemedicine visits in 2015[1]; and Teladoc alone recently reported in that in 2016 it provided over 950,000 visits, a 65% increase from 2015.[2] A recent survey of large employers indicated that 74% planned to offer a DTC telehealth option to their employees in 2016.[3] In this chapter we explore the rising popularity of DTC telemedicine, some of its unique features, and research on the quality and costs of the care provided.

HOW IS DTC TELEMEDICINE DIFFERENT FROM OTHER FORMS OF TELEHEALTH?

As suggested by its name, DTC telemedicine is distinct from other forms of telehealth in that the patient initiates the care. In most other forms of telehealth, a clinician initiates the visit. For example, if a patient arrives in an emergency department with strokelike symptoms, the emergency department physician initiates the telestroke system. Similarly, if a patient with schizophrenia needs specialty input from a psychiatrist, the community mental health clinic might initiate a telemental health visit. In contrast, DTC telemedicine visits are initiated by the patient, and there is no intermediary clinician. The actual mechanics of the visit are discussed next with several examples.

The DTC structure drives several other important differences in DTC telemedicine. DTC telemedicine visits are more likely to be provided in the patient's home. In contrast, many other forms of telehealth have regulations requiring the patient to present to a clinical setting such as a physician office or hospital. This difference can be important because in DTC telemedicine, no clinician is physically present with the patient as he or she interacts with the distant telemedicine clinician.

Although telehealth as a whole is composed of many for-profit companies, DTC telemedicine is dominated by for-profit companies, often venture capital funded and publicly exchanged, that only focus on telehealth. Their separation from the rest of the health system has raised concerns about their impact on the coordination of care.[4] However, the distinction between private DTC telemedicine companies and existing health systems has become blurred with "white labeling." In such a relationship, the private company provides the telemedicine platform and/or the providers, but an existing health system labels the care as its own. For example, Cleveland Clinic's new online video visits are marketed as Cleveland Clinic care but are actually delivered by American Well, a telemedicine company providing the technology platform and physicians.[5]

Payment for DTC telemedicine visits can also vary. Payors and employers increasingly provide coverage for these services, with different levels of patient cost-sharing (typically under $20). In addition, some companies market DTC services to the general public, including the uninsured. In cases where a patient does not have coverage through their payor or employer, they can generally pay out-of-pocket (typically $40 to $50 for urgent care visits).

MAJOR TYPES OF DTC TELEMEDICINE

As reflected in other types of telehealth, definitions are sometimes blurred, but the types of DTC telemedicine can be generally categorized by the following parameters. The first is whether the visit is synchronous or asynchronous. In synchronous visits, the interaction between clinician and patients is live and can use audio only or include a two-way video. Audio-only visits are common. In one prior study, the majority of synchronous DTC telemedicine visits at one company consisted of a simple telephone calls between patient and clinician.[6] Two-way video visits can be initiated on smart phones, tablets, or personal computers. In all cases, patients typically create an online account and enter information about their medical history to initiate a visit. The consulting clinician typically does not have any established relationship with the patient; however, the patient will be matched to a clinician licensed to practice in his or her state of residence. After evaluation, the clinician gives the patient a diagnosis and any recommended tests or prescriptions are sent electronically.

In asynchronous or "store-and-forward" visits, the transfer of information back and forth between patient and clinician is not in real time. With DTC telemedicine, asynchronous visits are generally called e-visits, although there is no consensus on this terminology. In an e-visit, patients log into their secure personal health record online portal with their health care provider or a company website and answer a series of questions about their condition. The questions are structured using a branching logic format so that an answer to one question will lead to subsequent questions asking for more details. This written information is sent to clinicians who make a diagnosis, prescribe the necessary care, include a note in the patient's electronic medical records, and reply to the patients often within several hours. E-visits are offered by numerous health systems and private companies such as Zipnosis. Zipnosis is another example of how the distinction between private companies and existing health systems is blurred; Zipnosis "white-labels" its e-visits for health systems such as Fairview Health.[7] Improvements in the interface for patients with asynchronous visits are being introduced. HealthTap's "Dr. AI service" converses with users to understand their complaints and has a more empathetic interface.[8]

One recent new distinction with asynchronous visits is whether the patient's responses are evaluated by a clinician or a computer algorithm. With the latter, the computer algorithm acts as a screen. If it is a straightforward scenario, then the diagnosis and treatment are decided by the algorithm. Only if there is something unusual or concerning with the clinical scenario does the physician become involved. For example, Lemonaid is a DTC company that uses such a model to treat conditions such as oral contraceptives, hair loss, and erectile dysfunction.[9]

WHAT CONDITIONS ARE BEING ADDRESSED BY DTC TELEMEDICINE

To our knowledge, there are no empirical studies that describe the national breakdown of DTC telemedicine visits. Therefore in this section we describe our general sense of the most common types.

Most DTC telemedicine visits appear to address "simple acute" problems including acute respiratory illnesses such as sinusitis, rashes, and urinary tract infections. The type of patient conditions addressed by one DTC telemedicine company in one study is described in Table 18-1.[6]

DTC telemedicine is also gaining popularity in dermatology and behavioral health. DTC telemedicine companies that focus exclusively on dermatology conditions include Direct Dermatology and DermatologistOnCall.[10,11] Visits are typically asynchronous where the patient submits both information about their condition and photographs to be reviewed by a dermatologist. A dermatologist then reviews the case and sends a report with any prescriptions, if needed, within two days. In at least one case, the DTC teledermatology company has "brick-and-mortar" sites where nurses help obtain a history and facilitate the taking of photographs.[12]

Although many telemental health visits are facilitated or initiated by a clinician, at least some companies are providing DTC telemental services such as cognitive behavioral therapy.[13] Because both teledermatology and telemental health are discussed in depth in other chapters, the rest of this chapter will focus only on DTC telemedicine for simple acute conditions.

EVIDENCE ON THE IMPACT OF DTC TELEMEDICINE

Although telemedicine is a promising avenue to improve health care access and patient satisfaction and to reduce costs, many concerns have been raised about the quality of health care provided.

▶ Quality

The Federation of State Medical Boards, state boards, and other physician organizations have expressed concern regarding the quality of DTC telemedicine.[14,15] The concerns with DTC telemedicine are driven by the lack of in-person physical exam, limited access to medical records, lack of follow-up, and barriers to diagnostic testing. Together these limitations may lead to poor quality of care, misdiagnosis, or higher rates of follow-up visits. Telephone visits have been flagged as particularly concerning given that such encounters involve no visual cues to assist with diagnosis.[16]

Assessments of the quality of DTC telemedicine to date are limited. Follow-up visits have been used as a rough proxy for quality. The logic is that higher rates of early follow-up after DTC telemedicine visits would suggest high rates of misdiagnosis and poor quality. Follow-up visits can occur at any site: emergency department, physician office, or DTC telemedicine companies. Studies have found that follow-up rates are similar among in-person office visits and DTC synchronous telemedicine visits[6] as well as e-visits.[17]

Another method of assessing quality has been to compare antibiotic prescribing across settings. For example, one study investigated antibiotic and

Table 18-1. Leading Reasons for Visits by Children and Adults at One DTC Telemedicine Company, April 2012–February 2013 Visits

Condition	Percent
Acute respiratory illnesses	31
Urinary tract infections and urinary symptoms	12
Skin problems	9
Abdominal pain, vomiting, and diarrhea	6
Back and joint problems	5
Influenza and general viral illnesses	5
General advice, counseling, and refills	5
Eye problems	4
Ear infections (internal and external)	4

broad-spectrum antibiotic prescribing rates for Teladoc and physician's offices, finding that the fraction of acute respiratory infection (ARI) visits at which an antibiotic was prescribed was similar for Teladoc (58%) and physician offices (55%). When antibiotics were prescribed, Teladoc physicians were more likely to prescribe a broad-spectrum antibiotic for ARI visits (86%) compared to 56% at the physician offices.[18] One assessment of e-visits in a health system found that antibiotic prescribing for sinusitis treatment was higher during e-visits than during physician office visits.[17] Another study highlighted that the training of the clinician may be an important factor; e-visits provided by nurse practitioners were associated with higher rates of prescribing medications than e-visits provided by physicians.[19] One limitation of these studies is that they assess the quality of antibiotic prescribing based on the diagnosis provided by the clinician; the underlying assumption is that the diagnosis is correct.

One method for assessing diagnostic accuracy and adherence to guidelines is to use secret shoppers. In a recent study, researchers used 67 trained standardized patients who presented to DTC telemedicine companies with the following six common acute illnesses: ankle pain, streptococcal pharyngitis, viral pharyngitis, acute rhinosinusitis, low back pain, and recurrent female urinary tract infection.[20] Conditions were misdiagnosed in 24% of visits and adherence to guidelines was only 54%. Although such rates are concerning, it is unclear how they compare to equivalent in-person visits. Given the ongoing debate on telephone visits, it was notable that there was no difference in quality between audio-only and video visits. Perhaps most importantly, the study also described significant variation in quality across the eight DTC telemedicine companies. Other research that studies the "average" DTC telemedicine misses this key point.

One consistent theme in evaluations is that DTC telemedicine clinicians are less likely to order tests. This is to be expected given the additional logistical hurdles in ordering a test. For example, whereas ordering a strep test in a physician office is relatively simple, in a DTC telemedicine encounter, the clinician must identify where the patient can get the test, follow up with the results, and then set up another interaction to discuss the results with the patient. Given this complexity, some DTC companies do not have the ability to order tests. If a test is needed, the patient is told to visit their primary care provider. Whether this lower rate of testing is "good" or "bad" depends on the clinical scenario: for instance, lower rates of testing in patients with back pain likely indicate higher-quality care because these tests are normally overused.[21] However, for conditions such as streptococcal pharyngitis or urinary tract infections lower rates of testing more likely indicate lower-quality care.[17]

In summary, studies assessing DTC telemedicine quality have been mixed. Some evidence supports that the care is equivalent to in-person care, whereas other research raises concern about the overuse of broad-spectrum antibiotics and misdiagnosis. Because lower rates of testing are consistently found with DTC telemedicine, there needs to be greater attention on how to facilitate appropriate testing. Finally, the care provided across DTC telemedicine providers is variable; some providers are providing higher quality care than others.

▶ Costs

DTC telemedicine visits are clearly lower cost than an equivalent in-person visit. One study found total costs (including prescriptions and testing) of $161 for DTC telemedicine visits and $219 for in-person primary care visits.[22] Thus, if patients substituted higher-cost physician office or emergency department visits with DTC telemedicine visits, there could be substantial savings.

The key to cost savings from DTC telemedicine therefore is substitution. However, it is also possible for DTC telemedicine visits to raise costs if they increase health care utilization by lowering the threshold for when patients seek care. A recent study quantified the relative fraction of DTC telemedicine visits that represented substitution versus new utilization. It found that 12% of DTC telemedicine visits were substitution and 88% represent new utilization. The net impact was an increase in health care spending.[23]

▶ Access

Patients who use DTC telemedicine tend to be both younger and healthier than the rest of the population.[6] More than one-third of e-visits are scheduled for the weekend and holidays, likely due to convenience.[6] The impact of DTC telemedicine on improving access to underserved communities remains poorly studied. One evaluation of Teladoc visits surprisingly found that users were not more likely to live in a rural community or a community with a shortage of clinicians.[21]

LEGAL AND REGULATORY ISSUES

As might be expected, the growth of DTC telemedicine has generated significant controversy. Organized medicine and state medical boards have expressed concern regarding both the quality and the impact on existing relationships between physicians and patients.

▶ Reimbursement

The reimbursement structure for DTC telemedicine is complex and depends on the payors' reimbursement policies and state regulations. Current Medicare payment policy does not cover DTC telemedicine because patients are not hosted at an existing health care site such as a physician's office or hospital. In contrast, private health plans have been much more enthusiastic about embracing DTC telemedicine. Aetna has covered visits by Teladoc since early 2011,[24] and Anthem has additionally white labeled a private DTC telemedicine company visits as Live Health Online.[25] Visits can be identified using modifier codes, and some health plans and Medicaid plans encourage use of Current Procedural Technology (CPT) codes designated for online visits such as 99444.

▶ Regulatory

One unique phenomenon in DTC telemedicine is a number of efforts by state regulators to restrict visits by requiring the clinician to have an existing relationship with the patient. Such a relationship is often defined as having a prior in-person visit with the patient. For example, Arkansas' regulations state, "A distant site provider will not use telemedicine to treat a patient located in Arkansas unless a professional relationship exists between the healthcare provider and patient," which means that "the healthcare professional has previously conducted an in-person exam and is available to provide appropriate follow-up care."[26] These regulations are often targeted at DTC telemedicine companies that only provide telehealth care. The rationale for these restrictions is that DTC telemedicine may be harmful because

of poor quality, because clinicians who provide the telehealth care do not have access to patient records, and because it may be difficult to set up appropriate follow-up care.

Likely the most contentious debate has been in Texas. In 2015, the Texas Medical Board voted to only permit telemedicine if the physician had a relationship with the patients before rendering a diagnosis or prescribing drugs.[27] This led to a protracted legal battle between Teladoc, a DTC telehealth company, and the Texas Medical Board. Teladoc sued the Texas Medical Board stating these rules violate antitrust laws, reduce access, and increase costs. They believed the Texas Medical Board was protecting existing Texas physicians from competition with private companies. The Federal Trade Commission has also expressed concern about the actions of the Texas Medical Board.[28]

This controversy was echoed in Mississippi. In 2015, the Mississippi Board of Medical Licensure proposed regulations that would have restricted out-of-state telemedicine companies from operating in Mississippi. As per the proposed regulation, companies operating in Mississippi were forced to establish a formal agreement with a Mississippi-based health care firm and to use only secured video conferencing when prescribing medication.[29] Teladoc rebutted that this regulation would preclude physicians from using telemedicine, and the videoconferencing requirements would reduce patient access and increase costs. The regulations were later withdrawn.

SUMMARY AND FUTURE DIRECTIONS

Although DTC telemedicine has already grown rapidly, that growth appears poised to accelerate both in problems addressed and number of visits. To date, the focus of DTC telemedicine has been primarily on treatment of low-acuity conditions, and we will likely see expansion of DTC telemedicine into other clinical areas. For example, DTC companies are beginning to offer services including tobacco cessation, breastfeeding support, chronic illness management, and sexual health. It is also a promising mechanism to provide medical care after a disaster.[30]

Several factors may fuel the growth in the number of visits. Many patients choose not to receive care because of the inconvenience of going to a physician office visit. As DTC telemedicine care becomes more common, it will appeal to new groups of patients who would not have otherwise sought care. Enrollment in high deductible health plans is increasing and patients in such plans may be particularly attracted to the lower-costs of DTC telemedicine. Other secular trends such as physician workforce shortages that limit the availability of timely primary care, greater penetration of smart phones, and greater reliance and comfort with health apps all may serve to increase demand for DTC services.

Although DTC telehealth is positioned for growth, a number of factors can slow its advance. First, the industry has not faced a serious malpractice lawsuit. DTC companies cite this as evidence that they are providing safe, high-quality care. However, given that DTC telemedicine is now reaching millions of patients, it is only a matter of time before litigation is brought forth for a medical error or adverse event. If such litigation becomes the subject of news stories, the industry will face additional scrutiny. Additional research that identifies quality concerns may also spur regulation and slow the growth of DTC telehealth. To date, research has been limited in part because there has been insufficient volume to conduct robust comparisons. There are some signs that industry players are taking active measures to address concerns about undertesting. Teladoc recently announced plans to support its providers in ordering lab tests and to incorporate follow-up into workflow.[31]

One unresolved question is how existing health systems will respond to DTC telemedicine. DTC telemedicine put pressure on traditional primary care settings to offer more convenient care that is lower cost. Many health systems have begun to offer some forms of DTC telemedicine, either creating the service on their own or white-labeling the care provided by private companies.[32] The latter is a new phenomenon in health care as health systems are "outsourcing" some of the care provided to the health system's patients. Health systems can offer non-DTC telemedicine options to increase convenience, including retail clinics and urgent care centers. Again, the distinctions between DTC telemedicine and these care sites may soon be blurred. For example, some retail clinics have begun to provide DTC telemedicine in some of their clinic locations.[33]

Although DTC telemedicine represents an exciting innovation in delivery, only time will tell if regulatory barriers and quality concerns will overshadow the convenience benefits or if this is indeed the dawn of a new era.

REFERENCES

1. Vesely R. Direct-to-Consumer Teleheath: The Sector Gets a New Diagnosis. May 16, 2016. http://healthjournalism.org/blog/?s=the+sector+gets+a+new+diagnosis. Accessed June 2, 2017.

2. *Teladoc Completes Record Visit Volume in 2016; Provides Preliminary Unaudited 2016 Results and 2017 Financial Outlook – Press.* January 25, 2017. https://www.teladoc.com/news/2017/01/09/teladoc-completes-record-visit-volume-in-2016-provides-preliminary-unaudited-2016-results-and-2017-financial-outlook/.

3. Pinsker B. Coming soon to a screen near you: Doctors. 2015. http://www.reuters.com/article/us-usa-health-telemedicine-idUSKCN0QH1S820150812. Accessed June 2, 2016.

4. Bodenheimer T. Coordinating care—a perilous journey through the health care system. *N Engl J Med* 2008;358(10):1064–1071.

5. American Well. *American Well, CVS Health and Cleveland Clinic Partner to Deliver On-Demand Care to Healthcare Consumers.* https://www.americanwell.com/press-release/american-well-cvs-health-and-cleveland-clinic-partner-to-deliver-on-demand-care-to-healthcare-consumers/. Accessed January 25, 2017.

6. Uscher-Pines L, Mehrotra A. Analysis of Teladoc use seems to indicate expanded access to care for patients without prior connection to a provider. *Health Aff (Millwood)* 2014;33(2):258–264.

7. Fairview Health Services. *Fairview Invests in Online Health Care Innovator Zipnosis.* January 6, 2015. http://blogs.fairview.org/blog/fairview-invests-online-health-care-innovator-zipnosis/. Accessed June 2, 2017.

8. HealthTap. *HealthTap Launches Dr. A.I.— Meet Your New, Personal AI-Powered Physician.* December 16, 2016. https://medium.com/@HealthTap/dr-a-i-80b4cf06be30#.680qwam4a. Accessed June 2, 2017.

9. Lemonaid Health. https://www.lemonaidhealth.com/. Accessed January 30, 2017.

10. Direct Derm. https://www.directderm.com/. Accessed January 25, 2017.

11. DermatologistOnCall. https://www.dermatologistoncall.com/. Accessed January 25, 2017.

12. Uscher-Pines L, Malsberger R, Burgette L, Mulcahy A, Mehrotra A. Effect of teledermatology on access to dermatology care among Medicaid enrollees. *JAMA Dermatol* 2016;152(8):905–912.

13. Doctor on Demand. *Mental Health*. https://www.doctorondemand.com/mentalhealth. Accessed January 25, 2017.

14. MobiHealthNews. *American Medical Association CEO Pans 'Ineffective' EHRs, D2C Digital Health, and Apps of 'Mixed Quality*. June 13, 2016. http://www.mobihealthnews.com/content/american-medical-association-ceo-pans-ineffective-ehrs-d2c-digital-health-and-apps-mixed. Accessed June 2, 2017.

15. Federation of State Medical Boards. *FSMB Survey Identifies Telemedicine as Most Important Regulatory Topic for State Medical Boards in 2016*. December 15, 2017. http://www.fsmb.org/Media/Default/PDF/Publications/20161215_annual_state_board_survey_sesults.pdf. Accessed June 2, 2017.

16. Modern Healthcare. *New Video Medicine Proposal Raises Telehealth Concerns*. http://www.modernhealthcare.com/article/20140425/NEWS/304259944. Accessed January 25, 2017.

17. Mehrotra A, Paone S, Martich GD, Albert SM, Shevchik GJ. A comparison of care at eVisits and physician office visits for sinusitis and urinary tract infections. *JAMA Intern Med* 2013;173(1):72–74.

18. Uscher-Pines L, Mulcahy A, Cowling D, et al. Antibiotic prescribing for acute respiratory infections in direct-to-consumer telemedicine visits. *JAMA Intern Med* 2015;175(7):1234–1235.

19. Bellon JE, Stevans JM, Cohen SM, et al. Comparing advanced practice providers and physicians as providers of e-visits. *Telemed J E Health* 2015;21(12):1019–1026.

20. Schoenfeld AJ, Davies JM, Marafino BJ, et al. Variation in quality of urgent health care provided during commercial virtual visits. *JAMA Intern Med* 2016;176(5):635–642.

21. Uscher-Pines L, Mulcahy A, Cowling D, et al. Access and quality of care in direct-to-consumer telemedicine. *Telemed J E Health* 2016;22(4):282–287.

22. Rohrer JE, Angstman KB, Adamson SC, et al. Impact of online primary care visits on standard costs: a pilot study. *Popul Health Manag* 2010;13(2):59–63.

23. Ashwood JS, Mehrotra A, Cowling D, Uscher-Pines L. Direct-to-consumer telehealth may increase access to care but does not decrease spending. *Health Affairs.* 2017;36(3):484–491.

24. *Aetna Members Now Have Access to Non-Urgent Care Consultations by Phone*. February 23, 2011. https://news.aetna.com/news-releases/aetna-members-now-have-access-to-non-urgent-care-consultations-by-phone/. Accessed January 25, 2017.

25. *Anthem Blue Cross Blue Shield Offers 'LiveHealth Online' App*. October 29, 2015. https://www.livehealthonline.com/en/news/2015/october/anthem-blue-cross-blue-shield-offers-livehealth-online-app/. Accessed January 25, 2017.

26. Center for Connected Health Policy. *State Telehealth Laws and Medicaid Program Policies*. http://www.cchpca.org/sites/default/files/resources/50%20State%20FINAL%20April%202016.pdf. Accessed June 2, 2017.

27. Modern Healthcare. *Texas Drops Appeal against Teladoc Lawsuit*. http://www.modernhealthcare.com/article/20161018/NEWS/161019900. Accessed January 25, 2017.

28. Federal Trade Commission. *Teladoc et al. v. Texas Medical Board et al*. https://www.ftc.gov/system/files/documents/amicus_briefs/teladoc-incorporated-et-al-v-texas-medical-board-et-al/teladoc_doj-ftc_amicus_brief.pdf. Accessed June 2, 2017.

29. *Proposed Mississippi Telemedicine Rule Goes Temporarily Offline*. http://watchdog.org/229825/proposed-mississippi-telemedicine-rule-goes-temporarily-offline/. Accessed January 25, 2017.

30. Uscher-Pines L, Fischer S, Chari R. The promise of direct-to-consumer telehealth for disaster response and recovery. *Prehosp Disaster Med.* 2016;31(4):454–456.

31. *Analyte Health and Teladoc Announce Partnership*. January 9, 2017. http://www.businesswire.com/news/home/20170109006115/en/Analyte-Health-Teladoc-Announce-Partnership. Accessed June 2, 2017.

32. NEJM Catalyst. *The Nuts and Bolts of Convenient Care Partnerships*. October 24, 2016. http://catalyst.nejm.org/the-nuts-and-bolts-of-convenient-care-partnerships/. Accessed June 2, 2017.

33. Polinski JM, Barker T, Gagliano N, et al. Patients' satisfaction with and preference for telehealth visits. *J Gen Intern Med.* 2016;31(3):269–275.

Telehealth in the Department of Defense

Ronald Poropatich, MD, Charles Lappan, MPA, MBA
and Gary Gilbert, PhD, MS

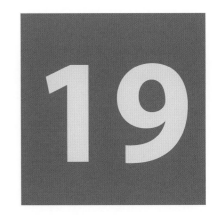

INTRODUCTION

The Department of Defense (DoD) comprises a complex health care system with a diverse beneficiary population and an annual budget that exceeds $52 billion. The Military Health System (MHS) seeks to offer high-quality and accessible health care services to its 10.6 million beneficiaries. It does this through a global direct care network composed of over 240 Military Treatment Facility (MTF) hospitals and clinics, supplemented by a purchased care network of community clinical providers. Access to care remains a challenge for the MHS, as many MTFs struggle to meet access standards and as the number of beneficiaries living distant from MTFs continues to grow. This has a significant financial impact on the managed care provider for the DoD called the TRICARE network.[1]

The DoD has identified telehealth (TH) as a potential means of achieving efficiencies and better care coordination by leveraging resources across MTFs, services, and agencies (eg, DoD/VA coordinated care) and by reducing reliance on purchased care through TH-mediated expansions to direct care services. The goal in providing TH services is to improve access to care and avoid beneficiaries being referred to civilian providers, thereby reducing purchased care costs.

DOD health care is managed at the triservice (Army, Navy, Air Force) level by the MHS, which provides programmatic funding and serves as the policy arm. Health care delivery is a service-specific responsibility.

This is important to understand as it affects delivery of a standardized TH solution across the DoD, with each service's active participation critical for success. To date, TH in the DoD has primarily been done by the U.S. Army, accounting for over 90% of all DoD TH activity and averaging over 5,000 TH consults/month across 22 time zones for more than 20 different medical specialties.[2]

Since 1992, TH and telemedicine (TM) have emerged as valuable components of the MHS in both garrison and deployed settings. The MHS has a worldwide mission of supporting active duty service members, retirees, and their beneficiaries in peacetime health care needs, including the continental United States (CONUS), as well as for deployed active duty service members and retirees outside the continental United States (OCONUS). In OCONUS, these technologies enable the MHS to project medical expertise to far-forward, remote and austere settings. In CONUS, these technologies can have comparable or even greater impact by improving access to care, readiness, quality, and in certain circumstances (such as enabling more home-based care), lower costs.[3] Expanding the use of TH in CONUS might enable the MHS to reduce reliance on expensive brick-and-mortar facilities; extend the impact and reach of its patient-centered medical homes; enable a declining number of MHS specialists to support providers engaged in primary care, psychological health, and prolonged field care; and directly engage the tech-savvy young adults who comprise the majority of the MHS beneficiaries.

OPERATIONAL TELEHEALTH IN SOUTHWEST ASIA

Background

In 1992, the U.S. Army began to explore the utility of TH to enhance medical operational support. The first use was in 1993 in Somalia[4] and was later expanded during the 1994 to 1995 Balkan conflicts.[5] The first U.S.-based military TH programs were started that same year, with Walter Reed Army Medical Center serving as the hub for teleconsultations across a 21-state region. With the onset of military operations in Afghanistan and Iraq in 2001 and 2003, respectively, the United States and partner nations found themselves in two sustained fights that would exceed a decade and half in length and lack clear exit strategies. Operation Enduring Freedom (OEF; Afghanistan) and Operation Iraqi Freedom (OIF; Iraq) required U.S. and coalition forces to carry on multiple simultaneous missions, including security and counter-insurgency operations, humanitarian assistance, nation building, and other activities. These activities were often performed by small, disaggregated units operating out of forward operating bases of various sizes and were conducted in a wide range of urban, rural, and austere settings in two nations separated by more than 1,400 miles. The complexity of supporting these operations, while simultaneously meeting the health care needs of other U.S. forces deployed on ships and in bases throughout the world and providing care to units garrisoned inside the CONUS, as well as millions of their dependents and military retirees, put a tremendous strain on the MHS.

To provide health support to sustain disaggregated military operations, medical planners sought to tailor the level and nature of clinical support using the organizations and resources available to them. The first major change occurred when the U. S. Army's Combat Support Hospitals (CSHs) were split-based to cover more ground and provide Role 3 (advanced echelon of care) medical capabilities over a broad geographic area. This shift was significant, because CSHs were not initially designed to be split. This change presaged many others that followed as medical support evolved to meet changing requirements of the line and evolving doctrine. The need to provide specialty backup to clinical providers staffing forward operating bases and other clinical sites "down range" opened the door to the adoption and rapid refinement of TH.

Although the bulk of innovation in military medical and surgical communities over the past 15 years has been directed at advancing combat casualty care, the bulk of health care delivery to deployed service members is not trauma related. This is especially true in long-term sustainment missions, where forces are deployed on an average of 6 and 12 months, and in some cases as long as 18 months. Medical care of this sort can be substantially enhanced if providers have ready access to the knowledge of experienced health care specialists, whether the consultation is provided in person or enabled via TH in its various forms. It is this kind of care, rendered in austere operational environments, that benefits most from the adoption of TH capabilities such as emailed TH consultation requests, tele-behavioral health (TBH), and teleradiology.

Military medicine has valued the clinical capability for reach-back teleconsultation to support remote providers in deployed settings as well as at U.S.-based health care facilities. The two main types of teleconsultation utilized are store-and-forward (asynchronous) and real-time (synchronous).

Based on encouraging results in Somalia in 1993, the Assistant Secretary of Defense for Health Affairs in 1994 officially chartered the U.S. Army Medical Research and Materiel Command (USAMRMC) Medical Advanced Technology Management Office (MATMO) as the DoD Telemedicine Test Bed and designated the Army as the DoD Executive Agent (http://www.tatrc.org/www/about/history.html). With MATMO (renamed Telemedicine and Advanced Technology Research Center [TATRC] in 1998) in the lead, TM services gradually expanded to additional overseas locations, including Croatia, Macedonia, and Bosnia (1994–1996); Haiti (1995); and Kenya (1998). These operations helped the U.S. military recognize that TM can significantly improve the delivery of care in remote settings.[6] TM was deployed more widely during OEF and OIF to support clinical care provided in Iraq, Afghanistan, and Kuwait. Expansion of TH services not only increased the breadth and capability of clinical services delivered in theater, it led to the creation of a more robust joint program.[6]

"Store and Forward" Telemedicine – the Email Teleconsultation Program: 2004–2016

In April 2004, the U.S. Army Medical Department (AMEDD) approved the use of the U.S. Army email system ("Army Knowledge Online" [AKO]) to provide teledermatology to deployed health care providers in Iraq, Kuwait, and Afghanistan.[7,8] This system has since been expanded to serve all overseas locations worldwide, including Navy ships at sea. Based on the initial success of teledermatology and TH support from other specialties, an overarching U.S. Army policy was established.[9] Through AKO, the services manage TH consultation requests in a secure, timely, and consistent manner to link deployed health care providers with rear-based consultants. To obtain a consult, the deployed health care provider submits an email request with a description of the patient's condition and any digital images necessary to illustrate the patient's problem. Upon transmission, the email is sent to the appropriate on-duty clinical specialist (eg, a dermatologist or a radiologist) who responds to the deployed provider within 24 hours of receiving a routine request. Emergent requests are handled more promptly.

The email teleconsultation program is not encrypted; therefore to remain within compliance with Public Law 104-19, the Health Insurance Portability and Accountability Act (HIPAA), these consultation requests must not include protected health information (PHI). This consultation service is designed for use by all DoD health care providers, with special emphasis on supporting deployed or geographically isolated health care providers serving an Army, Navy, Air Force, or Marine facility.

In-theater providers are responsible for following local policies regarding the electronic transfer of patient information and imagery, as well as documenting the consult they receive in the patient's electronic health record (EHR). Online training programs and reference materials are available to educate providers on its clinical use.

Between April 2004 and September 2016, more than 13,684 consults were completed, linking more than 3,400 remote providers with 20 different medical and dental specialties. The median response time over this 12-year period was just under 3 hours.[6] Data on average reply times from 2004 through 2016 are shown in Table 19-1, percentage usage by specialty in Table 19-2, location of remote provider in Table 19-3, and patient branch in Table 19-4. During this period, 39% of all consults were for dermatologic problems, followed by orthopedics (9%), infectious disease (7%),[10] neurology (6%), urology (5%), and ophthalmology (5%). Collectively, these

Table 19-1. Email Teleconsultation Program Reply Time History: April 2004–August 2016

Year	Average Reply Time	Median Reply Time
2004	5 hr 9 min	3 hr 55 min
2005	5 hr 16 min	3 hr 32 min
2006	5 hr 12 min	3 hr 30 min
2007	5 hr 8 min	3 hr 4 min
2008	4 hr 58 min	3 hr 11 min
2009	5 hr 11 min	3 hr 10 min
2010	5 hr 13 min	3 hr 23 min
2011	5 hr 12 min	3 hr 22 min
2012	5 hr 36 min	2 hr 57 min
2013	6 hr 54 min	3 hr 19 min
2014	4 hr 15 min	1 hr 23 min
2015	4 hr 37 min	1 hr 10 min
2016	4 hr 54 min	1 hr 47 min
Aug	4 hr 36 min	1 hr 57 min
Program	5 hr 13 min	2 hr 58 min

- 20 specialties with contact groups
- 13,684 teleconsultations
- 240 known evacuation were prevented
- 688 known evacuations were facilitated
- 3,404 different referring providers
- 1,331 teleconsultations on non-U.S. patients

six specialties comprised 72% of all teleconsultations (Table 19-2). U.S. Army providers generated more than half (53%) of the requests,[6] and the rest were evenly divided among Marine Corps (10%), Navy (10%), and Air Force (8%) providers as shown in Table 19-4.

The program improved the accuracy of decisions to initiate medical evacuation. Between 2004 and 2016, at least 240 needless medevacs were prevented (Table 19-1). At other times, tele-consultation facilitated timely recognition of a serious or life-threatening problem, prompting evacuation and contributing to a better outcome than would have otherwise been the case. Over the 12 year timespan of this review, a total of 688 evacuations were facilitated based on the advice of TH consultants.

Table 19-2. Program Summary by Specialty

	Total Consults By FV												2016												Program Totals	% Consults Program
	2004 Totals	2005 Totals	2006 Totals	2007 Totals	2008 Totals	2009 Totals	2010 Totals	2011 Totals	2012 Totals	2013 Totals	2014 Totals	2015 Totals	Oct	Nov	Dec	Jan	Feb	Mar	Apr	May	Jun	Jul	Aug	YTD		
Burn-Trauma		23	24	19	32	31	13	17	10	12	7	2	2	1			3	1	3		3	3	2	1	191	1%
Cardiology		2	67	41	61	67	84	51	32	30	36	34		1	3		3	5	3			3	2	25	530	4%
Dental						14	15	21	5	11	3	6	1	1		1	1	1			2			7	82	0.6%
Dermatology	321	543	528	468	562	526	560	543	281	231	291	215	18	15	17	13	22	23	21	21	21	18	27	216	5,285	38.6%
Infection Control						11	11	16	4	14	21	7	2							3				5	89	0.7%
Infectious Diseases		82	110	106	100	110	110	100	69	66	60	43	3	2		5	7		1	10	3	1		32	988	7.2%
Internal Medicine				34	50	57	64	70	53	29	24	19					1	1	2	1			1	6	406	3.0%
Microbiology				0		8	7	3	1	3	1	1												0	24	0.2%
Nephrology		13	18	33	30	29	20	19	19	6	9	14	2	3		1		1	1	1		2		10	220	1.6%
Neurology				78	123	145	123	129	69	40	28	27	3	2	4	5		4	1	3	2	5	3	32	794	5.8%
Ophthalmology	10	51	38	54	70	65	56	81	49	56	33	29	1	2	1	1	1	6	3	4	2	1	1	23	615	4.5%
Orthopedics				11	105	169	142	227	137	117	105	124	10	20	4	8	6	14	15	13	9	9	7	115	1,252	9.1%
Pain Management											3	6	1				1					1		3	12	0.09%
Pediatrics		8	21	27	24	20	15	7	6	2	2	1	1										1	1	134	1.0%
Prvt Med			3	13	13	25	26	25	23	14	12	4				1				2	1			5	163	1.2%
Rheumatology			13	26	20	21	32	35	19	16	17	10	1	2				1		1	2		1	9	218	1.6%
Sleep Medicine						12	5	16	4	3	3	5			1			1					1	4	52	0.4%
Toxicology		2	19	15	14	8	14	15	11	5	4	5						1		2			1	4	116	0.8%
Traumatic Brain Injury					8	42	63	74	34	8	16	8	3				1	2	2				2	9	262	1.9%
Urology				6	69	108	114	125	64	45	39	42	3	4	1	2	2	2		4	2		2	22	634	4.6%
Other Specialties	7		62	124	178	185	180	245	136	110	113	121	9	12	21	18	19	16	10	12	12	12	15	156	1,617	11.8%
Totals	331	731	903	1,055	1,459	1,653	1,654	1,819	1,026	818	827	723	60	64	52	55	63	79	60	77	59	52	64	685	13,684	

Table 19-3. Program Summary by Location

Location of Referring Physician	2004 Totals	2005 Totals	2006 Totals	2007 Totals	2008 Totals	2009 Totals	2010 Totals	2011 Totals	2012 Totals	2013 Totals	2014 Totals	2015 Totals	2016												Program Totals	% Consults Program
													Oct	Nov	Dec	Jan	Feb	Mar	Apr	May	Jun	Jul	Aug	YTD		
Major Facilities ≥ 100 Consults	286	682	827	1,008	1,378	1,586	1,570	1,745	936	696	667	617	48	55	47	48	47	63	48	53	49	41	54	553	12,551	94%
Afghanistan	6	80	127	131	160	346	610	744	496	316	276	129	6	3	3	2	15	6	7	13	5	1	8	69	3,490	26%
Bahrain						8	4	5		19	22	11		9	3	8	5	6						31	100	1%
CONUS		20	17	19	26	16	37	29	27	27	20	13	3	1	1	4			3	2				14	265	2%
Cuba (GTMO)			1		1				9	7	38	52	4	2	1	4	7	4	3	2	3	1	1	29	137	1%
Djibouti				18	20	46	10	49	68	56	9	18		1	4	4	3	3	5	2	6	1	2	31	325	2%
Egypt (MFO)	1	22	16	11	3	26	14	67	27	24	14	27	6	10	14	12	12	8	10	9	12	12	11	116	368	3%
Honduras		1			22	19	6	11	32	22	7	46	6	2	8	6	2	7	3	3	2	5	4	48	214	2%
Iraq	197	477	570	755	1,059	905	621	509	46	1	1	17				1					1	2	3	7	5,165	38%
Kuwait	64	52	32	20	15	62	65	99	77	83	153	111	13	9	8	7	1	12	7	12	7	8	17	101	934	7%
Kyrgyzstan		2	5		23	3	30	15	10	4	30														122	1%
Qatar	2	27	37	32	46	18	37	68	34	14	21	42	2	5	5	3	1	2	1	5	1	4	2	31	409	3%
US Navy Afloat	16	4	28	22	49	167	176	180	161	153	136	162	8	13	1	1	1	15	12	7	7	6	5	76	1,330	10%

Table 19-4. Program Summary by Branch of Service

	2004 Totals	2005 Totals	2006 Totals	2007 Totals	2008 Totals	2009 Totals	2010 Totals	2011 Totals	2012 Totals	2013 Totals	2014 Totals	2015 Totals	Oct	Nov	Dec	Jan	Feb	Mar	Apr	May	Jun	Jul	Aug	YTD	Program Totals	% Consults Program
																			2016 Patient Branch								
Air Force	11	62	85	95	142	96	124	105	56	66	102	76	3	4	7	8	7	3	2	7	4	4	3	52	1,072	7.8%
Army	252	405	431	540	751	888	905	1054	523	375	363	354	38	30	32	32	43	48	38	40	38	35	48	422	7,263	53.1%
Coast Guard						5	7	4	1	2	8	6												0	33	0.2%
Marine Corps	8	101	78	149	212	178	174	119	77	89	94	67	7	18	5	7	5	12	6	8	4	6	4	82	1,428	10.4%
Navy	18	8	37	30	71	191	161	218	173	139	129	145	5	8	4	2	1	12	6	3	5			46	1,366	10.0%
Contractor	6	27	30	24	40	36	56	47	34	11	11	8		3	1	1		1	1	7	2	1	2	19	349	2.6%
Detainee	3	13	23	33	15	27	14	2	3	8	10	3										1		1	155	1.1%
Non-Combatant	13	43	130	87	150	121	132	140	59	53	38	13			2	1	2	2	1	4	1		1	14	993	7.2%
Other	1	27	38	45	36	51	30	50	37	32	21	24	2	1	1	4	4	1	3	4	1	4	3	28	420	3.1%
Not Stated/NA	19	45	51	52	42	60	51	80	63	43	51	27	5				1		3	4	4	1	3	21	605	4.4%
Total	331	731	903	1,055	1,459	1,653	1,654	1,819	1,026	818	827	723	60	64	52	55	63	79	60	77	59	52	64	685	13,684	

The program benefitted U.S. allies as well, providing assistance to 1,331 non-U.S. patients, including local nationals and coalition forces (Table 19-1). The ready availability of expert clinical input via TM enhanced treatment by supplementing the limited medical resources on site.

▶ Tele-Behavioral Health: 2010 to 2016

Provision of behavioral healthcare (BH) in Forward Operating Bases is complicated by challenging or contested terrain, travel constraints and operational considerations. Under such circumstances, TBH offers the potential to increase access to care and enhance the delivery of BH services.

In contrast to the store-and-forward approach employed to secure assistance with reading X-rays and confirming visual diagnoses, TBH requires *real-time interaction* between the patient, their provider and the TH consultant. This requires use of secure, bidirectional video technology. In this way, BH experts can provide expert evaluation and treatment, even in locations that would otherwise lack access to these services.

TBH provides the following benefits:

- Improves access to BH providers for service members in need of emergency behavioral health evaluations

- Extends the reach of BH providers to far-forward deployed locations without incurring significant excess risk due to travel

- Allows BH providers located at remote outposts to continue to see patients at other outposts when unable to proceed with travel due to weather or hostile action

- Allows BH providers to make recommendations without the need of service member travel

- Assists in command directed evaluation (CDE) of service members by doctoral level BH providers without incurring the expense and risk of travel

To facilitate the rollout of TBH, the AMEDD Telehealth Office and the U.S. Army Medical Command Education and Training Workgroup of the Comprehensive Behavioral Health System of Care worked together in 2010 to craft clinical guidelines and adopt a joint Concept of Operations (CONOPS).

In August 2010, the first BH program, initially implemented on a pilot basis to evaluate its effectiveness, was placed in the Afghanistan theater of operations. Within the joint force's area of operations, four task forces were created. Each consisted of a central "hub" at a larger facility and three peripheral "spokes" in small forward operating bases (Figure 19-1).

To enable TBH consults to proceed at a modest per-unit cost, the program used repurposed DoD-issued laptops equipped with a commercial webcam, a pre-established secure Internet network (Centrix), and commercial software with a total cost of $355 per configured laptop. This enabled providers in Afghanistan to stream confidential video and audio over a secure military network (SIPRNet) to TBH consultants with Skype-like interactivity (see Figure 19-2 for system configuration in a deployed setting).

Preliminary results of TBH acceptance by troops in Afghanistan were encouraging for the first 100 soldiers evaluated (3.8 out of 5-point Likert rating). A majority of providers reported that TBH saved them travel time (43% report one to three days saved per encounter). The most common uses of TBH in Afghanistan included provision of psychodynamic therapy (69%) and management of medications (23%).

Based on the success of this pilot, TBH services were extended to Iraq in October 2011. By the end of that year, TBH providers were handling 20% of all in-theater mental health encounters. Over the next three years, TBH encounters accounted for over 2,000 visits per year through a network of 87 sites in the four regional commands. CENTCOM's mental health consultant provided clinical oversight of all TBH encounters in Iraq and Afghanistan, both face-to-face and TBH evaluations, and noted no significant differences in patient outcomes.

In 2011, the U.S. Army Public Health Command conducted a formal evaluation of the TBH program. Metrics included soldier perceptions; command acceptance; technical success and failures; total number of clinical sessions provided; estimated travel days saved; and a summary review of all tactics, techniques, or procedures (TTPs) that proved to be notably beneficial or detrimental to warfighters and their missions. The evaluation documented high satisfaction among providers, patients, and commanders. Importantly, it noted that "nearly 72% of theater TBH patients reported they would not have sought BH care if the telecare option had not been available."[11]

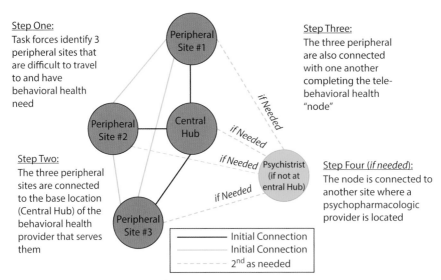

Step One:
Task forces identify 3 peripheral sites that are difficult to travel to and have behavioral health need

Step Two:
The three peripheral sites are connected to the base location (Central Hub) of the behavioral health provider that serves them

Step Three:
The three peripheral are also connected with one another completing the tele-behavioral health "node"

Step Four (if needed):
The node is connected to another site where a psychopharmacologic provider is located

Peripheral Site #1
Peripheral Site #2
Central Hub
Peripheral Site #3
Psychistrist (if not at entral Hub)

if Needed

Initial Connection
Initial Connection
2nd as needed

▲ **Figure 19-1.** Theater telebehavior health node design.

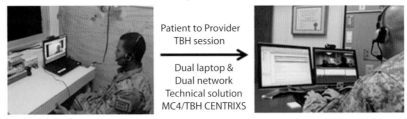

Requirement: To improve patient access to care at remote FOBs in an active combat theater. Also to reduce travel risk and extend virtual outreach by Behavioral Health Providers.

Patient to Provider TBH session

Dual laptop & Dual network Technical solution MC4/TBH CENTRIXS

Medical Impact: The TBH Pilot documented over 1,300 clinical care episodes during the last 9-months of FY12. Over 73% of these patients would not have been seen, without access to "tele", as reported by Public Health Command assessment. Providers documented encounters in AHLTA-Theater, the MHS electronic health record.

▲ **Figure 19-2.** Theater telebehavior health.

From FY12 to FY14, before the rapid draw-down of troop strength, the total number of TBH patients seen was 5,313. The program peaked in Afghanistan in 2012 with 87 operational sites in Afghanistan. In 2014, the average number of consults per month (102) was much lower than the preceding year (168).[6]

The value of TBH for patients includes a) prompt access to specialist consultations, b) helps reduce travel risk and wait time for appointments, and c) provides alternatives to long-term institutional care. The value of TBH to the clinician includes a) improves continuity of care and case management, b) provides timely and high-quality specialty clinics and applications through TH, c) reduces duplication of services or efforts, d) maintains consistency in clinical processes (medicine/laboratory), e) improves consistency and availability of training for practitioners engaged in TH, and f) reduces no-show rates in many cases.[12]

With the draw-down of troop strength in Afghanistan in 2015, the number of TBH sites fell to 12 sites, plus 2 satellite sites in Kuwait. There are plans to expand sites in Iraq from two to four in 2016. The current distribution of TBH assets in the CENTCOM area of responsibility is ideal and allows providers and patients to access subspecialty experts when needed to assist with psychotherapy, psychopharmacology, and administrative psychiatric evaluations. Communication with service members, professional colleagues, and commanders is achieved without the risk, expense, and disruption of prolonged travel. Each patient receives personalized care, and each episode is documented in their EHR. The success of these efforts suggests that TBH is an important capability in meeting the behavioral health care needs for service members deployed to combat zones.

▶ Teleradiology in Deployed Settings: 2005–2016

Teleradiology was first introduced into military deployments by the U.S. Army MATMO in the Bosnia conflict Operation Joint Endeavor in 1996.[13] In Iraq and Afghanistan, teleradiology has emerged as a critical medical capability on the battlefield. The proliferation of digital imaging in the CENTCOM area of operations, particularly computed tomography (CT) and magnetic resonance imaging (MRI), began in 2005. This created the opportunity to develop teleradiology capability using a commercial Picture Archiving and Communication System (PACS) rather than traditional radiographic film.

In 2005 and 2006, an Operational Needs Statements (ONS) authorized the procurement, deployment, and sustainment of a commercial teleradiology platform (Medweb; www.medweb.com) to support CSHs (Role 3 MTF) throughout the CENTCOM region. This facilitated the movement of digital images with radiologists in Iraq, Kuwait, and Qatar, as well as with consulting specialists based at the Landstuhl Regional Medical Center in Landstuhl, Germany. In the later years of the conflicts in Iraq and Afghanistan, falling clinical workloads in theater allowed deployed radiologists to reverse the flow of information and read/interpret digitized images taken at U.S. facilities where they are credentialed to support their home departments and maintain their clinical skills. In effect, they practiced "reverse TM" from their operational settings to their sustaining base.[14]

To enable transmission of images to Landstuhl, the MHS made use of deployable teleradiology systems (DTRS) and a theater image repository (TIR).[15] Digital images from theaters of operations in Afghanistan were transmitted to Germany, then sent on to the U.S. military treatment facilities. This way, each patient's images follow them through their transcontinental journey from a CSH in Afghanistan or Iraq to a Role 4 hospital in the United States.

An important related application in overseas sites is "remote diagnostic access" (RDA) that allows stateside technical experts to access the deployed radiology systems. This maintenance/monitoring capability allows CT and MRI technicians in the United States to quickly spot potential problems with forward-deployed scanning equipment and address them through a combination of remote patching and advice to technical support staff on the ground. Telemedical equipment maintenance has proven to be a vital component of a robust TH platform and for this reason should be included in all future TH implementation discussions.

As of December 2011, 13 teleradiology systems were deployed in Afghanistan and 22 additional sites were established in Iraq. Using images transmitted to Landstuhl and the United States, the U.S. Army is able to discuss the management of complex trauma cases with participating health care providers located at both deployed and stateside locations. They can even share clinical images from operating rooms during weekly trauma care conferences. Image sharing enriches the discussion of trauma management of battlefield wounds and ensures that lessons learned by experienced military trauma surgeons are passed on to new providers.

▶ Deployed Telehealth Summary

The last 15 years of sustained operations have provided DoD medical planners with ample evidence that TH in its various configurations is a valuable force multiplier.

Concept documents such as the U.S. Army's "Force 2025"[16] and Air Force "Military Operations in a Denied Environment"[17] detail its potential to support complex and disaggregated missions highlighted by long distances and more autonomy at the unit level.

Although few problem statements are totally solved with a singular solution, it is clear that in the future the U.S. military will need various medical capabilities to ensure mission success in a volatile world. Given the fiscal and manpower constraints imposed on the military health system and the infeasibility of supporting every forward operating base with a team of specialists, TH must be a large part of any future medical concept planning.

In addition to formulating new concepts and technologies to support tomorrow's warfighter, certain TH capabilities of demonstrated value should be matured into permanent solutions so medical units have them in their portfolio on day one of any future deployment. In addition, consideration should be given to expanding the scale and breadth of military medicine in CONUS, with an eye on using TH as an effective bridge between our sustaining bases in the United States and operationally deployed health care providers around the world. In summary, for the foreseeable future, TH in its various configurations will be a crucial component of care delivered throughout the MHS.

U.S.-BASED TELEHEALTH IN THE DEPARTMENT OF DEFENSE

▶ Background

Currently, the MHS uses numerous TH modalities in stateside facilities to deliver both synchronous and asynchronous care. Initial applications in the DoD stateside medical facilities were developed by the U.S. Army. The U.S. Army Medical Department Telehealth Network currently spans 50 countries and territories from America Samoa to Afghanistan, across 20 time zones.[6,8,18,19] A total of 22 service lines are available with BH constituting 55% of all TM services, followed by cardiology, dermatology, infectious disease, neurosurgery, pain management, and orthopedic surgery. Radiology is not counted in these 22 service lines because it is completely digital and considered standard of care. Thus, excluding teleradiology, approximately

50,000 TH encounters have been conducted per year since 2010.[6,8] There is increasing overall demand for the use of TM, especially in TBH. This service includes a variety of clinical programs across all regional medical commands and covering traumatic brain injury, psychiatry, psychology, and neuropsychologic care.[20–25] The U.S. Army Medical Command Telehealth Network Initiative that was started in 2008 has grown exponentially and has expanded to over 5,500 consults per month, from a handful of sites to greater than 90 in garrison (CONUS, Alaska, Hawaii, America Samoa, Pacific Islands, and Europe), and in Afghanistan to over 78 sites during the peak of the war in 2012. The DoD network has evolved from a U.S. Army–based program to a triservice network that is now working with the Air Force and Navy in sharing ideas and programs.

Using a web-based secure interface, teledermatology has been active in the CONUS by the U.S. Army since 1994.[26,27] Currently there are 22 active sites incorporating all three services. To date, over 40,000 teledermatology consults have been performed, and the Army accounts for the largest activity at over 75%. The primary method, a store-and-forward, has been in existence since 1999. For remote cardiology, tele-echocardiography using cardiac echo imaging takes place in the central part of the United States, with over 26,000 different consults conducted to date at seven sites. This service relies on contracted cardiologists for interpretation of the results. This well-established process has transitioned from core funding demonstrating a sustainable business service to a model for providing care in a peacetime environment on a regular basis.[28]

▶ Pacific Asynchronous TeleHealth

Tripler Army Medical Center (TAMC) located in Honolulu, Hawaii, serves as the DoD tertiary medical care facility for the Western Pacific MTFs in Japan, South Korea, and Guam, which have limited or no access to local specialty consultation services. The Pacific region spans five time zones and the International Date Line, making real-time TM impractical for cases that are nonurgent. This unique medical and geographic situation created the need for asynchronous TM capabilities between Western Pacific MTFs and TAMC.

In 2005, the Pacific Asynchronous TeleHealth (PATH) system was established to support hospitals and clinics in the Pacific theater (Japan, Korea, and Guam; https://path.tamc.amedd.army.mil). PATH is HIPAA compliant, operating on a secure platform and using encrypted passwords for provider authentication. PATH is a web-based, asynchronous platform and, when required, provides aeromedical evacuation case management. Hosted at TAMC, the PATH website enables remote providers to submit patient demographics, clinical data, and supplementary multimedia as dictated by the clinical scenario. Consultations are screened by physician managers at TAMC and forwarded to the appropriate specialists for input. If a specialist is not available at TAMC, other DoD providers can "electronically backfill" and provide consultative expertise as needed. In a similar fashion, patient movement requests are coordinated by both administrative and clinical personnel to ensure efficient, cost-conscious case management. All case discussion is done on the web-based platform, with notification of new case activity via HIPAA-compliant email. In 2005, the PacRim Teleconsultation Effectiveness Trial[29] demonstrated improved health care access and quality with significant cost savings. A retrospective review of 1,000 pediatric teleconsultations from 2006 to 2009 evaluated the PATH system's impact with regard to access, quality, and cost, demonstrating the benefits of incorporating asynchronous provider-to-provider teleconsultation into routine pediatric practice. The PATH System Review[30] of 1,000 pediatric teleconsultations in 2011 revealed a median response time of 14.5 hours (92% response < 1 week) with "Diagnostic" (72% of consults) and "Treatment" (21% of consults) cases. The referring provider's diagnosis and/or treatment plan was modified in 74% of the teleconsultations. PATH prevented air evacuation or referral to local subspecialist in 12% to 43% of all cases. PATH improved access to care in remote locales with quality subspecialty care to remote patients where local expertise is unavailable or limited. PATH also reduced costs by at least $200,000 per year by preventing unnecessary air evacuations and face-to-face consultations while also capturing workload credit for consultant providers. PATH is currently processing 3,500 cases/year from over 40 hospitals and clinics throughout the Pacific region, with over 45 different medical and surgical pediatric and adult specialties.

Health Experts onLine Portal

In 2014 the PATH team partnered with Naval Medical Center Portsmouth (NMCP) in Virginia to provide teleconsultation services to Navy Medicine East via the Health Experts onLine Portal (HELP) system (https://help.nmcp.med.navy.mil).

HELP is a web-based, HIPAA-compliant, secure, asynchronous system started by the NMCP in June 2014. NMCP serves as the DoD's tertiary medical care facility for Navy Medicine East MTFs in the eastern United States, Europe, the Middle East, and their regionally associated fleet and marine assets. Many have limited or no access to local specialty consultation services. This vast region spans 10 time zones, making real-time synchronous teleconsultation impractical. This unique medical and geographic situation created the need for asynchronous teleconsultation capabilities.

In February 2016, HELP demonstrated improved access and quality of care, while saving over $580,000 within its first year.[31] Other associated benefits include proper documentation in the patient's EHR, workload credit for specialty consultants, reduced testing, improved patient movement request coordination, and provision of continuing education to remote health care providers. Patient movement function was activated in February 2015 to allow outside MTFs and the Navy fleet improved visibility on their patients transferred to NMCP.

From initial summary data of the HELP System,[31] 1,755 cases involving 11,411 provider interactions have been completed. Of the 791 active users, 590 NMCP subspecialists in 57 different subspecialties have supported 67 ships and 28 other MTFs. The median response time is just over 7 hours with 75% of consults responded to within 24 hours, 58 medical evacuations prevented, and 245 network deferrals, saving a total of $1.19 million.

Teleaudiology Program

In Bethesda, Maryland, the Walter Reed National Military Medical Center (WRNMMC) Tele-audiology Program partnered the WRNMMC Audiology and Hearing Conservation clinics with the DiLorenzo TRICARE Health Clinic (DTHC) at the Pentagon for remote provision of hearing health services. From August 2015 to June 2016, it completed over 375 patient encounters.[32] Satisfaction survey results were extremely favorable from patients and providers. Furthermore, patients and their commands have benefited from reduced loss of productivity by eliminating lost duty time traveling to WRNMMC, with an estimated cost avoidance of $53,914.[32] The main challenges are the lack of resourcing of a permanent TH technician to sustain the current initiative at the DTHC, prolonged delay on completion of the Risk Management Framework (RMF) to expand services to locations across DoD, and lack of any administrative support to try to work these significant challenges. Based on these results, the tele-audiology team at WRNMMC is pursuing funding for expansion of the program across the DoD.

MOBILE HEALTH APPLICATIONS IN THE DEPARTMENT OF DEFENSE

▶ Mobile Health Background

In a 2015 Pew Research Center study, 64% of American adults own a smart phone, up from 35% in 2011.[33] In addition, 62% of Americans use a smart phone to access health care information.[33] As the use of smart phones continues to increase, its use in the day-to-day lives of end users to access medical information and engage with the medical health care team will subsequently increase. In addition, the smart phone will be an important tool to effect behavior change for unhealthy lifestyle choices (eg, smoking cessation programs) and real-time data capture to improve clinical outcomes (eg, hospital readmissions) for home-based care for chronic diseases (eg, diabetes, congestive heart failure). M-health use in the military and veteran population mirrors the civilian sector, with similar expectations planned for increased use in all settings with widespread technology insert in DoD/Veterans health care.[34]

Success in demonstrating improved access and quality of care, as well as the rapid advances in smart phone technologies, led to initial development in 2008 of m-health applications in the U.S. Army in both garrison and overseas operational bases. Initial efforts focused on standalone applications to improve coping skills with BH problems (stress, anxiety, and mood disturbance).[35,36] The National Center for Telehealth and Technology Program Office at the Defense Center of Excellence for Psychological Health and Traumatic

Brain Injury (DCOE) developed and tested applications focused on self-management tools, initially with breathing relaxation techniques (Breathe2Relax). Breathe2Relax was launched in 2011 and is a hands-on diaphragmatic breathing exercise app to help with mood stabilization, anger control, and anxiety management. Breathe2Relax can be used as a standalone stress reduction tool or can be used in tandem with clinical care directed by a health care worker.[36,37]

Other m-health applications evaluated include a self-management and education text message service for obstetric care outreach for pregnant and postpartum women called Text4Baby.[38] A randomized trial of Text4Baby was conducted among female military health beneficiaries at Madigan Army Medical Center, Tacoma, Washington. Participants provided consent, completed a baseline questionnaire, and then were randomized to enroll in Text4Baby or not. They were followed up at three time points thereafter through delivery of their baby. The main finding was a significant effect of high exposure to Text4Baby on self-reported alcohol consumption and quantities postpartum (OR 0.212, 95% CI 0.046-0.973, P = 0.046). This study, although limited in statistical outcomes, offers important lessons for future scalable m-health programs and suggests the need to study dose-response effects of these interventions (39).[39]

▶ Garrison Mobile Health Applications – "mCare"

Secure messaging (not to be confused with text messaging) is now implemented throughout the DoD to support numerous elements of health delivery, including consultations, appointments, delivering diagnostic results, and patient education.[40]

In response to unmet needs of service members in the U.S. Army Reserves, particularly those with BH problems, posttraumatic stress (PTS), or traumatic brain injury (TBI), in 2009 TATRC developed a mobile phone application called "mCare." The main goal was to augment the standard care provided throughout the geographically dispersed community-based clinics caring for soldiers across the United States in a rehabilitation medical hold status by adding secure messaging to/from patients and care team members. mCare was based on the ideas that a) patient engagement is active (as opposed to passive) with directed participation (as opposed to compliance) in the rehabilitation process and b) the treatment provider and his or her collaboration with the patient is essential to increasing patients' engagement.

From 2009 to 2011, AMEDD conducted an mCare pilot project to determine the requirements for coordination of care for Wounded Warriors across 18 states.[41] The primary objective was to determine if a secure m-health intervention would improve contact rates between patients and providers and positively affect the military health care system. Over 21 months, volunteers enrolled in a HIPAA-compliant mCare project, utilizing soldiers' own cell phones. The intervention included appointment reminders, health and wellness tips, announcements, and other relevant information to this population of rehabilitating wounded warriors exchanged between care teams and patients. The pilot project demonstrated the effectiveness and affordability of communicating with patients through their personal mobile devices with their care managers.[41] The initial intervention consisted of a performance improvement study that included validation and end-user assessment of the intervention.

To further evaluate the impact of mCare, a multi-center, prospective, randomized controlled trial (RCT) of U.S. Army soldiers between April 2011 and October 2012 measured recovery goal awareness, contact rates, symptom inventory severity, satisfaction, general well-being, and usability.[34] All service members receiving care had some type of illness or injury and therefore required long-term management as they progressed through the rehabilitation process and eventually transitioned into retirement, discharge, or returned to duty. Engagement with mCare among people with BH problems, PTS, and/or TBI were particularly of interest because these conditions can include debilitating cognitive (eg, deficits in attention, concentration, memory, speed of processing, new learning, planning, reasoning, judgment) and emotional (eg, depression, anxiety, agitation, irritability, impulsivity, aggression) signs and symptoms that make the monitoring and support provided by community-based providers simultaneously more difficult and more necessary. Data showed that participants' exposure to mCare declined systematically as they out-processed from rehabilitation, irrespective of presence or absence of a BH problem, PTS,

or TBI. The percentage of questionnaires study participants responded to was at least 60%, except for participants with BH problems plus PTS and/or TBI. Time to respond was generally 10 hours or less, and some weeks the average response time was less than 1 hour.[41] Mean response time was longer for participants with BH problems, with or with PTS and/or TBI. The regression analyses found that presence/absence of a BH problem, PTS, and/or TBI was not statistically related to total exposure, total percentage of questionnaires responded to, or total mean response time. Study results also showed a statistical difference in contact rates for soldiers, with the mCare group receiving seven times the contact rates compared to the "usual care" control group.[34] Altogether, these findings suggest satisfactory mCare adoption and use by service members in a community setting, even those with cognitive and emotional difficulties. As a result of this landmark research in mobile health, the mCare research team received the U.S. Army Greatest Inventions award in 2010.

Future analyses of the mCare RCT will address participant response to other components of mCare, as well as treatment group differences in health outcomes and traditional contacts with care team members. Follow-on studies are scheduled to evaluate specific elements of mCare where frequent provider contact and patient engagement could aid in the rehabilitation process. One study centers on pain and goal awareness in wounded service members. Another is an evaluation of the mCare system for chronic care management of people with diabetes. The latter study will expand mCare functionality to include biosensors and patient health record, allowing for a more informed picture of the patient's treatment compliance in the home environment.

▶ Home-Based Tele-Behavioral Health Using Mobile Devices

Evidence of feasibility, safety, and effectiveness of home-based TBH (HBTBH) needs to be established before adoption in the military health system. A recent randomized controlled noninferiority trial was performed to compare the safety, feasibility, and effectiveness of HBTBH to care provided in the traditional in-office setting among military personnel and veterans.[42] One hundred and twenty-one U.S. military service members and veterans were recruited at a military treatment facility and a Veterans Health Administration hospital. Participants were randomized to receive eight sessions of behavioral activation treatment for depression (BATD), either in the home via videoconferencing using mobile devices or in a traditional in-office (same room) setting. Participants were assessed at baseline, midtreatment (4 weeks), posttreatment (8 weeks), and 3 months posttreatment. Mixed-effects modeling results with Beck Hopelessness Scale and Beck Depression Inventory II scores suggested relatively strong and similar reductions in hopelessness and depressive symptoms for both groups; however, noninferiority analyses failed to reject the null hypothesis that in-home care was no worse than in-office treatment based on these measures. There were no differences between treatment groups with regard to satisfaction. Safety procedures were successfully implemented, supporting the feasibility of home-based care. The authors concluded that BATD can be feasibly delivered to the homes of active duty service members and veterans via videoconferencing.[42] Small-group differences suggest a slight benefit of in-person care over in-home TH on some clinical outcomes. This important study will serve as a catalyst to further study the role and opportunities for m-health use for in-home BH treatment among service members and veterans.

▶ Mobile Health Solutions on the Battlefield

Research in military medicine is revealing promising technologies that offer real-time electronic capture and transfer of data between the patient at point of injury (POI), point of care (POC), the medic, and providers, as well as enabling both the practice of TM in forward-deployed areas and the integration of algorithmic alerts and advice into patient monitoring and encounter documentation systems.[43]

With funding provided by the Assistant Secretary of Defense for Health Affairs Joint Program Committees for Informatics and Combat Casualty Care, TATRC has collaborated with the U.S. Army Communications & Electronics Research Development & Engineering Center (USACERDEC), the Army Product Manager Medical Communications for Combat Casualty Care

(PM MC4), the Marine Corps Warfighting Laboratory, and the U.S. Army Cyber Center of Excellence to evaluate integration of TM and medical information exchange technologies over tactical radio networks between ground and air ambulance vehicles and forward-deployed medical facilities on the battlefield.

Within U.S. and North Atlantic Treaty Organization (NATO) military forces, future missions aim to provide useful TM and medical informatics assistance to combat medics, capture accurate records of first-responder patient encounters, and communicate relevant patient information up the medical evacuation and treatment chain. The challenges in providing "operational medical data" without negatively affecting the medics' primary mission to provide quality field medical care have been elusive goals.[44]

Research is being conducted to evaluate enabling technologies for wireless acquisition and exchange of medical information over the current and future force tactical radio network to far-forward health care locations from dismounted medics and corpsman and from prehospital evacuation vehicles. In certain cases this has required exploration of "cross-domain" solutions to facilitate exchange of unclassified medical information over the SIPRNet with extension to unclassified systems operating on the nonsecure military internet (NIPRNET). Patient data included an electronic Tactical Combat Casualty Card (TCCC), imaging, and time-phased physiological monitoring and telemetry data, which in the case of dismounted medics, was captured wirelessly from soldier-worn monitors. Patient demographic data were wirelessly uploaded from patient ID cards and digital "dog tags" to the TCCC cards on Android mobile phones (referred to as end-user devices [EUDs]) using both radiofrequency systems (RFS) and near-field communications (NFC) technologies. TCCC cards could optionally be "bumped" using NFC or secure ultra-wideband transmission from the ground medics' EUDs to those of the evacuation vehicle medics. After being transmitted to medical treatment facilities, patient records were automatically uploaded through the DoD electronic medical record—Armed Forces Health Longitudinal Technology Application - Theater (AHLTA-T)—and the Theater Medical Data Store for posting to the service member's permanent military medical record. The range for remote monitoring and transmission of encounter documentation was significantly increased for both tactical radios and mobile 4G cellular networks by using an Aerostat airship, like those originally deployed in Afghanistan, as well as satellite communications. All user evaluations were conducted in the field at Fort Dix, New Jersey, during squad-level tactical operations.[45]

In 2013, the Joint Tactical Combat Casualty Care Committee revised the TCCC casualty cards to conform to the Joint Tactical Combat Casualty Care Guidelines and forwarded this to DoD leadership (Health Affairs) for staffing with the services and combatant commands as the proposed new prehospital casualty care card (DD Form 1380) for the U.S. military. The new card was immediately adopted in the Central Command region.[46] It was subsequently adjudicated and approved through all of the uniformed services, the combatant commands, and NATO and was thereby established as a standard for electronic patient encounter capture on the battlefield that is applicable to populating the Joint Trauma Registry as well as posting to the patient's permanent military EHR in both the current form (AHLTA/AHLTA-T) and the future MHS cloud-based EHR acquired from CERNER, the recently approved vendor for the new DoD EHR.[47]

TATRC-based research has incrementally advanced the state of the art in en route combat casualty care assessment, monitoring, and intervention using secure wireless communication capabilities. It is now technically possible and operationally feasible to combine physiological monitoring, encounter documentation, and telementoring technologies during en route care within and among various wireless EUDs over secure military tactical networks. The goal is to combine these capabilities in both form and function, thereby potentially reducing the footprints of both forward combat casualty care providers and their supporting equipment, potentially 1) making the medic's job easier to initiate POI/POC data capture to an electronic medical record while en route to higher roles of medical care, 2) reducing the number of redundant procedures, and 3) reducing the need for transport costs and personnel resources by providing real-time analysis of the patient's condition. This will allow for the triage of those patients that can be managed at or near the POI or point of medical evaluation, especially during periods of operationally necessitated prolonged field care.

Intelligent trauma registries are currently used for strategic medical purposes to enable determination of optimal practices that provide the best medical outcomes as opposed to having tactical utility. The Office of the Secretary of Defense/Health Affairs directed the services to implement the Joint Theater Trauma Registry (JTTR) in December 2004, which more recently evolved into the DoD Trauma Registry (DODTR).[48] The DODTR has had a major impact in documenting the types of wounds and treatments rendered, resulting in clinical process improvements and standardization of provider practice for hospital care. However, a comprehensive and integrated system for data collection and analysis to improve performance at the prehospital level of care is still lacking. Capture of the TCCC-based casualty cards, after-action reports, and unit-based prehospital trauma registries, linked with novel sensor biomarkers, need to be implemented globally and linked to the DoD Trauma Registry in a seamless manner that will optimize prehospital trauma care delivery.[49] The use of smart phones/EUDs at the POI/POC on the battlefield will enable this capability.

A future value of the data registry is to capture with EUDs/smart phones more granular medical data to determine the optimal protocol to perform for a specific polytrauma event. This could be called an "intelligent registry" where the product is a catalog for event-driven, goal-directed care using "operationalized" medical data (captured from POI to Role 3 CSHs) across the evacuation continuum and added to the JTTR. Such an intelligent registry would not only include current critical care physiologic data elements (ie, vital signs, treatments rendered) but also integrate novel biomarkers (ie, arterial vasoconstriction measurements) in a robust data set that over time can leverage machine learning approaches to enable predictive analytics and improved clinical outcomes. A critical requirement is the need to capture medical data at the POI/POC from interventions performed by the medic on the patient. Another important component of the intelligent data registry is the knowledge-building aspect that focuses on building a predictive capability for the efficacy of an intervention performed on a specific patient type exhibiting a specific clinical event. Development and sharing of civilian trauma registries with DoD operational medical data registries will accelerate the critical mass of evidence-based medical data needed to more rapidly refine the discriminatory accuracy of trauma events to achieve optimal interventional strategies.[50]

Based on a series of U.S. Army field exercises from 2010 to 2014 using EUDs, integration of patient monitoring, encounter documentation, and telementoring was shown to be feasible in tactical environments in support of dismounted medics as well as during prehospital evacuation.[45] Additionally, a reliable hands-free data entry method is nearly essential for effective medical information exchange during forward-combat casualty care. The research conducted by TATRC and coordinated with collaborating U.S. Army and joint research organizations has made rapid progress toward filling military health system gaps in medical information documentation and exchange at the POI, during prehospital evacuation, and at far-forward field medical settings. The DoD evaluations validated the research strategies of adopting and adapting both commercial and government-developed technologies rather than developing them from scratch, maximizing integration of convergent technologies to enable multiple applications within a single device, implementing medical applications on common user devices and networks, and exploiting operational technology assessment venues funded by nonmedical acquisition programs for evaluating operational and intelligence applications. Given the impending across-the-board cuts in defense research, this approach may be the only feasible way to accelerate development of deployed m-health solutions.

Continuing research conducted by TATRC in collaboration with other Army and DoD Joint Research Development Testing and Evaluation (RDTE) organizations is making rapid progress toward filling MHS gaps in patient monitoring, encounter documentation, medical information exchange, and TH for forward-deployed military forces.[51] Several prototype devices were evaluated against current service and Defense Health Program (DHP) capability gaps during a 2016 exercise conducted by the TATRC, the PM MC4, and the USACERDEC Ground Activity (CGA). Patient encounters were documented on Army Nett Warrior–type EUDs by combat medics at various points of care, including at the POI and during both ground and air evacuation, using software developed by or under the oversight of TATRC, the PM MC4, USACERDEC, and collaborating USAMRMC laboratories and integrated by CGA with the Army's current implementation of the Joint Tactical Radio System (JTRS). In order to validate the feasibility of the TATRC Medical Cloud Computing for Combat Casualty Care (MC5) project, a prototype "light" version of the military theater EHR AHLTA-T, called HALO (Health Application Light Operations), and a web-based server version of AHLTA-T, called Remote Data Services (RDS), were implemented by PM MC4 and USACERDEC at Aberdeen Proving Ground and at Fort Detrick and integrated into the CGA tactical network architecture in a simulated web-based approach to future cloud-based implementation of the Genesis EHR in theater.

The Tempus Pro patient monitoring, documentation, and telementoring system, modified under TATRC for military use, was also installed on both manned and unmanned ground evacuation vehicles and on an unmanned air vehicle and integrated with the CGA tactical network. Remote telemonitoring of patients during ground and air evacuation using the Tempus-Pro TM device and Iridium satellite communications was evaluated by the Navy/Marine Corps in the littoral battle space (land and sea areas in vicinity of the seashore) during the July 2016 Pacific Rim exercise called RIMPAC 16. Additional evaluations of air-to-ground telemonitoring during casualty evacuation missions using the Tempus-Pro system over the Army JTRS tactical networks were successfully conducted at the October 2016 Army Warfighting Assessment 17-1 conducted at Fort Bliss Texas, and White Sands Missile Range, New Mexico.

POLICY AND REGULATORY ISSUES

▶ Opportunities for Telehealth to Improve Military Health System Stateside Care

Although the MHS is a global leader in developing and deploying TH OCONUS, particularly in operational environments, it lags behind civilian health systems, including the Veterans Administration (VA), in adopting TH to support garrison and beneficiary care in CONUS. Based on the experience of these systems, the MHS should be able to achieve substantial improvements in access, quality, cost, and outcomes if it expanded adoption of TH services in CONUS. Current and potential benefits of TH include:

Improved patient experience

- Reduced wait times
- Improved access for persons with mobility issues or transportation challenges
- Dramatic time savings for patients who do not need to travel to clinic
- Increased efficiency of Medical Center (MEDCEN) specialty care clinics for in-person visits
- Improved access to specialist expertise
- Better outcomes and shorter lengths of stay (as through tele-ICU)
- In-home monitoring may reduce use of costly long-term care facilities
- Enables confidential delivery of BH services

Better population health

- Enhanced coordination of acute and trauma care for remote populations
- Promotion of better health management for tech-savvy young adults
- More effective monitoring of chronic conditions
- M-health apps may help management of addiction, chronic pain, and behavioral health issues
- M-health apps assist with maternal and child health, including vaccination reminders
- More effective tracking of health trends in populations
- Enhanced ability to do health systems research

Reduced per-capita costs

- Less reliance on costly brick-and-mortar facilities or in-person visits
- More efficient use of provider time
- Enables greater use of physician extenders
- Supports TH-enabled home visits and home health care that may reduce preventable emergency room visits, hospitalizations, and hospital readmissions
- Allows a small number of cognitive specialists to support a large number of primary care providers
- Reduces unproductive clinic downtime due to no-shows

- Earlier diagnosis and treatment may prevent costly disease progression and needless complications

Enhanced readiness

- Improved ability to support providers caring for rural populations. This capability also applies to military personnel in remote MTFs, aboard ships, and in theater
- Ready access to specialist consultation allows for better decision making at the POC and earlier initiation of needed treatment and reduces medically unnecessary medevacs
- Easy and confidential access to BH minimizes the stigma attached with seeking treatment for PTS

In the future, TH-enabled enlisted and other nonphysician providers (eg, physician assistants, nurse practitioners, combat medics, corpsmen) could support care in remote bases as well as disaggregated military operations. This capability may provide vital support for prolonged field care in austere settings.

The greatest short-term opportunities probably reside in BH and primary care. Improving teleconsultant support could also allow the MHS to increase the impact of a declining number of cognitive subspecialists. Integrating TH in ways that improve access, quality, and established relationships will be critical to its success. This would allow the MHS to offer patient-centered services (eg, BH, wellness, specialty consults, minor and urgent care) at times and in places that are convenient to service members, families, and retirees.

To ensure that such efforts meet regulatory and accrediting requirements, as well as applicable state and/or federal requirements, careful attention must be given to federal regulations that govern consent, protection of patient information, and ethical support for medical decision making. This includes processes for measuring outcomes, assuring safety, reviewing performance, and providing access to backup, in-person care when requested.

▶ Obstacles to Telehealth Expansion in the Continental United States

Despite the probable benefits and proven utility of TH, there are several real or perceived roadblocks to expansion. These fall into four general areas: administrative, technical, organizational, and quality-based.

- *Administrative* obstacles include issues related to difficulty coding and billing for TH services, confusion about clinical privileging, marked variability with state laws and lack of clarity in interpreting relevant federal regulations and policies.

- In the private sector, the majority of *technical* obstacles have been overcome, but the DoD has more stringent requirements for cybersecurity and the robustness of informational infrastructure than typically required of commercial devices.

- *Organizational* obstacles include those issues related to longstanding roles and clinical culture, the need for cooperation among different departments or branches, lack of an inter-organization cost accounting mechanism for telehealth personnel staffing across the services, and conflicting policies generated by various organizations.

- Finally, *quality-based* obstacles include selecting the proper cases to ensure appropriateness of care, and ongoing monitoring of telehealth clinical process and patient outcomes.

Some issues, such as the complex technical and security requirements that must be satisfied to connect DoD information systems, are far more challenging in the MHS than in civilian health systems. However, other considerations are easier. For instance, states laws vary with respect to TH practice, and most licensing boards limit provision of TH services by out-of-state providers. The sheer number of providers offering TH services may lead to "orphan events" and silos that prevent full integration of care.[52] The MHS can avoid such fragmentation by adopting DoD-wide policies that cross state lines. In addition, the DoD's existing AHLTA electronic medical records system tracks care across multiple specialties, as will its successor. The health services literature supports the idea that large, integrated systems such as Kaiser Permanente, the VA and the MHS provide an optimal context for adopting, expanding, and integrating TH into mainstream care.[53] Conversely, the multiple layers of review that DoD initiatives must navigate may impose transaction costs and regulatory hurdles that hinder expansion of TH. Identifying and overcoming these hurdles will be vital to enable TH expansion in the MHS.

▶ Policy Obstacles

TH technology and evidence of clinical effectiveness have substantially outpaced the legal and regulatory framework to enable it. In many states, medical societies and state licensing boards have erected regulatory barriers to keep practitioners in other states from offering TH services in state. Historically, third-party payors were reluctant to reimburse TH services, although this is beginning to change. To accelerate the adoption of TH, several bills and amendments are currently under consideration in the U.S. Congress, including:

The STEP Act (HR 1832) would allow military providers to practice TM outside the confines of MTFs, but it does not apply to TRICARE providers.[54] The act does allow for treatment of patients in their homes. The STEP Act would also:

- Expand DoD state licensure exemption so health care professionals can work across state borders. This applies only to licensing, not privileging, and includes civilians and personal service contractors with relevant credentials, but not nonpersonal services contractors or TRICARE providers.

- Requires the DoD and VA to submit plans for increasing patient access to TH.

National Defense Authorization Act (NDAA) 2017 S2943 (sponsored by Senator McCain, R-AZ).[55] (Note: The act has passed the Senate and is currently in reconciliation with the House NDAA.) It contains a number of notable provisions:

- Requires the Secretary of Defense to incorporate TH services into TRICARE direct and purchased care.

- Proposes that TRICARE must reimburse to the same level for TH visits as it does for in-person visits. Currently, the CMS reimbursement schedule followed by TRICARE does not treat all forms of TH according to the type of treatment provided.

- Reimbursement rates must incentivize purchased care providers to use TH; copays or cost-sharing for patients should be reduced or eliminated.

- Specifies that location of service is with the provider, not the patient (ie, providers not subject to multistate laws for licensing, etc. This is contrary to the current standard, which defines the point of origin is always with the patient).

- Sect. 726 stipulates new competition for all private-sector support contracts to the MHS and that "new" partners must maximize real-time TH and have a standard payment structure for TH providers.

The Veterans E-Health & Telemedicine Support (VETS) Act of 2012 (H.R. 6107)

Although the language in the act was not specifically directed to the MHS, it was introduced in July 2012 by House members Glenn Thompson (R-Pa.) and Charles Rangel (D-N.Y.) to enable providers affiliated with the Department of Veterans Affairs to deliver TM services across state lines and eliminates requirements that providers be licensed in the same state as their patients. Unfortunately, the bill was not passed. It was reintroduced in 2015 by Congressmen Thompson and Rangel as the "Veterans E-Health & Telemedicine Support Act of 2015." This legislation would allow health care providers to treat veterans using TM, even if the veteran is located in a state where the health care professional is not licensed. Specifically, the VETS Act would allow any health care professionals employed or under contract with the VA—even those located outside of federal facilities—to use TM to provide treatment to veterans, irrespective of any other provision of law. Although the VETS Act's prospects for passage are uncertain, it reflects ongoing interest in Congress to use TM to efficiently deliver care in federal health care programs (http://thompson.house.gov/press-release/thompson-and-rangel-introduce-veterans-e-health-telemedicine-support-act-2015).

TELEMEDICINE DEVELOPMENT WITH THE NORTH ATLANTIC TREATY ORGANIZATION AND THE DEPARTMENT OF DEFENSE

▶ Background

As NATO has evolved its doctrine from that of strictly national medical support during operations to that of multinational medical support, the importance and need for TM and the standardization thereof have become apparent. In 2000, NATO created the Telemedicine Expert Panel (TMED EP) when few nations had deployed TM systems to support military field operations. This group and its successor, the Telemedicine Expert Team (TMED ET), have been encouraging the nations to deploy TM in support of their forces and have continued developing the doctrine and technical standards which will facilitate the use of TM within NATO. This has been a highly successful effort, and TM is increasingly being used within the military medical structures of some NATO and Partnership for Peace (PfP) nations to provide medical care to deployed military personnel.

The NATO reality today is that of multinational operations, with an increasing likelihood of multinational medical support structures. Fiscal and operational constraints in recent years have mandated a decrease in the size of the logistics "footprint" in a deployed theater of operations. This fact, combined with the decreasing size of the military medical services of most NATO and partner nations, has made it increasingly difficult for health care providers "to provide a standard of medical care as close as possible to prevailing peacetime medical standards" during field operations as required by NATO doctrine.[56,57] Effective use of teleconsultation may, to some degree, alleviate this difficulty, as has been demonstrated in recent operations, including those in Afghanistan.

NATO identified as early as 1995 a significant "capability gap" in multinational medical communications capabilities, which even today hinders full and effective implementation of multinational teleconsultation across national boundaries. To be fully effective in a multinational environment, they must be fully integrated into an overarching NATO Medical Information Management System (MIMS) architecture. The development of the required architecture is the responsibility of the Medical Information Management Systems Working Group (MIMS WG), of which the TMED ET is now a subgroup, and to which it provides input concerning operational requirements for teleconsultation as well as the unique technical and communications requirements.[58-60]

▶ North Atlantic Treaty Organization Telemedicine Expert Panel and Expert Team

The lack of adequate interoperability for medical data and interoperable TM systems has been identified since 2000 by the NATO Committee of the Chiefs of the Military Medical Services (COMEDS), the Allied Command Operations (ACO), and the Medical Standards Working Group (Med Standards WG) as a significant capability gap. In 2000, the General Medical WG established a TM subcommittee to address these needs. This subcommittee was converted to the TMED EP and was established in June 2001 as a subgroup of the Medical Information Management Systems (MIMS) Working Group. It then began to address the technical and clinical aspects of TM. After the TMED EP was successful in developing a series of TM-specific technical and policy/standardization documents, it was converted into an ET as part of the NATO Medical Communications Information Systems (MedCIS) WG, so as to ensure that the TMED-specific work done previously could be successfully integrated into the future development of NATO-wide medical communications doctrine.

The goals of the TMED ET are to 1) develop TM interoperability standards for use among deployed NATO forces, 2) assist in the development of doctrine to support TMED use, and 3) coordinate medical information management efforts with the MedCIS.

The TMED ET continues to meet on a regular biannual basis and is working closely with the MedCIS Panel on numerous medical informatics initiatives (patient tracking, medical disease surveillance, and medical logistics) in support of other NATO panels and expert teams. The accomplishments of these groups have been reported in detail.[58]

Key Accomplishments of the Telemedicine Expert Team

The following is a list of TMED ET accomplishments:

1. Developed and submitted in 2004 a Tele-Consultation Standardization Agreement (STANAG #2517), which was ratified among NATO nations in May 2005 with TMED metrics and business practices incorporated.

2. STANAG has been repeatedly updated and improved. STANAG 2517, edition 4, was ratified and then was converted to AMEDP-37 in 2011.

3. A teleconsultation CONOPS was developed in 2009 and has been distributed to all NATO and PFP nations.

4. TM definitions were developed and incorporated into AMEDP-13 alpha (NATO Medical Glossary) in 2011.

5. In 2005 the TMED ET planned and completed a Telemedicine Interoperability Study (TIOpS), which compared telemedical diagnoses and recommendations for a set of standardized case studies among four NATO nations (United States, UK, Netherlands, and Spain) in a nonwartime setting that proved the feasibility and clinical acceptability of multinational teleconsultation diagnoses and advice.

   a. The results of this study showed that even across national professional borders, diagnoses of the TM-transmitted test cases and recommendations as to their management were of an acceptable quality across national boundaries.

6. The U.S. Army deployed a strictly national field TM system with its forces in Iraq and then in Afghanistan,[61-63] and it rapidly became evident that other deployed nations had a need for this capability. Rather than encouraging each nation to develop its own system, it was recommended that the U.S.-only system could be made available to other deployed NATO-related forces in Afghanistan. A teleconsultation memorandum of understanding (MOU) between NATO and the AMEDD was completed in November 2008. This capability was deployed to the International Security Assistance Force (ISAF) in Afghanistan during February 2009. The program was utilized on a regular basis among three NATO nations (Canada, Netherlands, and Spain), with Canada being the most frequent user. This provided a real-time multinational use of teleconsultation.[62,63]

The primary result of the TMED ET effort was the publication of STANAG 2517, which was developed through Edition 4, and which has proven useful to several nations newly establishing teleconsultation systems. With the publication of Allied Administrative Publication (AAP-3), it was decreed that the contents of this STANAG should be continued, but that it had to be converted to a covering STANAG and an Allied Medical Publication (AMEDP) in accordance with new NATO guidance regarding standardization hierarchies. This document was subsequently issued bearing the number AMEDP-37, which is currently in effect.[64,65]

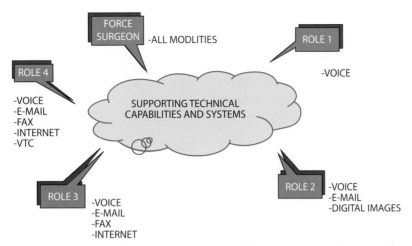

▲ **Figure 19-3.** A schematic view of the telecommunications modalities required at a given role of care and visibility of the situation by the force surgeon.

▶ Standardization Agreement 2517/ AMedP-37

The aim of this agreement is to register national acceptance of interoperability assistance and guidance to be used by nations wishing to develop teleconsultation systems for deployment in support of NATO or NATO-led missions. Participating nations agreed to utilize the guidelines and recommendations included during the development of national teleconsultation systems for deployment in a multinational NATO environment, if they determined they wished to deploy such systems.

Although there are multiple definitions of TM, TH and teleconsultation, there is no "official" TH standard. The following definitions were used in this STANAG:

Telemedicine – The use of advanced telecommunication technologies to exchange health information and provide healthcare services across geographic, time, social and cultural barriers.

Telehealth – The use of telecommunication techniques for the purpose of providing TM, medical education, and health education over a distance.

The provision of specialty services (eg, dental, mental health, cardiology, and dermatology) by health care specialists to patients and/or other physicians. Teleconsultation may employ a wide range of technologies from simple voice communication to real-time media conferencing facilities, along with the ability to handle medical specialty–specific data streams (eg, heart and lung sounds, echocardiograms, video and still images) captured with the use of specialized equipment.[64,65]

The STANAG identifies the need to create standard operating procedures for NATO teleconsultation in support of medical operations. In addition, each nation is required to ensure that operational medical support plans consolidate and integrate standard operating procedures. Such procedures should include:

a. Standardization of consultation priorities (routine, priority, or emergency) with expected response times for each priority

b. Definition of preferred referral patterns

c. Definition of standard reporting formats and clinical guidelines as they emerge

d. Definition of practices to ensure patient privacy, confidentiality, and integrity of medical data

e. Consideration of the requirement for MOUs that detail the legal authorities, responsibilities, and legal status of clinicians engaged in teleconsultation

▶ North Atlantic Treaty Organization Science for Peace and Security Telemedicine Project in Ukraine

The NATO Science for Peace and Security (SPS) Telemedicine Project is developing and demonstrating a multinational TM system to improve access to health services and increase survival rates in emergency situations, including in remote areas.[66,67] The technology was successfully live tested during a field exercise in Lviv, Ukraine, in September 2015, attended by NATO Secretary General Jens Stoltenberg and the president of the Ukraine, Petro Poroshenko.

Co-organized by the *Euro-Atlantic Disaster Response Coordination Centre* (*EADRCC*) and the State Emergency Service (SES) of Ukraine, the field exercise involved 1,100 rescue workers from 34 countries. It was the first time that independent national TM systems interacted to provide medical support in a disaster scenario.[68]

Once developed, this multinational TM system could have a dual use for both civilian and military application, including crisis situations. Portable medical kits would allow first responders to connect to the system to receive advice from medical specialists in case of an emergency, even in remote areas. Through the use of modern communications technologies, an international network of medical specialists would be able to assess the patient, determine the diagnosis, and provide real-time recommendations. *The TM project has high-level political backing and involves an incredible pool of scientists and experts. It aims to save lives in emergency situations as well as in military operations.*

TM supports the teams on the ground in remote areas with expertise that is not present at the scene of the disaster. This will quickly allow getting the right medical support to those who need it most, having the potential to save many lives on the battlefield as well as in disasters. Against the background of the current conflict in the Ukraine, this multinational system has the potential to increase survival rates in remote areas, including for wounded Ukrainian soldiers.

Supported by the SPS Program, this cooperation between allied countries, Romania, and the United States, as well as NATO partners Finland, the Republic of Moldova, and the Ukraine, will also provide advanced equipment and training for users of the system. The partner countries involved contribute experience and knowledge to this project. Finland, for instance, has an advanced national TM capability in place, which brings related subject matter expertise. Moldova and Ukraine are providing highly qualified medical and communication technology personnel with a particular focus on emergency situations. The creation of a set of guidelines is envisioned based on existing standards so that in the future, other countries may be able to connect their national TM systems into the wider multinational capability.[68]

SUMMARY

Since 1993, the DoD has been a leader in the development and use of TH technologies across the broad spectrum of health care beneficiaries in diverse geographic settings. The influence of the DoD in expanding the role of TH in overseas military operations and in NATO has been noteworthy.

Despite initial advances in development of TH across the MHS, current efforts for stateside TH advances need a more comprehensive approach to address the clinical, technical, and administrative DoD TH issues. The DoD will need to commit greater resources and structure for a TH program that includes the needs of the services in cooperation with the Defense Health Agency. Leveraging the experience and lessons learned from the VA and successful civilian programs will be beneficial for success. Identifying and assembling the key DoD agencies that need to organize into a DoD WG is an important step. This will require an understanding from senior leaders that a shared vision with financial commitment will be needed for large-scale implementation and sustainment of TH across the DoD. Only through a shared common vision and commitment to excellence in health care delivery, augmented with technology, will the desired results that our service members and their families deserve be achieved.

REFERENCES

1. Department of Defense: Military Health System. http://www.health.mil/. Fairfax, VA, 2016.
2. Poropatich R, Lai E, McVeigh F, Bashshur R. The U.S. army telemedicine and m-health program: making a difference at home and abroad. *Telemed J E Health* 2013;19(5):380–386.
3. National Academies of Science: The Role of Telehealth in an Evolving Health Care Environment – Workshop, Summary. http://www.nationalacademies.org/hmd/Reports/2012/The-Role-of-Telehealth-in-an-Evolving-Health-Care-Environment.aspx. Washington, DC, November 2012.

4. Crowther JB, Poropatich RK. Telemedicine in the US Army: case reports from Somalia and Croatia. *Telemed J* 1995;1(1):73–80.

5. Gomez E, Poropatich RK, Karinch MA, Zajtchuk J. Tertiary telemedicine support during global military humanitarian missions. *Telemed J* 1996;2(3):201–210.

6. Poropatich RK, Lai E, McVeigh F, Bashshur R. The U.S. Army telemedicine and m-health program: making a difference at home and abroad. *Telemed J E Health* 2013;19(5):1–7.

7. OTSG/MEDCOM Policy Memo 04-003. Use of Tele-Dermatology Consults Prior to Patient Evacuation from Operation Iraqi Freedom (OIF) and Operation Enduring Freedom (OEF) Locations. https://onestaff.amedd.army.mil/medcom/. May 2004.

8. Poropatich RK, DeTreville R, Lappan C, Kohuth C. The United States Army telemedicine program – general overview and current status in Southwest Asia. *Telemed J E Health* 2006;12(4):396–408.

9. OTSG/MEDCOM Policy Memo 05-004. Use of Army Knowledge Online (AKO) Email in Support of Electronic Telehealth Medical Consultation by Deployed Providers. https://onestaff.amedd.army.mil/medcom/. March 2005.

10. Schmidt T, Lappan CM, Hospenthal DR, Murray CK. Deployed provider satisfaction with infectious disease teleconsulation. *Mil Med* 2011;176(12):1417–1420.

11. Winters M. Department of Defense: Telemedicine in the Iraq War. http://www.militaryspot.com/news/telemedicine-in-the-iraq-war. December 2012.

12. Garcia MM, Lindstrom KJ. Telebehavioral health: practical application in deployed and garrison settings. *US Army Med Dep J* 2014;Oct-Dec:29–35.

13. Clyburn CA, Gilbert GR, Cramer TJ, Lea RK, Ehnes SG, Zajtchuk R. Development of emerging technologies within the department of defense: a case study of operation joint endeavor in Bosnia. *Acquisition Review Quarterly* 1997;4(1):101–121.

14. Gilbert GR, Meade K, Rapp T, Detreville R. An Emerging web-enabled radiology business practice within the U.S. Army. Proceedings of American Telemedicine Association Annual Meeting. Presentation: http://www.atmeda.org/conf/annualmeet.htm. 2004.

15. Department of Defense: Defense Health Agency: Deployed Tele-Radiology System (DTRS)/Theater Imaging Repository (TIR). http://www.Health.mil/Deployed. Tele-Radiology System (DTRS)/Theater. Imaging Repository (TIR)/PIA. November 2008.

16. U.S. Army Training and Doctrine Command: Force 2025 and Beyond Unified Land Operations Win in a Complex World. http://www.arcic.army.mil/app_Documents/tradoc_ausa_force2025andbeyond-unifiedlandoperations-wininacomplexworld_07oct2014.pdf. October 2014.

17. Department of Defense - U.S. Joint Chiefs of Staff: Joint Concept for Entry Operations. http://www.dtic.mil/doctrine/concepts/joint_concepts/jceo.pdf. April 7, 2014.

18. Mahnke CB, Jordan CP, Bergvall E, Person DA, Pinsker JE. The Pacific Asynchronous TeleHealth (PATH) system: review of 1,000 pediatric teleconsultations. *Telemed J E Health* 2011;17(1):35–39.

19. Doarn CR, Shore J, Ferguson S, et al. Challenges, solutions, and best practices in telemental health service delivery across the pacific rim-a summary. *Telemed J E Health* 2012;18(8):654–660.

20. Jones MD, Etherage JR, Harmon SC, Okiishi JC. Acceptability and cost-effectiveness of military telehealth mental health screening. *Psychol Serv* 2012;9(2):132–143.

21. Stetz MC, Folen RA, Yamanuha BK. Technology complementing military behavioral health efforts at tripler army medical center. *J Clin Psychol Med Settings* 2011;18(2):188–195.

22. Gros DF, Strachan M, Ruggiero KJ, et al. Innovative service delivery for secondary prevention of PTSD in at-risk OIF-OEF service men and women. *Contemp Clin Trials* 2011;32(1):122–128.

23. Doarn CR, McVeigh F, Poropatich R. Innovative new technologies to identify and treat traumatic brain injuries: crossover technologies and approaches between military and civilian applications. *Telemed J E Health* 2011;16(3):373–381.

24. Nieves JE, Candelario J, Short D, Briscoe G. Telemental health for our soldiers: a brief review and a new pilot program. *Mil Med* 2009;174:12–13.

25. Girard P. Military and VA telemedicine systems for patients with traumatic brain injury. *J Rehabil Res Dev* 2007;44(7):1017–1026.

26. Vidmar DA. The history of teledermatology in the department of defense. *Dermatol Clin* 1999;17(1):113–124.

27. Pak HS, Datta SK, Triplett CA, et al. Cost minimization analysis of a store-and-forward teledermatology consult system. *Telemed J E Health* 2009;15(2):160–165.

28. Mahnke CB, Mulreany MP, Inafuku J, Abbas M, Feingold B, Paolillo JA. Utility of store-and-forward pediatric telecardiology evaluation in distinguishing normal from pathologic pediatric heart sounds. *Clin Pediatr (Phila)* 2008;47(9):919–925.

29. Callahan CW, Malone F, Estroff D, Person DA. Effectiveness of an Internet-based store-and-forward telemedicine system for pediatric subspecialty consultation. *Arch Pediatr Adoles* 2005;159:389–393.

30. Mahnke CB, Jordan CP, Bergvall E, Person DA, Pinsker JE. The Pacific Asynchronous TeleHealth (PATH) system: review of 1,000 pediatric teleconsultations. *Telemed J E Health* 2011;17(1):1–5.

31. Lin AH, Cole JH, Chin JC, Mahnke CB. The Health Experts online at Portsmouth (HELP) system: one-year review of adult and pediatric asynchronous telehealth consultations. *SAGE Open Med* 2016;4:2050312115626433.

32. Department of Defense – USAMRMC: AAMTI Project Spotlight: Net-Centric Audiology Program Enables Wide Area Persistent Hearing Surveillance. http://www.tatrc.org/www/about/Nsltr/TATRC_Nsltr_16_6_Q3.pdf. June 2016.

33. U.S. Smartphone Use in 2015. http://www.pewinternet.org/2015/04/01/us-smartphone-use-in-2015/. 2015.

34. Pavliscsak H, Little JR, Poropatich RK, et al. Assessment of patient engagement with a mobile application among service members in transition. *J Am Med Inform Assoc* 2016;23(1):110–118.

35. Department of Defense. http://t2health.dcoe.mil/news/new-mobile-app-helps-troops-self-manage-behavior-stress. 2011.

36. Shore JH, Aldag M, McVeigh FL, et al. Review of mobile health technology for military mental health. *Mil Med* 2014;179(8):865–878.

37. Luxton DD, Hansen RN, Stanfill K. Mobile app self-care versus in-office care for stress reduction: a cost minimization analysis. *J Telemed Telecare* 2014;20(8):431–435.

38. Evans WD, Abroms LC, Poropatich R, Nielsen PE, Wallace JL. Mobile health evaluation methods: the Text4baby case study. *J Health Commun* 2012;17 (suppl 1):22–29.

39. Evans W, Nielsen PE, Szekely DR, et al. Dose-response effects of the text4baby mobile health program: randomized controlled trial. *JMIR Mhealth Uhealth* 2015;3(1).

40. Byrne JM, Elliott S, Firek A. Initial Experience with patient-clinician secure messaging at a VA medical center. *J Am Med Inform Assoc* 2009;16(2):267–270.

41. Poropatich RK, Pavliscsak HH, Tong JC, Little JR, McVeigh FL. mCare: using secure mobile technology to support soldier reintegration and rehabilitation. *Telemed J E Health* 2014;20(6):563–569.

42. Luxton DD, Pruitt LD, Wagner A, et al. Home-based telebehavioral health for U.S. military personnel and veterans with depression: a randomized controlled trial. *J Consult Clin Psychol* 2016;84(11):923–934.

43. Poropatich RK. TATRC's Strategy for the Research and Development of Mobile Health Applications, Presented to the Fed Communications Commission, July 12, 2010. http://reboot.fcc.gov/c/document_library/get_file?uuid=8ac18153-1b96-4e14-958c-9538a7fc272c&groupId=19001. 2010.

44. Manemeit C, Gilbert GR. "Joint Medical Distance Support and Evacuation JCTD, Joint Combat Casualty Care System Concept of Employment" NATO HFM-182-33 paper. http://ftp.rta.nato.int/public/PubFullText/RTO/MP/RTO-MP-HFM-182/MP-HFM-182-33.doc. 2010.

45. Gilbert GR, Manemeit C. Remote Patient Monitoring, Encounter Documentation, and Telementoring Over Secure Mobile Tactical Networks NATO STO-MP-HFM-231 paper. https://www.cso.nato.int/pubs/rdp.asp?RDP=STO-MP-HFM-231. 2013.

46. US Forces Fragmentation Order 13-138 Directs Changes to TCCC System, DoD US Army, Deployed, Afghanistan, USFOR-A (MC), July 13, 2013.

47. Meeting Minutes Committee on Tactical Combat Casualty Care, MacDill AFB, FL: 4-5 February 2014.

48. Combat Trauma Lessons Learned from Military Ops of 2001-2013.Defense Health Board, Office of Assistant Secretary of Defense; Health Affairs 2015.

49. Kotwal RS, Butler FK, Montgomery HR, et al. The tactical combat casualty care casualty card TCCC guidelines - proposed change 1301. *J Spec Oper Med* 2013;13(2):82–87.

50. Berkow J, Poropatich R. Trauma Care in a Rucksack (TRACIR), a Disruptive Technology Concept. *Small Wars Journal* http://smallwarsjournal.com/jrnl/art/%E2%80%9Ctrauma-care-in-a-rucksack%E2%80%9D-tracir-a-disruptive-technology-concept. 2016.

51. Gilbert GR. DoD Executive After Action Report - Patient Monitoring, Encounter Documentation, Medical Information Exchange and Telemedicine Technology Field Evaluations at Roles I-III conducted by USAMRMC TATRC in conjunction with Army CERDEC Ground Activity 2016 Telemedicine Prototype Field Evaluations. USAMRMC TATRC, September 9, 2016.

52. Daniel H, Sulmasy LS. Policy recommendations to guide the use of telemedicine in primary care settings: an American College of Physicians position paper recommendations for the use of telemedicine in primary care settings. *Ann Intern Med* 2015;163(10):787–789.

53. Bashshur RL, Shannon G, Krupinski EA, Grigsby J. Sustaining and realizing the promise of telemedicine. *Telemed J E Health* 2013;19(5):339–345.

54. Janos E, Roll C. U.S. Department of Defense Expands Telemedicine Access for Military Members. https://www.healthlawpolicymatters.com/2016/03/08/u-s-department-of-defense-expands-telemedicine-access-for-military-members/. March 2016.

55. Center for Connected Health Policy. S2943-- National Defense Authorization Act for Fiscal Year 2017. http://cchpca.org/sites/default/files/resources/S%202943%20%E2%80%93%20National%20Defense%20Authorization%20Act%20updated.pdf. June 2016.

56. MC 0326/3 "NATO Principles And Policies Of Medical Support", para 4A(2); September 26, 2011.

57. AJP 4.10 (A), Allied Joint Medical Support Doctrine, March 2006.

58. Lam DM, Poropatich RK. Telemedicine deployments within NATO military forces: a data analysis of current and projected capabilities. *Telemed J E Health* 2008;14(9):946–951.

59. Lam DM, Poropatich RK, Gilbert GR. Telemedicine standardization in the NATO environment. *Telemed J E Health* 2004;10(4):459–465.

60. Lam D, Poropatich RK, Gilbert GR. Telemedicine standardization in the NATO Environment. In: Klapan I, Cikes I, eds. *Telemedicine*. Telemedicine Association Zagreb; 2005:444–451.

61. Poropatich RK, Morris TJ, Gilbert GR, Abbott KC. The United States army program for deployment telemedicine. In: Klapan I, Cikes I, eds. *Telemedicine*. Telemedicine Association Zagreb; Zagreb, Croatia; 2005:427–435.

62. Poropatich RK, Lappan C, Lam DM. Operational use of U.S. army telemedicine information systems in Iraq and Afghanistan – consideration for NATO operations. In: Latifi R, ed. *Telemedicine for Trauma, Emergencies, and Disaster Management*. Norwood, MA: Artech House; 2011:173–182.

63. Meade K, Lam DM. A deployable telemedicine capability in support of humanitarian operations. *Telemed J E Health* 2007;13(3):331–340.

64. Lam DM. Force protection and its potential utilization of telemedicine and medical information system modalities. Chapter in Force Health Protection RTO-EN-HFM-137(2008). NATO Research and Technology Organisation. Paris, France. November 2008.

65. Lam DM. NATO multinational medical operations and the requirement for interoperability and data exchange, chapter in *Force Health Protection* (RTO-EN-HFM-137, AC/323(HFM-137)TP/67): NATO Research and Technology Organisation, Paris, France, March 2007, pp. 4-1–4-12.

66. Lam DM, Mackenzie CF, Hu FP, et al. Challenges to remote emergency decision-making for disaster or homeland security. Proceedings of the Human Factors & Ergonomics Society 49th Annual Meeting; Zagreb, Croatia; 2005; 544–547.

67. Latifi R, Peck K, Porter J, et al. Telepresence and telemedicine in trauma and emergency care mangement. In: Latifi R, ed. *Establishing Telemedicine in Developing Countries: From Inception to Implementation*. Amsterdam, The Netherlands: IOS Press; 2004:193–199.

68. NATO. EADRCC consequence management field exercise in Ukraine. http://www.nato.int/cps/en/natohq/news_118671.htm. September 21, 2015.

The Role of Telehealth in International Humanitarian Outreach

Dale C. Alverson, MD, FAAP, FATA

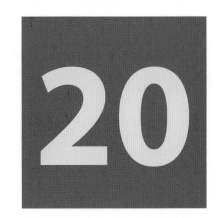

INTRODUCTION

The dynamic evolution of information and communication technologies (ICT) is allowing the exploration and implementation of the use of telehealth for the underserved, particularly in developing low- and middle-income countries (LMIC).[1,2] By definition, "humanitarian" efforts are concerned with or are seeking to promote human welfare, involving an event or situation that causes or involves widespread human suffering. Certainly this applies to addressing health issues in these developing countries throughout the world.[3–6] Telehealth offers the tools to provide humanitarian support in the global community to address disparities in health care at many levels, including sharing knowledge, education, training, research, and direct health care services.[7,8] To be effective, the telehealth applications must address the needs of those countries and their communities in a manner that is appropriate, realistic, and collaborative, as well as meets reasonable standards of care.[9]

The world can be considered one community, with mankind its citizens. The needs for health care are universal, and these types of efforts should rise above political, cultural, religious, and historical differences. Telehealth and ICT offer tools to improve access to care, share knowledge, and ultimately improve the health and quality of life of all people in the global community, including regions where health disparities can be profound. Using advances in ICT, telemedicine and e-health are offering a means to transform systems of care for people throughout the world by not only providing greater access to clinical service, consultation, and sharing knowledge, but also addressing education and training, health systems development, public and community health, epidemiology and research.

Leap-frogging over prior barriers, rapid advances in ICT, computing, and wireless networks are offering greater continuity in access to these services in both developed and developing countries. The use of telehealth must be put in the context of the critical health needs in each country, cultural perspectives, current and future communication infrastructure, other supportive resources, and likelihood for sustainability. Furthermore, these telehealth efforts should be aimed at improving the local capacity in providing ongoing health services in each country and blending into that country's health care strategies.

In combination, these communication technologies and health-related applications constitute the concept of telehealth. As defined by the World Health Organization (WHO), telehealth is providing a broad spectrum of health services over distance and the integration of telecommunications systems into the practice of protecting and promoting health.[3]. Global development and integration of communication systems and networks, wireless, and broadband are creating opportunities for international collaboration using telehealth and a platform for exchange, with the potential for formation of a true "network of networks" and "virtual collaboratory" that can be used worldwide. A network of this magnitude represents far more than a communication infrastructure because it facilitates partnerships and collaboration between health care providers and educators, public health workers, investigators, and other international organizations and stakeholders.

The time is now for open and constructive dialogue designed to facilitate that coordination between key stakeholders and other international organizations. These types of international exchange experiences enhanced with telehealth offer significant opportunities for understanding the common denominators, as well as unique differences, related to global health among countries and cultures around the world. These programs can promote international understanding and mutual respect in a manner that can improve the health of the entire global community.

STEPS IN DEVELOPING AN INTERNATIONAL TELEHEALTH PROGRAM

The following represents recommended steps that should be considered when planning, developing, and implementing an international telemedicine program.

1. **Define the country or region with which one desires to work**

   Because overall global needs are significant, it is important to clearly define the country or countries and region of the world with which you plan to collaborate and provide services. Often this is related to an existing relationship an organization has with these countries or region. In this regard, if not already done, identify a "champion" within that country or region with whom you will work who understands their culture, political landscape, and health perspectives, building upon existing relationships within that country. Also consider interactions and collaborations with government entities, such as the ministry of health, and other national academic medical centers or other health care provider systems within the country so that telemedicine can be appropriately integrated in their health care initiatives.

2. **Survey what other telehealth-related programs may already be in place in that country**

   Determine whether there are other telemedicine initiatives in the countries of interest and explore opportunities to collaborate, complement those programs, and avoid unnecessary duplication of effort. Often, one finds there are or have been telemedicine-related programs in a country. Attempts should be made to contact those involved in those existing telemedicine programs or understand why a past program is no longer active or wasn't sustained so that future similar efforts can be successful, learning from prior challenges.

3. **Perform a needs assessment**

   It is critical to determine what health needs can be realistically addressed through telehealth and integrated into their health care system. This may require prioritizing those needs and focusing on those that are of the highest priority. Often the first need to address is education, sharing knowledge and training so that any investment in managing those health care needs can be adequately addressed with a trained and knowledgeable workforce. Putting in technology and expending financial resources without addressing these workforce issues make it difficult to implement a telehealth program and to see a return on investment in those efforts that can lead to sustainability.

4. **Define together the overall vision, mission, goals, and objectives of the telehealth initiative in the country**

   It is important to clearly articulate and agree upon the goals and objectives of the program so that all participants involved are engaged in the effort. Sharing a common vision and mission can lead to a sustained effort, which leads to successful implementation and sustainability, as well as create a platform for achieving support from other stakeholders, both within and outside the country.

   An example of how this might be articulated is demonstrated as follows:

   Vision:
   Telehealth will be fully integrated into the health systems of the country or region of interest and improve the health of its people.

   Mission:
   To use telehealth as a set of tools to address the health issues and needs of the region and improve health outcomes of their citizens.

   Goals:
   - Develop a telehealth infrastructure that addresses the needs in the region as defined by their health leaders.
   - Develop specific programs using telehealth as tools to share knowledge, education, and access to needed health services.

- Determine the most appropriate telehealth technologies and platforms to meet defined needs.
- Develop a means to determine improvements and measures that demonstrate impact.
- Develop a realistic business plan for implementation and sustainability.

5. **Develop a technical plan**

   a. Determine the spectrum of telehealth technologies that could be realistically applied in that country.

   b. Determine the network infrastructure and connectivity available or that could be developed to support the technologies deployed.

   c. Plan for training and education in using the technologies.

6. **Develop the operational plan**

   a. Determine the workforce and staff availability to support the specific telehealth application at both hubs and spokes and both within country or with other countries providing health care services.

   b. Integrate the telehealth program into the workflow.

   c. Determine how telehealth encounters and activities will be documented, such as integration into electronic health records (EHRs).

   d. Determine needs for credentialing, privileging, and licensing telehealth providers, as well as compliance with that country's rules and regulations, along with international standards.

   e. Perform a risk management assessment and determine if there is adequate protection of patients and providers and support in case of any adverse events.

7. **Develop the business plan**

   Determine what resources and finances are needed for implementation and ongoing support and sustainability. Define the return on investment (ROI); consider a cost-benefits analysis; and develop the value proposition that can respond to the decision makers and funders, assuring that the support will be used appropriately, effectively, and efficiently, as well as align with their strategic direction.

8. **Develop an evaluation plan**

   a. Determine the metrics or measures of success that will demonstrate the benefits of the telehealth initiative.

   b. Determine, design, and implement the methods for data collection and analysis and who will be responsible for those efforts.

   c. Generate reports that demonstrate the impact and consider publications of those efforts.

9. **Plan for continued quality improvement (CQI) of the telehealth program**

   Develop systems and methods to respond to challenges in the telehealth program in order to receive periodic feedback from all participants so that the program can make any needed improvements. CQI efforts can assist in sustainability and provide opportunities for expansion, as well as integration of new applications or technologies that will likely continue to evolve over time.

EXAMPLES OF SUCCESSFUL OR PLANNED INTERNATIONAL HUMANITARIAN TELEHEALTH EFFORTS

The programs described in this section represent only a sample of established or developing international telemedicine humanitarian initiatives. These programs use a spectrum of ICT, telehealth platforms, and models, applying possible collaborations with nonprofit and for-profit entities, nongovernmental organizations (NGOs), and governmental agencies, along with panels of health care provider volunteers and experts. These programs may provide consultation, case reviews, education, and knowledge sharing, as well as augment in-person provision of health services. These services can be synchronous (real time), asynchronous, or a combination of both. The platforms may use wireless systems connected to the Internet; be web-based; include text and images; utilize mobile devices such as smart phones or tablets; or use specialized equipment, carts, and peripheral devices to support consultation.

▶ Swinfen Charitable Trust

The Swinfen Charitable Trust (http://www.swinfencharitabletrust.org/) based in the United

Kingdom was started in 1998 by Lord and Lady Swinfen as a nonprofit organization to provide asynchronous consultation to health care providers in developing countries. It uses a secure web-based platform that operates 24 hours, 7 days a week throughout the year and allows an authorized health care provider in a participating developing country to request a consult about a specific patient using text and attaching images as needed. A large panel of specialty volunteers has been recruited and continues to be recruited. These individual volunteer specialists are contacted via email based upon the type of consultation requested. When a consult is requested, the appropriate specialist is asked to log into the website and respond within 48 hours, providing possible diagnoses and management options. On average each case is answered within 12 hours. Health care providers can also request additional information from the referring provider and ask other specialty consultants to participate as needed. These consults may reinforce current diagnosis and treatment; suggest other possible diagnoses, additional testing, procedures, or treatments within the context of the local resources available; or, if feasible, suggest transfer of the patient to a higher-level facility for further evaluation, management, or procedures such as surgery that cannot be done locally. Swinfen Charitable Trust has 335 hospital links in 76 countries involving nearly 600 referring providers and over 700 consultants in over 120 specialties. They have examined nearly 5,000 cases since 1998 and use four medically trained system operators: three in the UK (two voluntary) and one in New Zealand.

The following is a compelling case example managed through the Swinfen Charitable Trust and one of their certified pediatric specialists that led to a positive outcome without which this child would likely not have received the care that was needed. A 4-month-old infant was referred to the Swinfen Charitable Trust by a team staffing an orphanage for children with medical needs for evaluation of growth failure and cyanosis. Her birth weight was 2.0 kg, and at 4 months she weighed 3.7 kg. Her vital signs were pulse (P) 150, respiratory rate (RR) 40, and oxygen saturation 80% in room air. Cardiac examination showed a grade III/VI continuous murmur at the upper-right sternal border. Peripheral pulses were normal. Chest X-ray showed levocardia, cardiomegaly, decreased pulmonary vascularity, and a right-sided stomach bubble. A limited echocardiogram showed a complete atrioventricular (AV) canal defect. After discussion with colleagues at a children's hospital more than 750 miles away, at 6 months of age, she was transferred and found to have asplenia syndrome, pulmonary atresia, imbalanced complete AV canal, double outlet right ventricle, right-sided patent ductus arteriosus, aorticopulmonary collaterals, and a diaphragmatic hernia. The infant was begun on amoxicillin prophylaxis. She underwent repair of the hernia, followed by a bidirectional Glenn procedure. Postoperatively, she did very well and returned to her orphanage receiving antibiotics, baby aspirin, and diuretics. She was adopted soon thereafter, and has since undergone a Fontan procedure with an excellent hemodynamic result. She is developmentally normal at age 4.

Medecins Sans Frontieres

Medecins Sans Frontieres (MSF), Doctors Without Borders, has been providing humanitarian health care in many developing countries, particularly after natural disasters or during wars and conflicts resulting in manmade disasters. Recently they have developed a web-based platform, similar to the Swinfen Charitable Trust, for asynchronous consults for providers in those countries being served and provided by a panel of specialty volunteers.

ECHO

The ECHO (Extension for Community Health Outcomes) Project founded by Dr. Sanjeev Arora at the University of New Mexico in 2003 (http://echo.unm.edu/about-echo/) uses telehealth ICT to provide primary care providers with education and case reviews of patients with common complex diseases that started with the need for care of patients with hepatitis C.[10,11] Demonstrating success, ECHO has rapidly expanded to other diseases and health issues.[12–29] This model is being replicated throughout the United States and other regions, such as Canada, India, Vietnam, Ireland, Mexico, South American countries, parts of the Caribbean, Australia, Egypt, and countries in Africa, with the hope of touching 1 billion lives worldwide by 2025.[30,31] As stated on their web page, "The ECHO model™ does not actually 'provide' care to patients. Instead, it dramatically increases access to specialty treatment in rural and underserved areas by providing front-line clinicians with the knowledge and support they need to manage patients with complex conditions." These ECHO sessions often include multiple providers at different locations and create "learning loops" for group education and knowledge sharing through case discussions and reviews. See also https://www.statnews.com/2016/09/12/doctors-primary-care-specialists-project-echo/ and https://www.stepsforward.org/modules/project-echo.

Shriners

Shriners provides free orthopedics, cleft lip palate repair, burn care and reconstruction, orthotics, prosthetics, plastic surgery, and spinal cord surgery for children (http://www.shrinershospitalsforchildren.org/). They are committed to providing the best care for children in their specialty areas regardless of a family's ability to pay. Telemedicine provides screening and follow-up care for children being served from around the world at Shriners facilities (http://www.shrinershospitalsforchildren.org/search?q=telemedicine). For example, the telemedicine burn clinic at Shriners Hospital for Children – Mexico City is now in operation to provide follow-up care for the burn patients that were treated at Shriners Hospitals for Children in Galveston. The goal of the telemedicine clinic is to follow up with these patients by optimizing resources and avoiding the stress of travel for patients and relatives. The Shriners' coordinators have noted in orthopedics, telemedicine is used routinely. For many patients, being able to connect with telemedicine services has actually made their treatment possible. For example, a growing child with an orthopedic problem is often at risk for recurrent deformity. As a bone grows, it may not grow correctly, even after surgery to correct the alignment. Health care providers often need to follow their patients closely until they are done growing to treat any recurrent deformity before it becomes more severe.

Other Academic Programs

Children's Hospital Colorado's telehealth program supports the University of Colorado (CU) Center for Global Health, with their primary telehealth usage occurring at a clinic in Guatemala.[32] They support a weekly tele-education conference between experts at CU and the community health nurses in Guatemala, and the topics are designed to increase the nurses' capacity to provide evidence-based care in their community. One of the most successful projects has been breastfeeding education with the nurses now feeling more confident in their abilities to support breastfeeding moms locally. They also have residents rotating at this site who present cases on a monthly basis during morning report or noon conference in Denver via videoconferencing. This helps them stay connected to their home program while working internationally and brings global health education to the other residents who don't go to the Guatemala clinic. They've also been trialing a Helping Babies Breathe (HBB) course taught via telehealth at this clinic. It is still a pilot project, but preliminary data suggest that passing rates and knowledge/skills teaching are quite good. The model uses a lead instructor in Denver who teaches the didactic sessions, monitors skills practice, and tests the students via teleconferencing, and local staff and residents rotate in Guatemala and help with the course execution. They've taught two telehealth courses with plans to retest the students later this year to assess skill retention.

Telehealth is also being used to facilitate global health research at the University of Colorado. Thus telehealth can be used to facilitate large-scale global research projects that otherwise tend to be expensive and difficult from a logistic perspective. For example, discussions with the American Academy of Pediatrics (AAP) have the goal of generalizing the HBB teaching model to other locations once it's established enough to move beyond the pilot stage. In addition, one of their global health researchers is exploring use of the telehealth system to facilitate his projects with less travel time and costs. One of these projects would be assessing efficacy of the pneumococcal vaccine in the Philippines, and the telehealth component would capture tympanic membrane exams with digital otoscopes/tympanograms using local research assistants; then pediatric ear/nose/throat (ENT) specialists would interpret the results in the United States. They use their system to do mortality case review for a hospital in India.

The Children's National Health System at George Washington University School of Medicine and Craig Sable, MD, Director, Echocardiography and Telemedicine, have been providing pediatric cardiology telehealth services to countries, such as Morocco, United Arab Emirates (UAE), Uganda, and Brazil.[33,34] These have included evaluation of patients with rheumatic heart disease, and as the participants have noted: "The global burden of rheumatic heart disease is nearly 33 million people. Telemedicine, using cloud-server technology, provides an ideal solution for sharing images performed by non-physicians with cardiologists who are experts in rheumatic heart disease." The program coordinators have described their experience in using telemedicine to support a large rheumatic heart disease outreach screening program in the Brazilian state of Minas Gerais. The program uses cloud-based sharing of echocardiographic images with expert support between the sites in Brazil with Washington, DC. Secondary goals included (a) developing and sharing online training modules for nonphysicians in echocardiography performance and interpretation and (b) utilizing a secure web-based system to share clinical and research data. Their efforts included 4,615 studies that were performed by nonexperts at 21 schools and shared via cloud technology. Latent rheumatic heart disease was found in 251 subjects (4.2% of subjects: 3.7% borderline and 0.5% definite disease). Of the studies, 50% were performed on fully functional echocardiograph machines and transmitted via Digital Imaging and Communications in Medicine (DICOM) and 50% were performed on handheld echocardiograph machines and transferred via a secure Dropbox connection. The average time between study performance date and interpretation was 10 days. There was 100% success in initial image transfer. Less than 1% of studies performed by nonexperts could not be interpreted. As the project coordinators stated: "A sustainable, low-cost telehealth model, using task-shifting with non-medical personnel in low and middle income countries can improve access to echocardiography for rheumatic heart disease."

Another project from the Children's National Medical Center has used telemedicine for neurologic disorders.[35] The authors state: "A telemedicine program was developed between the Children's National Medical Center (CNMC) in Washington, DC, and the Sheikh Khalifa Bin Zayed Foundation in the United Arab Emirates (UAE)." A needs assessment and a curriculum of onsite training conferences were devised preparatory to an ongoing telemedicine consultation program for children with neurodevelopmental disabilities in the underserved eastern region of the UAE. Weekly telemedicine consultations are provided by a multidisciplinary faculty. Patients were presented in the UAE with their therapists and families. Real-time (video over Internet Protocol; average connection, 768 kilobits/s) telemedicine conferences were held weekly following previews of medical records. A full consultation report followed each telemedicine session. They report that between February 29, 2012, and June 26, 2013, 48 weekly one-hour live interactive telemedicine consultations were conducted on 48 patients (28 males, 20 females; age range, 8 months to 22 years; median age, 5.4 years). The primary diagnoses were cerebral palsy, neurogenetic disorders, autism, neuromuscular disorders, congenital anomalies, global developmental delay, systemic disease, and epilepsy. Common comorbidities were cognitive impairment, communication disorders, and behavioral disorders. Specific recommendations included imaging and DNA studies; antiseizure management; spasticity management (including botulinum toxin protocols); and specific therapy modalities including taping techniques, customized body vests, and speech/language and behavioral therapy. Improved outcomes were reported in terms of clinician satisfaction, achievement of therapy goals for patients, and requests for ongoing sessions. The project coordinators concluded that weekly telemedicine sessions coupled with triannual training conferences were successfully implemented in a clinical program dedicated to patients with neurodevelopmental disabilities by the Center for Neuroscience at CNMC and the UAE government. International consultations in neurodevelopmental disabilities utilizing telemedicine services offer a reliable and productive method for joint clinical programs.

The Harvard Global Mental Health Program and Program in Refugee Trauma and their director of telemedicine, Eugene F. Augusterfer, and colleagues have been using telemedicine to provide support to victims of disaster in Haiti and refugees in Syria in collaboration with Yale University School of Medicine.[36,37] As the author states: "Telemental health (TMH) is an important component in meeting critical mental health needs of the global population. Mental health is an issue of global importance; an estimated 450 million people worldwide have mental or behavioural disorders, accounting for 12% of the World Health Organization's (WHO) global burden of disease. However, it is reported that 75% of people suffering from mental disorders in the Developing World receive no treatment or care. In this paper, the authors review global mental health needs with a focus on the use of TMH to meet mental health needs in international and post-disaster settings. Telemedicine and TMH have the capacity to bring evidence-based best practices in medicine and mental health to the under-served and difficult to reach areas of the world, including post-disaster settings." The authors reported on the mental health impact of the Haiti 2010 earthquake and on the limited use of telemedicine in postdisaster Haiti. They underscore the point that published papers on the use of TMH in postdisaster settings are lacking and reviewed considerations before working in TMH in international and postdisaster settings. As they also note, given the scarcity of mental health resources available for refugees in areas of conflict, it is imperative to investigate interventions that would be accepted by the refugees. In this study they surveyed 354 Syrian refugees using the HADStress screening tool and asked about their openness to referral to psychiatry and telepsychiatry. Of the surveyed sample, 41.8% had scores on HADStress that correlate to posttraumatic stress disorder. However, only 34% of the entire sample reported a perceived need to see a psychiatrist, and of those only 45% were open to telepsychiatry.

NIH-Fogarty

The NIH Fogarty program includes the Global Health Research and Research Training eCapacity Initiative (R25) with the purpose to develop innovative educational approaches that enhance research capacity at LMIC institutions by expanding the use of ICT in global health research and research training (https://www.fic.nih.gov/Programs/Pages/ecapacity.aspx). In addition, participants in the programs should develop into adaptable users of ICT who are able to sustain such activities as changes arise in technology. This program aims to leverage the research capacity established by current or former Fogarty International Center research and training grants through direct links with these awards (https://www.fic.nih.gov/Pages/Default.aspx).

Telehealth Associations

The American Telemedicine Association (ATA) (http://www.americantelemed.org/home) has several members involved in international telemedicine activities, including the International Special Interest Group (SIG) and the ATA Latin American and Caribbean Chapter (ATALACC) and the Pacific Islands Chapter of ATA (PICATA). ATA has developed memoranda of agreement with many partner countries and their telemedicine initiatives and/or associations, including Armenia, Australia, Canada, China, Nepal, Netherlands, India, France, Iran, Korea, Pakistan, and the United Kingdom. This is enabling the exchange of ideas, experience, and expertise related to telehealth in the global community. For example, a two-day symposium on electronic hospitals and telemedicine held at the Tehran University of Medical Sciences (TUMS) occurred on October 12, 2010. The symposium was attended by academics from Iran and some guests from the United States. The event brought about a memorandum of understanding (MOU) which was signed between the university and the ATA. This MOU will serve to establish cooperation between the two institutions and will include educational, research, and scholarly activities along with operational plans in telemedicine, as well as holding joint symposia. Both the TUMS chancellor and the president of the association hope this agreement will help improve the health system and act as a starting point for sharing information and experience in this field.

The International Society for Telemedicine and eHealth (ISfTEH) also has several international partners represented in 93 countries and territories, and their mission is to facilitate the international dissemination of knowledge and experience in telemedicine and e-health, providing access to recognized experts in the field worldwide (https://www.isfteh.org/).

Company Donation Collaborative Programs

Other initiatives have worked with companies to foster telehealth programs in other countries, such as in Guatemala, Guam, Mexico, Philippines, Pakistan, Bhutan, and Jordan.

Telemedicine has the potential to bring medical expertise to patients located anywhere in the world.

Unfortunately, history suggests that telemedicine systems are often abandoned after the completion of a demonstration or pilot project and are never fully adopted for long-term use—often because standard procedures and workflows within the health care organization are never examined and modified to support the routine use of telemedicine. A telemedicine implementation in Jordan was supported by Cisco Systems.[38] The principal participant developers addressed the organizational adoption of telemedicine technologies based on an example case study drawn from an implementation in two hospitals in Jordan. Three types of specialty consults were offered: dermatology, cardiology, and nephrology based upon high-priority needs identified by health care individuals in Jordan. The Cisco systems equipment could support delivery of images and data needed by these specialists, including high-resolution skin images and heart and lung sounds. Each participating specialist was able to provide one hour per week of teleconsultations. There were two participating cardiologists, two nephrologists, and one dermatologist, for a total of five hours of consultations per week. A fixed schedule was created, with each consultation hour for a specialist occurring at the same time each week. They identified the organizational challenges and the potential benefits. Cisco Systems and the project coordinators state that they hope their efforts will encourage anyone who develops or donates telemedicine systems to consider not only how challenging organizational barriers to use can be, but also how easily they can be overcome.

AMD Global Medicine has provided humanitarian support in Guatemala, where 40% of the Guatemalan population faces a future without adequate health care.[39] For many indigenous families, Mayan Families is their only access point for affordable and quality health care. The Charlie Gomez Medical Clinic provides preventive and primary health care, education, and follow-up to the families they work with. The telemedicine equipment allows them to deliver these services to patients in their local communities with specialists from various partner organizations in the region, including WINGS Guatemala, Opal House Guatemala, and Wuqu' Kawoq – Maya Health Alliance.

Another recently launched AMD-supported telemedicine program works with the underserved patient population on the island of Guam, with cost-effective,

real-time access to secure medical consultation services from specialists an ocean away.[40] The Department of Public Health and Social Services and Good Samaritan Hospital have partnered to connect patients in Guam with medical staff in Los Angeles. There is also collaboration between Hospital Infantil De Las Californias and Tiopa Santuario de Luz and a community health clinic in the village of Autlan de Navarro. The Hospital Infantil De Las Californias is the only pediatric specialty hospital in the Tijuana region of Mexico, with 25 specialties in a 56,000-square-foot facility. Sixty percent of the staff serve in a volunteer capacity. No child is ever turned away because of the family's inability to pay. The Tiopa Santuario de Luz was created by music legend Carlos Santana and Dr. Martin Sandoval. Since 2005 Santana and his family's Milagro Foundation have provided the operating funds. The Santana Telehealth Project was formed to connect Hospital Infantil De Las Californias and Tiopa Santuario de Luz. The project will include primary care and specialist referrals over live video, as well as remote patient monitoring. Once established, the program will be a telehealth model that can be used for expansion into other underserved communities.

Disaster logistics relief focused on bringing humanitarian health care to patients in the Philippines after the destruction of Typhoon Haiyan. Telemedicine was used to perform onsite examinations of patients while communicating live back to physicians and specialists in the United States for consult.

The Paul Chester Children's Hope Foundation provides vital assistance to improve the lives and well-being of families in developing countries such as in rural Kenya. Their medical outreach programs bring critical health resources and treatments to remote communities, harnessing the expertise of their volunteer medical professionals. In order to treat patients, they leveraged telemedicine technology to set up video consults with U.S. doctors from the middle of Narok or from the coast of Malindi.

Medical Mission for Children uses telemedicine to help critically ill children all over the world. Medical Mission for Children's Telemedicine Outreach Program (TOP) is a cost-efficient way for health care professionals to consult on unique cases where one doctor may have more specialized training and can discuss a case more thoroughly than a general practitioner. The telemedicine equipment takes a medical consultation from speculation to diagnosis and treatment. Remote diagnostic instruments such as a telephonic stethoscope allow a doctor in the United States to accurately assess the auscultation of a child's heart even though they are thousands of miles apart.

Comsats is a telecommunications provider in Pakistan that offers health care services to rural citizens via telemedicine in the areas of Gokina, Mehra Behri, Dagai, Swabi, Quetta, Maraka, Muzaffarabad, Chak Faiz, Sangu, Shadoband in Gwadar, and Ubhri. They have set up 14 rural clinics in these small towns, providing 100% free service to patients. To date, they have completed 40,000 telemedicine consults. This telehealth initiative was necessary to help people save the cost of transportation and paid visits to the doctors.

Bhutan Ministry of Health brings health care access to communities more than 14 hours away from major medical facilities. For example, the ministry set up a telemedicine clinic in a remote mountainous community to connect the members with health care services provided by the Royal University of Bhutan.

OTHER INDIVIDUAL AND PRIVATE ASSOCIATIONS/TEAM EFFORTS

Health Information Associates International (http://www.healthinformationinternational.com/) has assisted in the development of telemedicine networks in Ecuador in collaboration with the University of New Mexico (UNM) and Universidad Tecnologica Equinoccial in Quito.[41,42] This has also entailed working on the development of telemedicine in Nepal, Nigeria, and other countries to effectively integrate telehealth.

Boats in the Amazonian region are currently being configured as mobile floating clinics on the Rio Aquarico, Rio Napo, and Rio Morona, which are major tributaries in Ecuador connecting to the Amazon. These boats could have telehealth links connected to medical experts in Ecuador, or anywhere in the world, through wireless telecommunication connections, providing exciting opportunities for cultural exchange and knowledge sharing, as well as opportunities for international faculty and student interaction in a variety of disciplines (see Figures 20-1 and 20-2). Formal agreements for these projects have been established between Universidad Tecnologica Equinoccial (UTE)

in Quito and other universities, Ministry of Public Health Ecuador, University of New Mexico School of Medicine, and the Iberoamerican Science, Technology, and Education Consortium (ISTEC). The Ecuadorian Air Force has donated broadband satellite connectivity throughout the country, as well as links to international networks. Some connections are also being provided through other commercial telecommunication networks. This telehealth network is already establishing links between universities in Ecuador and remote communities in the Ecuadorian jungle, the Andes, and the Galapagos. Several Latin American countries are expressing an interest in participating in these telehealth projects or have developed telehealth programs, including Mexico, Venezuela, Colombia, Peru, Bolivia, Argentina, and Brazil. These efforts will be coordinated in collaboration with the ATALACC. As health problems become more global, telehealth can assist in forming bridges between all countries to address critical health issues in even the most remote areas. Medical students from UNM have been traveling to Ecuador to conduct preliminary surveys regarding the health knowledge, attitudes, beliefs, and behaviors of the local people and providers in-country, including a recent survey related to Chagas disease. The remote sites can serve as "base camps" for ongoing field research, such as further investigation related to tropical diseases such as malaria, dengue fever, leishmaniasis, and others. Using Ecuador as an international model, telehealth technologies create a means of maintaining virtual continuity in addressing global health issues, education, and research. These types of international exchange experiences offer significant opportunities for understanding the common denominators, as well as unique differences, related to global health among countries and cultures around the world. These programs can promote international understanding and mutual respect in a manner that can improve the entire global community.

In Nepal, such efforts are aimed at creating a partnership between counterparts in medical schools and other universities and U.S. telehealth centers to enhance the understanding of telehealth technology, management, and general implementation and apply it to the target cluster of villages and then replicate this experience in other parts of the country. Some wireless microwave networks have been developed in Nepal by individuals such as Mahabir Pun (see Figures 20-3 and 20-4) to

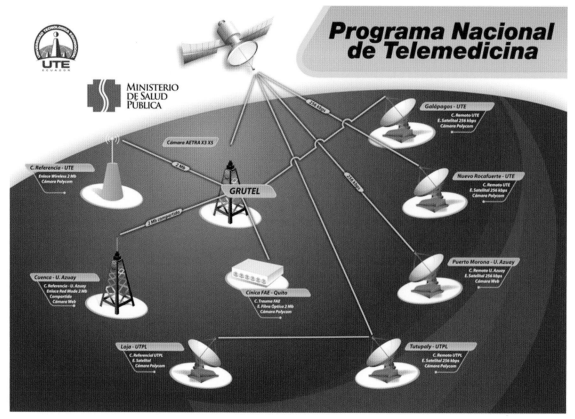

▲ **Figure 20-1.** Telehealth network in Ecuador; demonstrating existing and proposed sites.

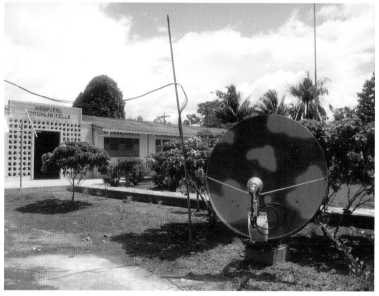

▲ **Figure 20-2.** Satelite dish outside hospital in the jungle of Ecuador to support telehealth.

Mustang Network

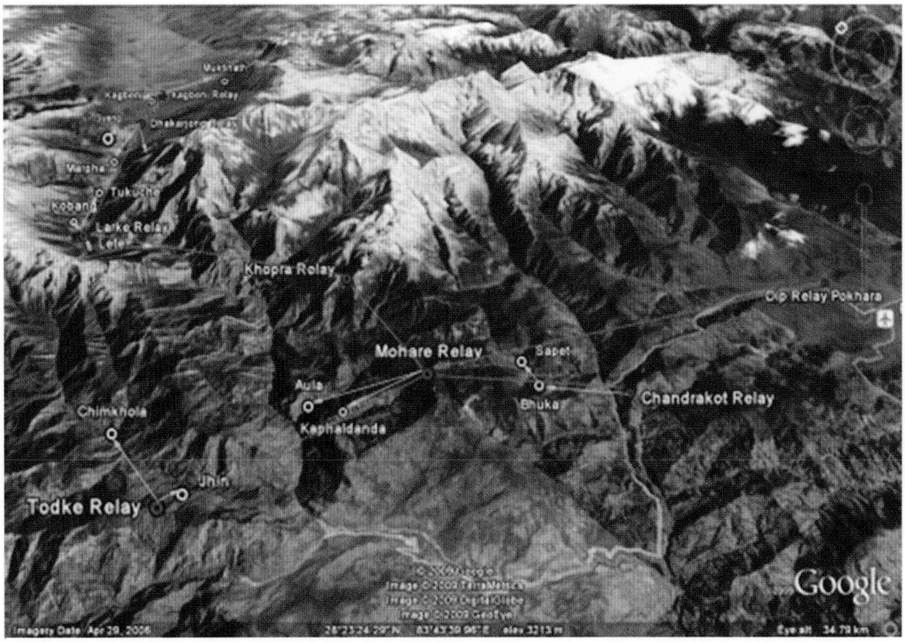

![Example of one of the wireless microwave networks in Nepal]

▲ **Figure 20-3.** Example of one of the wireless microwave networks in Nepal. (Courtesy of Mahabir Pun.)

create connections to other urban centers and hospitals that connect through the mountain passes to remote villages, and even to the base camp at Mt. Everest (Figure 20-5). These efforts are also supported by the America Nepal Medical Association (http://www.anmf.org/), many other health care provider systems, health care professionals, and telecommunication initiatives in Nepal.

In addition, partnership can be created with academic institutions (eg, graduate programs in policy research, development, and the environment) in Nepal to help develop and implement school curriculum to collect and analyze environmental data (forest, vegetation, river, stream, pollution, hydrology, insects) and share it internationally with similar programs in places like Albuquerque, New Mexico, and Ecuador. Also, these efforts will help in publishing and disseminating reports and data through electronic portals (journals and newsletters). In addition these initiatives promote telemicrofinancing in and around the cluster of villages to fund small businesses and encourage investments, whenever possible, in skills training and products that are pro-health and environmentally friendly (eg, green investment). For

Putting a Grid Antenna

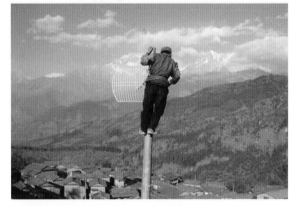

▲ **Figure 20-4.** Example of placing a microwave antenna to provide line-of-site connections through the mountain passes. (Courtesy of Mahabir Pun.)

further information on the Nepal Study Center please go to http://nepalstudycenter.unm.edu/.

There have been efforts to connect to the Global Medical Network in Kyiv, Ukraine, with support from Children of Chernobyl Relief and Development

Chhukung Relay at 5,100 m

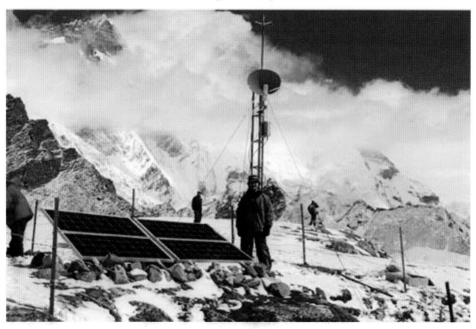

▲ **Figure 20-5.** Wireless network connection at base camp at Mt. Everest. (Courtesy of Mahabir Pun.)

Fund and the Ukrainian Children's Cardiac Centre. Objectives include the following: 1) Through the use of real-time video consultation, create a forum for doctors in Ukraine to recognize and understand the maximum potential of telemedicine within their respective fields of medicine; 2) Provide a comprehensive understanding of what telemedicine is, how to use it, and what is the extent of the potential for doctors and patients; 3) Through the use of various examples, explain how telemedicine is coordinated and managed in the international medical community, with the potential to adopt these protocols in Ukraine; and 4) Construct an opportunity for networking between international lecturers and doctors in Ukraine, as well as among the domestic medical community.

Several telehealth initiatives are taking place in Africa, including Nigeria, Ghana, Zambia, Kenya, Uganda, South Africa, and others.[14] There has been a greater level of interest in using telehealth for education and knowledge sharing as opposed to using telemedicine clinical services which is consistent with early telehealth experiences in the developing world.[43] This is due in part due to a significant health care workforce shortage and the need for more education and training. Africa has 24% of the world's disease burden, but only 3% of the health care workers and less than 1% of world health expenditure.[44] If telehealth is implemented effectively and appropriately in these developing countries, it can play an important role in addressing these critical health care issues in Africa.[45–47]

The AFHCAN Program (Alaska Federal Health Care Access Network) at the Alaska Native Tribal Health Consortium in Anchorage, Alaska, began its international efforts in 2003. The initial efforts were funded and supported through the Northern Forum, a nonprofit international organization composed of subnational or regional governments from eight northern (Arctic) countries. AFHCAN was initially involved in a number of Arctic nations meetings focused on telehealth planning and technical assistance, particularly in two regions of Russia (Yakutsk and Khanty-Mansiysk). These efforts included AFHCAN hosting an International

Telehealth Conference in Anchorage at which special sessions focused on the needs and options to expand telehealth in rural Arctic areas. Due to the high interest in AFHCAN's technologies, the program developed a multilingual version of the software that provides a "store-and-forward" platform. The software is now available in English, Spanish, Danish, and Greenlandic. The latter languages were part of a sales effort through AFHCAN's distributor to provide telemedicine carts and software throughout Greenland. AFHCAN software has also been installed and used in a wide variety of countries, including Australia, Bhutan, Bolivia, Brazil, Canada, China, Ethiopia, Greece, Iceland, Maldives, Mexico, Panama, Russia, Spain, United Kingdom, and Vietnam. AFHCAN leadership continues to collaborate with other countries on design, development, and training on telehealth technologies. This includes many years of teaching in an annual program hosted by the United States Telecommunications Training Institute (USTTI), which brings students from foreign countries to the United States for training in telehealth. AFHCAN has also been a leader in developing and reviewing telehealth technologies and has been consulted by experts from China, Canada, Finland, and other countries.

Another organization providing international telemedicine support is called SALUS Telehealth (http://salustelehealth.com/). It was founded by Ms. Paula Guy, who has several years of leadership experience in building telemedicine networks in the state of Georgia. She has served as CEO for SALUS Telehealth. Under her direction and in collaboration with several partners, Georgia, Alabama, and Global Partnership for TeleHealth have become a robust, comprehensive telehealth network. There are several examples of their international telemedicine initiatives.

In Guatemala, while serving as CEO for Georgia Partnership for Telehealth (GPT), Ms. Guy worked with the Louisiana State University Health Science Center (LSU) and Casa Para Ninos Aleluya (CASA) to launch its first international telemedicine program. The new partnership was formed through an ongoing relationship with Guy and the former Louisiana senator and family medicine practitioner, Dr. Donald Hines. The mission of the collaboration was to deliver much needed primary and specialized medical care to the children of the CASA orphanage through the use of telemedicine technology. The orphanage is home to over 400 abused, orphaned, and mistreated children and is located just outside of Guatemala City. Started in 1988 by missionaries Mike and Dottie Clark, CASA's vision is for the kids they serve to have a chance in life by bringing pediatric specialty care to the clinic in order to change the futures of these children. The medical needs of hundreds of the children at CASA are met daily through a few nurses that manage a clinic onsite. The new technology will greatly aid caregivers' capabilities in providing quality medical care to the children. The new technology has become a magnet for other missions who are struggling to serve the estimated 200,000 orphaned children across Guatemala. The clinic was up and online within 24 hours, and the nursing staff at CASA was trained and certified as telemedicine presenters and supported by GPT as they continue to serve Cuidad de Los Ninos. AcuteCare Telemedicine (ACT) recently donated their time and expertise to make telemedicine a reality at CASA. Dr. James M. Kiely, a partner in Atlanta Neurology, P.C., ACT, and medical director of the Neurophysiology Departments at Northside Hospital and St. Joseph's Hospital of Atlanta, recently demonstrated the benefits of telemedicine capabilities at the orphanage. As a specific case example, Dr. Kiely remotely treated a 19-year old CASA patient with a history of intractable epilepsy. The young patient was on numerous medications but continued to experience recurring seizures. By using a high definition audiovisual connection provided by GPT, Dr. Kiely was able to interview the patient's parents and examine the patient remotely. The imaging results, hemiparesis, and description of seizures allowed him to determine that the likely type and cause was attributed to porencephaly, the failure of one hemisphere of the brain to develop. Kiely was able to recommend appropriate medications to onsite doctors and to suggest additional steps to take if the patient's epilepsy remained intractable. The process worked extremely well and marked the beginning of a new relationship between the missions and medical providers across the region.

In Zambia, the American International Health Alliance (AIHA), Zambian Department Force, and Salus Telehealth have worked together to develop and implement a telemedicine program for the Zambian military and Zambian citizens located in neighboring villages.

Salus has worked with AIHA to build a telemedicine program that includes establishing telemedicine presentation sites at five military bases. These rural bases connect to Maina Soko Military Hospital located in the capitol of Lusaka. The telemedicine program has been designed to afford the smaller, more rural hospitals access to specialty physician care. The military bases utilize telemedicine to present Zambian citizens in bordering villages to medical professionals throughout the country. Their team has met with the U.S. Embassy to work on expanding the telemedicine footprint to all Zambian citizens. Salus plans to continue cultivating a relationship with key business leaders, Zambian government officials, and the U.S. Embassy to bring quality health care throughout the country.

In Honduras, Ms. Guy and her team worked with the Jackson Healthcare Foundation to implement telemedicine at three Predisan Good Samaritan Clinics in Honduras. The goal is to determine the efficacy of this system in a remote, international setting. The primary interest is in its clinical applications, but also testing the technology as it applies to biomedical equipment maintenance and repair. Dr. Roger Madrid, family practice physician; Dr. Pedro Meza, OB/GYN; and Dr. Amanda Madrid were trained on the telemedicine technology, including the peripherals, software, and portable ultrasound system. Visits were made to very remote clinics, including Culmi-Cesamo Clinic, Culmi-El Cerro Clinic, Las Cabas Clinic, and Agua Caliente. Dr. Meza performed an ultrasound with the portable system and transmitted it back to the main clinic and was amazed at the quality. Doctors at Predisan now have the capability of seeing patients in the most remote areas using the telemedicine equipment. They also have instant access to physicians in the United States for consultations. Since the installations have been completed, over 30 consultations have been successfully conducted. Dr. Amanda Madrid, a native of Honduras, came to Predisan in 1987, one year after the ministry began. She is the mission's founding medical director and the founder of CEREPA addiction treatment center. In Macedonia, a telemedicine system was installed at University Children's Hospital in Skopje and Northside Hospital in Georgia to allow colleagues in neonatal intensive care units (NICUs) at both institutions to collaborate remotely. This technology will allow physicians on an ongoing basis to present cases, share best practices, and sustain professional relationships—all in an effort to improve patient outcomes and advance the standard of care.

This effort appears to be the first application of telemedicine to connect a Macedonian hospital to another hospital abroad. This project was possible because of the collaboration with a neonatologist from Northside, Dr. Larry Wallin, and Ms. Guy and the Telemedicine International Partnership, which is providing the technology and service. Dr. Wallin was joined by telemedicine expert Matt Jansen and health technology expert Tom Judd to assess the NICUs in Skopje and to install the telemedicine system at University Children's Hospital. Physicians from both institutions have connected several times to discuss the care of their NICU patients, which brings better health outcomes to babies. This project is part of LinkAcross' broader effort to address the issue of infant mortality in Macedonia, which is 2.5 times higher than the European Union (EU) average.

The Syrian American Medical Society (SAMS) is a nonprofit, nonpolitical, medical, and humanitarian relief organization that represents thousands of Syrian American health care professionals in the United States. SAMS has been on the frontlines of crisis relief in Syria and neighboring countries to alleviate suffering and save lives. SAMS operates 106 medical facilities throughout Syria that provide general and specialized medical care for Syrians in need. Programs range from primary care to more specialized treatment in order to provide effective and needs-based health care. SAMS is already using telemedicine inside of Syria and in refugee settlements in Turkey and supports hundreds of thousands of Syrian refugees in Jordan, Lebanon, Greece, and Turkey. SAMS provides refugees with medical and dental care, winterization support, and psychosocial programs. It operates the largest medical facility in Za'atari Camp in Jordan, and SAMS's members lead frequent medical missions to volunteer their skills for the care of refugees.

CONCLUSION

The evolution of ICT in terms of telehealth now offers increasing opportunities to bring critical health care services to people around the world in a manner that can improve the health and quality of life in the global community. These humanitarian telehealth initiatives can promote human welfare and assist in alleviating widespread human suffering where it may be most needed in a timely manner. Challenges remain regarding development of plans for ongoing sustainability, finding adequate resources, and demonstrating the positive impact on health outcomes and an ROI. Opportunities to use telehealth meaningfully will continue to increase and allow many stakeholders to play a role in these efforts and complement the global health efforts around the world. These important telehealth humanitarian efforts can address global health, share knowledge, enhance mutual understanding between countries and cultures, and enhance collaboration around the world.[48]

REFERENCES

1. Wootton R, Patil NG, Scott RE, Ho K, eds. *Telehealth in the Developing World*. London: Royal Society of Medicine Press and Ottawa: International Development Research Center; 2009.

2. Mills A. Health care systems in low- and middle-income countries. *N Engl J Med* 2014;370(6):552–557.

3. World Health Organization. *Health-for-all Policy for the Twenty First Century (Document EB101/INF. DOC./9)*. Geneva: WHO; 1998.

4. World Health Organization. *WHA58.28 e-Health*. Geneva: WHO; 2005.

5. World Health Organization. *Strategy 2004-2007. E-health for Health Care Delivery*. Geneva: WHO; 2004.

6. United Nations. Millennium Development Goals. Available at www.un.org/millenniumgoals/.

7. Wootton R, Craig J, Patterson V, eds. *Introduction to Telemedicine*. 2nd ed. London: Royal Society of Medicine Press, Ltd.; 2006.

8. Pushkin D, Johnston B, Speedie S. American Telemedicine Association White Paper: Telemedicine, Telehealth, and Health Information Technology. http://www.americantelemed.org/files/public/policy/HIT_Paper.pdf. Verified September 18, 2009.

9. Alverson DC, Mars M, Rheuban K, et al. International pediatric telemedicine and eHealth: transforming systems of care for children in the global community. *Pediatr Ann* 2009;38(10):579–585.

10. Arora S, Kalishman S, Thornton K, et al. Expanding access to hepatitis C virus treatment—Extension for Community Healthcare Outcomes (ECHO) project: disruptive innovation in specialty care. *Hepatology* 2010;52(3):1124–1133.

11. Arora S, Thornton K, Murata G, et al. Outcomes of treatment for hepatitis C virus infection by primary care providers. *N Engl J Med* 2011;364(23):2199–2207.

12. Arora S, Geppert CM, Kalishman S, et al. Academic health center management of chronic diseases through knowledge networks: Project ECHO. *Acad Med* 2007;82(2):154–160.

13. Arora S, Thornton K, Jenkusky SM, et al. Project ECHO: linking university specialists with rural and prison-based clinicians to improve care for people with chronic hepatitis C in New Mexico. *Public Health Rep* 2007;122(suppl 2): 74–77.

14. Arora S, Kalishman S, Dion D, et al. Partnering urban academic medical centers and rural primary care clinicians to provide complex chronic disease care. *Health Aff (Millwood)* 2011;30(6):1176–1184.

15. Arora S, Kalishman S, Dion D, et al. Knowledge networks for treating complex diseases in remote, rural, and underserved communities. In: McKee A, Eraut M, eds. *Learning Trajectories, Innovation and Identity for Professional Development*. The Netherlands: Springer; 2012:47–70.

16. Arora S, Boyle J, Comerci G, Katzman J, Olivas C. Project ECHO: the force multiplier for pain education and management. *Painview* 2013;9(4):4–7.

17. Arora S, Thornton K, Komaromy M, et al. Demonopolizing medical knowledge. *Acad Med* 2014;89(1):30–32.

18. Carey EP, Frank JW, Kirsh SR. Implementation of telementoring for pain management in Veterans Health Administration: spatial analysis. *J Rehabil Res Dev* 2016;53(1):147.

19. Catic AG, Mattison ML, Bakaev I, et al. ECHO-AGE: an innovative model of geriatric care for long-term care residents with dementia and behavioral issues. *J Am Med Dir Assoc* 2014;15(12):938–942.

20. Chand P, Murthy P, Gupta V, et al. Technology Enhanced Learning in Addiction Mental Health: Developing a Virtual Knowledge Network: NIMHANS ECHO. In *Technology for Education (T4E), 2014 IEEE Sixth International Conference on Technology* (pp. 229–232). IEEE; December 2014.

21. Colleran K, Harding E, Kipp BJ, et al. Building capacity to reduce disparities in diabetes training community health workers using an integrated distance learning model. *Diabetes Educ* 2012;38(3):386–396.

22. Zigmond J. Teaching by telementoring. Project ECHO advancing physicians' skill sets. *Mod Healthc* 2013;43(37):28–29.

23. Salgia RJ, Mullan PB, McCurdy H, et al. The educational impact of the specialty care access network–extension of community healthcare outcomes program. *Telemed J E Health* 2014;20(11):1004–1008.

24. Scott JD, Unruh KT, Catlin MC, et al. Project ECHO: a model for complex, chronic care in the Pacific

Northwest region of the United States. *J Telemed Telecare* 2012;18(8):481–484.

25. Katzman JG, Comerci G Jr, Boyle JF, et al. Innovative telementoring for pain management: project ECHO pain. *J Cont Educ Health Prof* 2014;34(1):68–75.

26. Gordon SE, Dufour AB, Monti SM, et al. Impact of a videoconference educational intervention on physical restraint and antipsychotic use in nursing homes: results from the ECHO-AGE Pilot Study. *J Am Med Dir Assoc* 2016;17(6):553–556.

27. Komaromy M, Duhigg D, Metcalf A, et al. Project ECHO (Extension for Community Healthcare Outcomes): a new model for educating primary care providers about treatment of substance use disorders. *Subst Abus* 2016;37(1):20–24.

28. Lewiecki EM, Baron R, Bilezikian JP, et al. Proceedings of the 2015 Santa Fe Bone Symposium: clinical applications of scientific advances in osteoporosis and metabolic bone disease. *J Clin Densitom* 2016;19(1):102–116.

29. Socolovsky C, Masi C, Hamlish T, et al. Evaluating the role of key learning theories in ECHO: a telehealth educational program for primary care providers. *Prog Community Health Partnersh* 2013;7(4):361–368.

30. Dubin RE, Flannery J, Taenzer P, et al. ECHO ontario chronic pain & opioid stewardship: providing access and building capacity for primary care providers in underserviced, rural, and remote communities. *Stud Health Technol Inform* 2015;209:15–22.

31. Tahan V, Almashhrawi A, Kahveci AM, Mutrux R, Ibdah JA. Extension for community health outcomes-hepatitis C: small steps carve big footprints in the allocation of scarce resources for hepatitis C virus treatment to remote developing areas. *World J Hepatol* 2016;8(11):509.

32. Asturias EJ, Heinrichs G, Domek G, et al. The center for human development in Guatemala: an innovative model for global population health. *Adv Pediatr* 2016; 63(1):357–387.

33. Sable C, Roca T, Gold J, Gutierrez A, Gulotta E, Culpepper W. Live transmission of neonatal echocardiograms from underserved areas: accuracy, patient care, and cost. *Telemed J* 1999;5(4):339–347.

34. Sable C. Telemedicine applications in pediatric cardiology. *Minerva Pediatr* 2003;55(1):1–13.

35. Pearl PL, Sable C, Evans S, et al. International telemedicine consultations for neurodevelopmental disabilities. *Telemed J E Health* 2014;20(6):559–562.

36. Augusterfer EF, Mollica RF, Lavelle J. A review of telemental health in international and post-disaster settings. *Int Rev Psychiatry* 2015;27(6):540–546.

37. Jefee-Bahloul H, Moustafa MK, Shebl FM, Barkil-Oteo A. Pilot assessment and survey of Syrian refugees' psychological stress and openness to referral for telepsychiatry (PASSPORT Study). *Telemed J E Health* 2014;20(10):977–979.

38. Branagan L, Chase LL. Organizational implementation of telemedicine technology; methodology and field experience. In 2012 IEEE Global Humanitarian Technology Conference. Seattle, Washington USA, 2012; 271–276.

39. Charlie Gomez Medical Clinic. https://www.mayanfamilies.org/page/medicalclinic.

40. Losinio L. Telemedicine program launched. *Minerva Pediatr* June 9, 2016. https://www.postguam.com/news/local/telemedicine-program-launched/article_c9b4d502-2d62-11e6-96d8-934e206312a5.html

41. Hidalgo R, Alverson DC, Cartagenova G, Maldonado L. Development of a Collaborative Telehealth Network in Ecuador: Programa Nacional de Telemedicina. American Telemedicine Association National Annual Meeting, Seattle, WA, April 6-9, 2008. *Telemedicine J E Health* 2008;14(supp 1):51.

42. Hopkins KS, Alverson DC, Hidalgo RO, Cartagenova G, Johnson-Moser S. Integrating Cross-Cultural Indigenous and Western Healing with Modern Technology Update. American Telemedicine Association National Annual Meeting, Seattle, WA, April 6-9, 2008. *Telemedicine J E Health* 2008;14(supp 1):52–53.

43. Bashur RL, Shannon GW. *History of Telemedicine: Evolution, Context, and Transformation*. New Rochelle, NY: Mary Anne Liebert; 2009.

44. World Health Report 2006. http://www.who.int/entity/whr/2006/whr06_en.pdf. Accessed 4 July, 2009.

45. Olusanya BO, Ruben RJ, Parving A. Reducing the burden of communication disorders in the developing world: an opportunity for the millennium development project. *JAMA* 2006;296:441–444.

46. United Nations Department of Economic and Social Affairs, Population Division (2009). World population prospects: the 2008 revision, Highlights, Working Paper No. ESA/P/WP.210. 2009; 1–109.

47. Achieving the Millennium Development Goals in Africa. Recommendations of the MDG Africa Steering Group, June 2008. http://www.mdgafrica.org/pdf/MDG%20Africa%20Steering%20Group%20Recommendations%20-%20English%20-%20LowRes.pdf. Accessed 4 July, 2009.

48. Wootton R. Telemedicine support in the developing world. *J Telemed Telecare* 2008;14:109–114.

Patients, Their Physicians, and Telehealth

Jack Resneck, Jr., MD, Sylvia J. Trujillo, MPP, JD
and Kristin Schleiter, JD, LLM

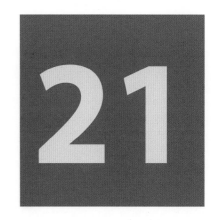

INTRODUCTION AND PROMISE OF TELEMEDICINE

Physicians have embraced innovation in health care delivery for decades and recognize that digital health, including high-quality telemedicine, holds great potential to improve patient access to care and care coordination. An expanding evidence base in many medical specialties is elucidating the clinical situations in which various telemedicine technologies can be deployed with high efficacy and safety for patient care, as well as highlighting scenarios in which these technologies or their uses have not met our expectations. This important evidence base is informing a growing body of clinical guidelines and position statements on best practices.

Physicians have been pioneers in the development and deployment of telemedicine technologies, as well as rigorous evaluation and publication of their outcomes. Although telehealth affects how care is delivered and how patients interact with physicians, the profession of medicine has recognized that the fundamental professional and ethical responsibilities to deliver high-quality, coordinated care are unchanged by these evolving technologies. Physicians have, therefore, engaged deeply to advance the development of evidence-based guidelines, ethical standards, licensure frameworks, legislative and regulatory patient protections, insurance coverage, physician education opportunities, and reliable digital tools to advance the use of appropriate telemedicine to provide quality care for our patients.

AMERICAN MEDICAL ASSOCIATION TELEMEDICINE POLICY

The American Medical Association's (AMA's) physician and medical student members have played a central role in the development of medicine in the United States since 1847.[1] Scientific advancement, standards for medical education, launching a program of medical ethics, and improved public health were the goals of the AMA's founders and remain central to the AMA's focus today.[1,2] Through the process outlined later, the AMA plays a pivotal role in advancing best practices, processes, and policies for integrating telemedicine into medical practice.

Telemedicine constitutes the practice of medicine. Given the rapid rate of technological innovation, this area of medicine has the potential to accelerate transformations in medical care. However, telemedicine also has significant implications for altering established patterns and methods of patient care and associated policies that require informed and thoughtful engagement and leadership from the physician community and other health care stakeholders. The range of ethical and health policy considerations have been far-ranging and will continue to evolve through an established process within the AMA designed to accommodate advancements in medical practice.

The AMA's telemedicine initiatives and advocacy reflect the input and deliberation of the broadest group of physicians in the nation. The AMA House of Delegates (House or the HOD) is the principal policy-making body of the AMA.[3] The HOD represents the views and interests of physician delegates from more than 170 state medical associations and national medical specialty societies.[4] The HOD delegates meet twice per year at annual and interim meetings to deliberate and cast votes that establish policy on health, medical, professional and governance matters, as well as the principles within which the AMA's business activities are conducted. Members of the AMA Board of Trustees (Trustees) are elected by the HOD and are responsible for setting AMA priorities and initiatives consistent with AMA policy. In addition, the House, Trustees, and AMA staff benefit from the perspective and expertise of a number of physician leadership councils that have contributed to the development of AMA reports that inform the HOD's and the Trustees' deliberation, policy adoption, advocacy, and strategic initiatives.[5] The leadership councils that have contributed to the most recent telemedicine policies include the Council on Ethical and Judicial Affairs (CEJA), the Council on Legislation (COL),[6] the Council on Medical Service (CMS), the Council on Medical Education (CME), and the Council on Science and Public Health (CSAPH).

In addition to recommendations made by the COL to the Trustees, the policy recommendations contained in the following reports have been adopted by the House and currently guide AMA telemedicine strategic initiatives and advocacy:

- CME Report 6, Annual Meeting 2010, Telemedicine and Medical Licensure (CMS Report 06-A-10)[7]
- Board of Trustees (BOT) Report 22, Annual Meeting 2013, Professionalism in Telemedicine & Telehealth (BOT Report 22-A-13)[8]
- CSAPH Report 5, Annual Meeting 2014, Guidelines for Mobile Medical Applications (CSAPH Report 5-A-14)[9]
- CMS Report 7, Annual Meeting 2014, Coverage and Payment for Telemedicine (CMS Report 7-A-14)[10]
- BOT Report 3, Interim Meeting 2014, Facilitating State Licensure for Telemedicine Services (BOT Report 3-I-14)[11]
- CEJA Report 1, Annual Meeting 2016, Ethical Practice in Telemedicine (CEJA Report 1-A-16)[12]
- CMS Report 5, Annual Meeting 2016, Virtual Supervision of "Incident to" Services (CMS Report 5-A-16)[13]

- CME Report 6, Annual Meeting 2016, Telemedicine in Medical Education (CME 06-A-16)[14]
- CMS Report 6, Interim Meeting 2016, Integration of Mobile Health Applications and Devices into Practice (CMS Report 06-I-16)
- Over a period of six years, the AMA HOD has adopted sweeping telemedicine policy to address funding to support research and clinical validation, medical practice standards and patient protections, medical ethics, oversight of telemedicine technologies (devices and software), insurance coverage and payment, liability, infrastructure and technology interoperability, and medical education and training. As this area of medicine continues to advance, it is expected that the AMA's Trustees and House will continue to consider emerging issues in this area.

Two of the telemedicine reports—CEJA Report 1-A-16, Ethical Practice in Telemedicine and CMS Report 7-A-14, Coverage and Payment for Telemedicine—contain seminal policies that are foundational policies and ethics guidance for physicians providing telemedicine.

CEJA Reports, once adopted by the House, interpret the AMA Code of Medical Ethics to provide practical ethics guidance on timely topics for physicians, residents, medical students, and others in health care. AMA physician members must adhere to the AMA's Code of Medical Ethics,[15] and it is widely referenced as an authoritative source of medical ethics. CEJA Report 1-A-16 establishes the ethical parameters physicians are expected to practice within, and the Opinion serves as the foundation for physicians offering telemedicine services. The AMA's Code of Medical ethics provides that physicians' fundamental ethical responsibilities don't change when providing telemedicine. CEJA Report 1-A-16 specifies that any physician engaging in telemedicine must:

- Disclose any financial or other interests in particular telemedicine applications or services
- Protect patient privacy and confidentiality

As adopted, CEJA Report 1-A-16 outlines broad obligations physicians have when providing telemedicine, including:

- Informing patients about the limitations of the relationship and services provided

- Encouraging telemedicine patients who have a primary care physician to inform them about their online health consultation and ensure the information from the encounter can be accessed for future episodes of care

- Recognizing the limitations of technology and taking appropriate steps to overcome them, such as by having another health care professional at the patient's location conduct an exam or obtaining vital information through remote technologies

- Ensuring patients have a basic understanding of how telemedicine technologies are used in their care, the limitations of the technologies, and ways the information will be used after the patient encounter.

CMS Report 7-A-14, Coverage and Payment for Telemedicine, covers a broad range of policy and practice requirements. A valid physician–patient relationship must exist before telemedicine services are provided.[16] Once that relationship is established, physicians may use telemedicine technologies with their patients at their discretion consistent with their ethical obligations. CMS Report 7-A-14 reaffirmed AMA policy that physicians who deliver telemedicine services must be licensed in the state where the patient receives services, and the delivery of care must be consistent with the state's scope-of-practice laws. Additional patient protections are specified in the policy, including adherence to laws to protect privacy and security of patient information, patient choice of treating physician, and notice of patient cost-sharing responsibilities. The policy also outlines AMA support for expanded telemedicine research and pilots, national medical specialty society development of clinical practice guidelines, verification of liability coverage, and

engagement with other stakeholders to advance quality telemedicine.

Because this area of medicine is likely to continue to present novel clinical practice issues and questions, it is important that physicians and telemedicine stakeholders remain abreast of existing AMA policies and track the adoption of new telemedicine policies. AMA policies are available on the organization's webpage and can be searched through the online Policy Finder.[17]

CLINICAL INNOVATION TO CLINICAL INTEGRATION

Medical innovation may be iterative or transformative, but in either case there is a path to clinical integration. This path does not necessarily follow a predictable succession from one category to the next, as pictured below. Nonetheless, addressing the challenges and barriers that emerge in the categories in Figure 21-1 (Innovation/Validation, Regulation/Quality Assurance, Payment, Liability, Infrastructure, Professional Development/Education) is often necessary to scale integration. The AMA's telemedicine policy development and adoption cover each of the categories outlined in Figure 21-1. The AMA's strategic initiatives and advocacy at the federal and state level address and support the modernization required in each category to support patient-centered adoption and integration of telemedicine.[18]

To enhance strategic initiatives and advocacy consistent with AMA policy, the AMA contracted with Kantar TNS to survey physicians in order to investigate physician motivations, current usage, and expectations for integrating digital health tools into their practice (The Digital Health Study: Physicians' motivations and

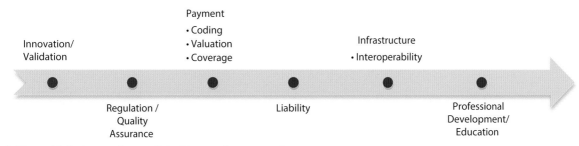

▲ **Figure 21-1.** Innovation to clinical integration categories.

requirements for adopting digital clinical tools, 2016 [Digital Health Study]).[19] The Digital Health Study includes specific questions concerning telemedicine as well as others related to mobile health, remote monitoring, and mobile health applications, among other categories of digital health. The Digital Health Study findings validate that AMA telemedicine policy development and adoption are timely. The survey has been a critical tool to further inform AMA strategic initiatives and advocacy activities.

The Digital Health Study found that physicians are optimistic about digital health innovation and the potential to transform medical practice and improve patient care utilizing these digital health tools. At time of the survey, physicians reported using a few digital tools and expected to use more in the future. Furthermore, surveyed physicians in large and complex practices tended to use digital health tools more, and age was less of a factor than practice size and setting for physician adoption. According to the study, however, telemedicine has not yet "crossed the chasm of adoption," and there is not across-the-board enthusiasm for telemedicine. The surveyed physicians ranked in order of importance the key issues that must be addressed to support their adoption of digital health tools, including:

- Standard liability insurance coverage
- Data privacy and security
- Workflow integration with electronic medical record (EHR) systems
- Insurance coverage and payment.

The AMA has invested significant resources to provide guidance and to develop solutions in these critical areas to support widespread clinical integration.[20]

PATIENT PROTECTIONS AND MEDICAL PRACTICE ACCOUNTABILITY

▶ Valid Relationship

A valid patient–physician relationship must be established for a telemedicine service to take place. In addition to being a legal requirement in most states, the establishment of this relationship triggers important ethical obligations physicians have to patients, such as the responsibility to respect patient privacy and confidentiality, and the obligation to provide help so patients understand their medical condition and options for treatment.[21]

In most states, a telemedicine encounter itself can establish a patient–physician relationship through real-time audiovisual technology. However, some states require a prior in-person visit before a patient exam via telemedicine, require that a patient site presenter be present with the patient for an initial exam via telemedicine, or require the patient to be at an established medical site for an initial exam via telemedicine. Some states also require a prior in-person visit before issuing a prescription based on a telemedicine exam.

AMA policy[22] provides that a valid patient–physician relationship must be established before the provision of telemedicine services through:

- A face-to-face examination, if a face-to-face encounter would otherwise be required in the provision of the same service not delivered via telemedicine; or
- A consultation with another physician who has an ongoing patient–physician relationship with the patient, so long as the physician who has established a valid physician–patient relationship must agree to supervise the patient's care; or
- Meeting standards of establishing a patient–physician relationship included as part of evidence-based clinical practice guidelines on telemedicine developed by major medical specialty societies, such as those of radiology and pathology.

Exceptions to the foregoing include on-call, cross-coverage situations; emergency medical treatment; and other exceptions that become recognized as meeting or improving the standard of care. The AMA also believes that if a medical home does not exist, telemedicine providers should facilitate the identification of medical homes and treating physicians where in-person services can be delivered in coordination with the telemedicine services.

Several specialty societies have concurred that it can be clinically appropriate to establish a patient–physician relationship via telemedicine. For example, the American College of Physicians believes that a valid patient–physician relationship can be established through a telemedicine encounter using real-time audiovisual technology so long as the standard of care required of an in-person visit is met, or so long as the physician is consulting with another physician who has an established relationship with the patient and oversees that patient's care.[23]

In addition, the Federation of State Medical Boards has weighed in with the Model Policy on the Appropriate Use of Telemedicine Technology in the Practice of Medicine.[24] This model policy highlights the fundamental nature of the patient–physician relationship to the provision of care and clarifies that physicians must take steps to establish this relationship. The model policy states that the physician–patient relationship "tends to begin when an individual with a health-related matter seeks assistance from a physician who may provide assistance. However, the relationship is clearly established when the physician agrees to undertake diagnosis and treatment of the patient, and the patient agrees to be treated, whether or not there has been an encounter in person between the physician (or other appropriately supervised health care practitioner) and patient."

▶ Licensure

In the United States, medicine is a licensed profession regulated by the individual states. The nation's medical boards license both allopathic (MD) and osteopathic (DO) physicians.

Most states require that the telemedicine practitioner be licensed in the state where the patient is located at the time of the encounter. A handful of states have mechanisms for special telemedicine registration for physicians who are providing care to patients of the state via telemedicine but lack a brick-and-mortar practice in the state. A few others provide reciprocity agreements between states whereby a physician need not obtain an additional license or register in order to treat patients in the state.

AMA policy provides that physicians and other health practitioners delivering telemedicine services must abide by state licensure laws and state medical practice laws and requirements in the state in which the patient receives services.[25] At the same time, the AMA supports mechanisms for greater reciprocity between state licensing jurisdictions, has supported pluralistic approaches to credentials verification and validation of physician credentials (such as the Federation Credentials Verification Service), and has encouraged increased uniformity in acceptance of examination scores and in other requirements for medical licensure. The AMA has also long encouraged medical boards to modernize and streamline the medical licensure system. One such mechanism through which to streamline and modernize the medical licensure system is the Interstate Medical Licensure Compact (Compact).

Interstate Medical Licensure Compact

The Compact offers a new, voluntary expedited pathway to licensure for qualified physicians who wish to practice in multiple states, increasing access to health care for patients in underserved or rural areas and allowing them to more easily connect with medical experts through the use of telemedicine technologies.

While making it easier for physicians to obtain licenses to practice in multiple states, the Compact strengthens public protection by enhancing the ability of states to share investigative and disciplinary information. The Compact is being implemented in a growing number of states, with others expected to adopt it soon.

The Compact is a reasonable approach to license portability that builds on the existing system of state medical licensure while not otherwise changing a state's existing medical practice act. Notably, the Compact is consistent with AMA policy that physicians delivering telemedicine services must be licensed in the state where the patient receives services, or provide these services as otherwise authorized by the state's medical board, and that such physicians should abide by the licensure and medical practice laws and requirements of the state in which the patient receives services.

At the date of publication, 18 states were participating in the Compact, with many more slated to join the Compact in the coming years. The Compact is in the process of establishing its administrative process for expedited licensure. As such, expedited licensing is not yet available but will be soon. The Compact's website is a great place to monitor developments in the rulemaking, administrative meetings, and progress toward launch.[26]

Federal Preemption Efforts

A number of telemedicine stakeholders have attempted to secure passage of federal legislation that would preempt the ability of states to regulate health and safety for individuals receiving services in their state. The AMA continues to vigorously oppose federal bills and regulations that would eviscerate the essential patient protections afforded by state-based licensure. The impetus ostensibly for federal preemption is to reduce the compliance costs for telemedicine companies and health systems that employ physicians providing services in multiple states, but does not account for the important patient protections state-based licensure provides or the cost and difficulty associated with establishing and complying with national registration programs (such as the difficult and time-consuming registration process for the Physician Open Payments Program administered by the Centers for Medicare & Medicaid Services[27]).

After initial efforts to secure passage of federal bills to create a national license failed, another troubling strategy to federally preempt state licensure and medical practice laws has emerged in more recent congressional sessions. Language has been included in federal bills that would permit a single license issued in any state to be effective in all states. Preemption of states laws under either approach would hobble the ability of states to investigate complaints; enforce any disciplinary measures on behalf of patients and the public; or ensure compliance with state laws and regulations governing prescribing, minor consent requirements, reproduction, and end of life. A single state license that would allow a physician to practice in all states would deprive state legislatures and medical boards of the legal authority to compel physicians licensed out of state to submit to the jurisdiction of the state or the medical board for purposes of investigations, hearings, and disciplinary actions. Patients with complaints and concerns would face substantial hurdles and costs securing recourse from state legislatures and medical boards if the state where the physician is licensed is not the same state as where the patient is located, particularly where substantial geographic distances are involved. The widespread adoption of the Compact will address the compliance and cost concerns of those seeking to preempt state laws while preserving the essential patient protections afforded by state-based oversight of state licensure and state medical practice laws.

STATE MEDICAL PRACTICE LAWS

State medical practice acts provide an important road map for the practice of telemedicine. Medical practice acts commonly include provisions on informed consent—including whether informed consent specific to telemedicine is required by state law, how to establish a relationship with a new patient via telemedicine, any restrictions on prescriptive authority based on exams conducted via telemedicine, privacy laws, medical recordkeeping requirements, and state-specific prohibitions on fraud and abuse. Although many of these provisions simply confirm that state laws apply to telemedicine practice as they would in-person treatment, it is important for physicians to understand what areas of state law apply equally and what telemedicine-specific laws need to be followed.

COVERAGE AND PAYMENT

Physicians and health systems consistently cite lack of coverage and payment for services delivered via telemedicine as one of the obstacles to its adoption. Progress is being made at the state and federal level to ensure appropriate coverage, but there is still work to be done.

▶ Parity

State

Laws addressing payment and coverage for telemedicine services at the state level fall into three areas: private insurance, Medicaid, and state employee health plans. Before adopting telemedicine into practice, it is important to find out where your state falls on the spectrum of state laws. At the time of publication, 31 states had laws requiring private payors to cover telemedicine, 26 states provide coverage under state employee health plans, and nearly all state Medicaid programs cover telemedicine services.

The scope of each state's laws varies greatly. State laws or coverage policies can restrict coverage based on provider, technology, condition being treated, or patient setting. Some state Medicaid programs, for example, reimburse only for physician services, not those provided by nurses or physician assistants. State Medicaid programs can also limit the modalities that are covered, for example, excluding store-and-forward or remote patient monitoring of patient vital signs from covered services. Further, some Medicaid policies restrict coverage to certain patient care settings, like hospitals or doctor's offices, thereby preventing coverage of telemedicine services provided to the patient at school, at home, or in other settings. Still other state laws include geography or distance requirements for coverage of telemedicine, although those remaining laws appear to be falling out of favor, with 86 states covering telemedicine services without distance restrictions or geographic designations.

The AMA has advocated at the state level for coverage of telemedicine services to the same extent that those services would be covered in person. The AMA model Telemedicine Act can be used as the basis for a comprehensive telemedicine coverage law that ensures that physicians and other health care professionals are adequately compensated for the care provided to their patients via telemedicine.

Federal Health Care Programs

The AMA continues to strongly support expanded coverage and payment of telemedicine by federal health care programs. The telemedicine policies of the various federal health care programs are varied and run the full continuum. Currently, the Veterans Health Administration (VHA) and the Medicare program play the most influential role in the area of coverage and payment.

On one end of the continuum is the VHA which has been an early adopter and innovator of telemedicine[28] service delivery modalities and covers a comprehensive range of telemedicine services.[29] The VHA's deployment of telemedicine is aided by:

- A shared EHR system
- Health care providers, including physicians, employed by a single entity
- Professional development and training capacity
- Control of and funding for infrastructure to enable telemedicine, including computers, peripheral devices, software, and technical support

The AMA has urged Congress to provide increased funding and support to further expand access to VHA telemedicine services. In addition to meeting the needs of the nation's veterans, the VHA contributes to telemedicine efficacy research, pilots, and model programs that grow the evidence base in a manner that benefits patients and physicians outside of the VHA. Telemedicine advocates are able to rely on the VHA best practices as a road map to implementation, and the telehealth clinical evidence is utilized to urge other payors to offer telemedicine services as a covered health benefit.

In contrast to the VHA, the Medicare program has lagged substantially behind in terms of coverage and payment of telemedicine services, largely, though not exclusively, due to restrictive provisions of the federal law governing the program. Although certain telemedicine services are covered and paid by Medicare, these are limited to a short list of live video interactive services where an eligible Medicare beneficiary is located in a qualifying geographic location and facility (originating site) with extremely limited exceptions.[30] The Centers for Medicare & Medicaid Services, the federal agency that administers the Medicare program, annually proposes and considers public requests to expand the list of covered telemedicine services, yet the agency faces statutory restrictions that prevent it from expanding beneficiaries eligible for such services to include, for instance, underserved beneficiaries in urban areas.[31] The law also limits store-and-forward telehealth service coverage to demonstration projects in Alaska and Hawaii.[32]

Although support for expanded access for all Medicare beneficiaries has grown rapidly among major health care providers and many policy makers over the past couple of years, passage of federal bills have been stymied due to the Congressional Budget Office (CBO) estimates of the budgetary effect.[33] The CBO is responsible for providing nonpartisan analyses of budgetary and economic issues to support the congressional budget process. The CBO has scored legislation that would expand Medicare beneficiary access to telemedicine as increasing spending as opposed to decreasing or having a cost-neutral impact on Medicare spending relative to the current law. The AMA is working with a broad group of health care stakeholders to develop a framework and proposed methods consistent with

CBO general specifications[34] that would be utilized by nationally regarded researchers to conduct analyses and develop reports that could be relied upon or used by the CBO in future scoring exercises.

In addition to supporting federal legislation that would expand Medicare coverage, the AMA has continued to urge the CMS to exercise (1) discretionary authorities to waive statutory restrictions or (2) general grants of authority to manage the Medicare program in order to:

- Remove the current geographic and originating site restrictions that prevent delivery of what would otherwise be covered services in urban and suburban areas

- Permit coverage for dually eligible Medicare–Medicaid beneficiaries who currently are not able to benefit from the same telehealth services as Medicaid-only beneficiaries

- Permit telehealth and remote monitoring services in all existing alternative payment and shared savings model programs, including one-sided and two-sided risk-sharing tracks

For fiscal year 2016 and 2017, the Centers for Medicare & Medicaid Services has exercised increasing levels of flexibility to allow expanded access to telehealth services, but overall the agency remains cautious and decidedly incremental.

▶ National Solutions: Coding, Valuation, Coverage, and Program Integrity

National adoption of telemedicine has been advanced by the AMA through two additional initiatives that remove barriers to coverage and payment. The AMA's Current Procedural Terminology® (CPT) Editorial Panel[35] established a Telehealth Services Workgroup (TSW), and the AMA convened a Digital Medicine Payment Advisory Group (DMPAG) composed of 14 leading experts, primarily practicing physicians, with substantial expertise in coding, valuation, coverage, and/or telehealth.

Current Procedural Terminology® Editorial Panel Telehealth Services Workgroup

Physicians typically submit electronic claims to payors to obtain payment for medical services. CPT® descriptive terms and identifying codes are the most widely accepted medical nomenclature used to electronically report medical procedures and services under public and private health insurance programs.[36] It is important to note that having a CPT® code (or any other code) does not mean that payors will cover a service or pay the amount sought for the service. Payors may have benefit designs that exclude coverage of the service, or a payor may determine that a service may not otherwise meet applicable coverage criteria. The CPT® code set is also used for other activities such as developing guidelines for medical care review.

To ensure that the code set reflects current medical practice, the CPT® Editorial Panel hosts meetings open to interested stakeholders three times annually to consider updates to the CPT® code set. In 2015 the CPT® Editorial Panel established the TSW and charged the workgroup with:

- Recommending solutions for the reporting of current nontelehealth services when using remote telehealth technology (to include but not be limited to evaluation and management (E/M) services). Considerations will include potential new codes, use of current codes without or with modifier, and add-on code(s).

- Addressing the accuracy of the current code set in describing the services provided when telehealth data are reviewed and analyzed, including potential code set revisions and/or education for:

  - Appropriate code use (eg, E/M versus data analysis codes).

  - Potential code development to report analysis of transmitted data.

  - Definition of data types whose interpretation will require differentiation and consideration of separate reporting of current E/M services/codes.

  - Potential new E/M services codes based on emerging new patterns for sites of service.

- Recommending whether any other telehealth service codes should be developed based upon services currently being provided.

- Developing new introductory language or modifying existing introductory language to guide coding of telehealth services.

- Facilitating discussions with key stakeholders who may wish to bring forward telehealth services applications for consideration.[37]

In February 2016, the CPT® Editorial Panel approved an application based on a TSW recommendation to establish a modifier (95) for reporting synchronous (real-time) telemedicine services effective January 1, 2017.[38] In May 2016, the panel accepted guidelines, instructions, and definitions to define synchronous services for the CPT® modifier.[39] In addition, the CPT® Editorial Panel approved a code change application whereby 79 CPT® codes were approved to utilize the modifier (95).

Digital Medicine Payment Advisory Group

In early 2017, the DMPAG was established to provide expert advice on the complex interlocking issues of coding, valuation, coverage, and program integrity to AMA staff, leadership, councils, committees, and the CPT® Editorial Panel.

The DMPAG includes prominent, national experts in telemedicine who are trained and practice in varied medical specialties, geographic locations, and practice settings. The DMPAG is positioned to provide insight and information on the impact of telemedicine across medical practice settings and specialties. In addition to experts who practice telemedicine and oversee large health system telemedicine programs, the DMPAG includes physicians with substantial coding, valuation, and coverage expertise. The DMPAG also includes industry representatives with technology expertise and will inform the AMA's views on the barriers experienced by innovators new to medical practice.

The DMPAG current charge provides that consistent with AMA policy, the DMPAG will provide input and expertise to support the development of strategies that ensure access to telemedicine services by addressing:

- Research and data needs to support the use of digital medicine technologies and services in clinical practice
- Existing code sets (with an emphasis on CPT and Healthcare Common Procedure Coding System Level II code sets administered by CMS) and the level to which they appropriately capture these services and technologies
- Program integrity concerns of payors, including but not limited to, appropriate code use and other perceived risks unique to digital medicine
- Factors that affect the fair and accurate valuation for services delivered via telehealth

- Public and private health insurance coverage of telemedicine and remote patient monitoring, including greater transparency of services covered by payors and advocacy for enforcement of parity coverage laws

The charge may change after consideration of recommendations and suggested revisions offered by DMPAG members. The DMPAG will provide the AMA with a window into optimal strategies and opportunities to fundamentally transform established medical practice along a range of issues that affect whether a physician and other health care providers are paid for telemedicine services.

AMERICAN MEDICAL ASSOCIATION INNOVATION ECOSYSTEM

The AMA has a broad portfolio of strategic digital medicine initiatives as part of an innovation ecosystem that supports clinical validation, quality assurance through industry-supported guidelines, scaling infrastructure and interoperability, and professional development. Recent AMA efforts to advance digital health innovation that is patient centered, evidence based, interoperable, and outcomes focused include:

- Serving as a founding partner to Health2047, a health care innovation company that combines strategy, design, and venture disciplines, working in partnership with leading companies, physicians, and entrepreneurs to improve health care.[40]
- Partnering with MATTER, Chicago's health care technology incubator, to allow entrepreneurs and physicians to collaborate on the development of new technologies, services, and products in a simulated health care environment.[41]
- Partnering with Omada Health, a telemedicine platform, and Intermountain Healthcare to scale evidence-based, technology-enabled care models that are key to addressing the more than 86 million Americans who currently have prediabetes.[42]
- Developing a beta version of the AMA Physician Innovation Network—a platform to connect physicians to provide feedback to health technology entrepreneurs for improved solutions.
- Serving as one of four initial founding members of Xcertia, a new, multistakeholder collaboration

dedicated to improving the quality, safety, and effectiveness of mobile health applications (apps).[43]

- Offering an online telemedicine module as part of the AMA's *StepsForward* online learning community to support physicians interested in incorporating telemedicine into their clinical practice.[44]

The AMA will continue to leverage collaborations with external partners to maximize impact and to increase the opportunity for success through complementary matching of reach and expertise. As a result, the AMA's enterprise-wide digital medicine ecosystem is expected to expand so that physicians are positioned to lead technology-enabled transformations and to ensure that such advances deepen physician satisfaction, strengthen the patient–physician relationship, and improve patient-centered health outcomes.

REFERENCES

1. https://www.ama-assn.org/ama-history.
2. https://www.ama-assn.org/about/our-vision.
3. https://www.ama-assn.org/about-us/house-delegates-hod.
4. https://www.ama-assn.org/content/ama-house-delegates.
5. https://www.ama-assn.org/about-us/councils.
6. The COL reviews proposed federal legislation and recommends appropriate action in accordance with AMA policy. It also recommends changes in existing AMA policy when necessary to accomplish effective legislative goals and recommends to the Trustees new federal legislation and legislation to modify existing laws of interest to the AMA. The COL is appointed by the AMA Trustees, and the COL's reports and recommendations are confidential and solely for consideration by the Trustees, although the COL also advises and collaborates with other AMA leadership councils.
7. http://ama.nmtvault.com/jsp/viewer.jsp?doc_id=ama_arch%2FHOD00006%2F00000002&query1=&recoffset=0&collection_filter=All&collection_name=1ee24daa-2768-4bff-b792-e4859988fe94&sort_col=publication date&CurSearchNum=-1
8. https://www.ama-assn.org/sites/default/files/media-browser/public/hod/a13-bot-reports_0.pdf.
9. https://www.ama-assn.org/sites/default/files/media-browser/public/hod/a14-csaph-reports_0.pdf.
10. https://www.ama-assn.org/sites/default/files/media-browser/public/about-ama/councils/Council%20Reports/council-on-medical-service/a14-cms-report7.pdf.
11. https://www.ama-assn.org/sites/default/files/media-browser/public/hod/i14-bot-reports_0.pdf.
12. https://www.ama-assn.org/sites/default/files/media-browser/i16-ceja-reports.pdf.
13. https://www.ama-assn.org/sites/default/files/media-browser/public/about-ama/councils/Council%20 Reports/a16-cms-reports-final-update.pdf.
14. https://www.ama-assn.org/sites/default/files/media-browser/i16-cme-reports.pdf.
15. https://www.ama-assn.org/content/council-ethical-and-judicial-affairs.
16. Coverage of and Payment for Telemedicine H-480.946.
17. AMA Policy Finder. https://www.ama-assn.org/about/policyfinder.
18. https://www.ama-assn.org/practice-management/improving-digital-health.
19. https://www.ama-assn.org/sites/default/files/media-browser/specialty%20group/washington/ama-digital-health-report923.pdf.
20. https://www.ama-assn.org/delivering-care/digital-health-your-practice.
21. AMA Code of Medical Ethics Opinion. https://www.ama-assn.org/sites/default/files/media-browser/code-of-medical-ethics-chapter-1.pdf
22. AMA Policy H-480.946(2), Coverage of and Payment for Telemedicine.
23. Annals of Internal Medicine. Policy Recommendations to Guide the Use of Telemedicine in Primary Care Settings: An American College of Physicians Policy Paper. 2015. http://annals.org/aim/article/2434625/policy-recommendations-guide-use-telemedicine-primary-care-settings-american-college
24. Federation of State Medical Boards. Model Policcy for the Use of Telemedicine Technologies in the Practice of Medicine. www.fsmb.org/Media/Default/PDF/FSMB/Advocacy/FSMB_Telemedicine_Policy.pdf.
25. AMA Policy D-480.999.
26. Interstate Medical Licensure Compact. www.license portability.org.
27. Shut Down: Open Payments Registration Site Temporarily Closed to Physicians, AAFP, August 13, 2014. http://www.aafp.org/news/government-medicine/20140813openpayglitch.html
28. Statement of Kevin Galpin, MD, Acting Executive Director for Telehealth, Veterans Health Administration, Department of Veterans Affairs Before U.S. House of Representatives Committee on Veterans' Affairs, Subcommittee on Health, August 9, 2016.
29. VHA Telehealth offerings. https://www.telehealth.va.gov/
30. Medicare Learning Network, Telehealth Services, ICN 901705, November 2016. https://www.cms.gov/

Outreach-and-Education/Medicare-Learning-Network-MLN/MLNProducts/downloads/TelehealthSrvcsfctsht.pdf

31. Id.

32. Id.

33. Payers Urge CBO to Give Telemedicine a Fair Shake, *mHealth Intelligence*, October 24 2016. https://mhealth-intelligence.com/news/payers-urge-cbo-to-give-telemedicine-a-fair-shake

34. Congressional Budget Office Blog, Telemedicine, July 29, 2015 https://www.cbo.gov/publication/50680

35. The AMA Trustees appoint the 17-member CPT Editorial Panel, which exercises independent authority to maintain and update the code set. Eleven physicians are selected from physicians nominated by national medical specialty societies. Four physician representatives are appointed based on nomination by Blue Cross Blue Shield of America, the American Hospital Association, the American Health Insurance Plans, and the Centers for Medicare & Medicaid Services. Two health professionals are selected from the Health Care Professionals Advisory Committee (composed of representatives of allied health professionals).

36. https://www.ama-assn.org/sites/default/files/media-browser/specialty%20group/washington/ama-digital-health-report923.pdf

37. CPT Telehealth Services Workgroup.

38. Tab 51, Telehealth Services Appendix ZZ, CPT Editorial Summary of Panel Actions, February 2016.

39. Tab 38, Telehealth Services Definitions, CPT Editorial Panel Summary of Panel Actions, May 2016.

40. AMA Launches Silicon Valley Integrated Company, Health2047, AMA Press Center, January 11, 2016.

41. AMA, MATTER to Create Tech-enabled "Physician Office of the Future," AMA Press Center, February 4, 2015.

42. AMA, Omada, Intermountain Healthcare Partner Against Type 2 Diabetes, AMA Press Center, July 26, 2016.

43. Alliance Forms to Develop Guidelines for Evaluation of mHealth Apps, AMA Press Center, December 21, 2016.

44. StepsForward: Adopting telemedicine in practice.

The State Policy Framework of Telehealth

Latoya S. Thomas, Digital Health Policy Expert

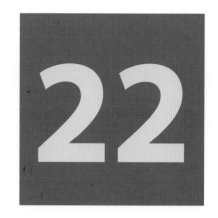

INTRODUCTION

In Federalist Papers No. 45, President James Madison stated that "[t]he powers delegated by the proposed Constitution to the federal government are few and defined. Those which are to remain in the State governments are numerous and indefinite."[1] Neither he, nor other visionaries of our founding government, could have foreseen the impact this position would have on the health and well-being of a technologically advanced society 200 years later.

Innovations in health care, such as telehealth, have elevated the influence of state-level policies in the larger health ecosystem. States are playing a significant role to ensure that nontraditional health care delivery models such as telehealth are accessible, secure, equitable, and worth merit. For example, agencies with regulatory oversight of health professionals, health facilities, utilities, public health and welfare services, insurance, commerce, and business can all shape regulatory policies that affect telehealth adoption and utilization.

Lawmakers also look beyond their own state borders to align policies that facilitate interstate collaboration. Health care workforce shortages coupled with more mobile societal lifestyles find patients, providers, and caregivers seeking advice, treatment, and consultations in another state. The concepts of where health care is rendered and received when telehealth intervenes challenge the ethical and regulatory boundaries of states' rights and state borders.

Although policies related to telehealth are varied and nuanced, they provide a necessary framework to enable existing and new manners for which telehealth is permitted, delivered, and financed. However, the nature of these policies is sometimes caught between competing interests and technological evolution. How does a state entity allow room for innovation and mobility while defining standards for telehealth development, adoption, and utilization that protect business and public interest?

INSURANCE COVERAGE AND REIMBURSEMENT OF TELEHEALTH

Telehealth providers who rely on the health insurance market for a revenue stream and sustainability must navigate a system that is not always clear on eligibility, coverage, and payment. Traditionally, lack of coverage and payment for telehealth has been a barrier to adoption by providers and patients across the health care spectrum. The enforcement of billing practices by some insurers would indiscriminately permit coverage and payment for telehealth-provided services such as radiology but deny payment for other covered health care services provided remotely.

Over the past few decades states have tried to correct this loophole by developing and promoting statutory and regulatory insurance frameworks that encourage telehealth adoption and utilization statewide. The progress in states' acceptance of telehealth has been incremental yet significant. In 2005, 24 state Medicaid programs covered telehealth-provided services and only two reimbursed for telehealth in the home.[2] Twelve years later, 50 state Medicaid programs and the District of Columbia cover telehealth-provided services and 39 reimburse for telehealth in the home.[3]

Whereas the states are incubators of innovations with decades of experience embracing telehealth, conversely, federal programs like Medicare have found very little adoption of telehealth. This is largely due to statutory restrictions that prohibit telehealth coverage to approximately 80% of Medicare beneficiaries because they live in nonrural communities.[4] Other policy areas that stifle telehealth growth for Medicare include limits on designated patient settings, eligible provider types, and restraints on permissible modalities (eg, remote patient monitoring).[5]

On the other hand, Medicaid, which is another federal program that covers 20% of the U.S. population, administers insurance coverage to eligible low-income beneficiaries and is not bound by the same federal restrictions as Medicare. In fact, the Centers for Medicare & Medicaid Services (CMS) encourages states to use telemedicine to satisfy federal requirements for efficiency, economy, and quality of scale.[6] CMS also does not require states to submit a state plan amendment (SPA) to cover telehealth for the delivery of services already agreed to by the state and federal entity.

Although states have latitude to comprehensibly cover services regardless of the delivery method, no two states are alike in their approach to use telehealth as a means of addressing public health concerns. The Pennsylvania Department of Public Welfare initiated Medicaid coverage of telehealth in 2007 to enhance access to mental health services and improve the quality of care for expectant mothers due to the shortage of specialists.[7] This included reducing neonatal intensive care unit (ICU) stays, unnecessary hospital stays, and avoidable patient medical transportation. During an office visit, enrolled beneficiaries were provided remote access to maternal-fetal specialists and psychiatrists using interactive audio-video equipment or telephone. Studies have shown the value of using telehealth to reduce costs and alleviate the complications of high-risk pregnancy.[8-10] The effectiveness of Pennsylvania's program led to the expansion of telehealth to include home-based telecare activity, sensor, health status, and medication monitoring for the elderly or adults with disabilities, as well as other specialty services.[11-13]

The approach to regulate telehealth coverage varies by state and may require approval or action by more than one agency. Some states have chosen to enforce changes in their health plan terms and conditions of coverage through regulation or bulletin/notice, whereas others enact legislation. Guidance may include a new section on telehealth comprehensively, or may include a subtle mention in each benefit design. For example, coverage and payment conditions for telehealth may vary depending on the type of health professional providing services, place of service/location of the patient, types of services, and modality used.

Twenty-three states and the District of Columbia allow Medicaid coverage of telehealth in schools. States have many options to improve school-based telehealth, which include enacting legislation, proposing changes in administrative regulations, or applying for a federal block grant under Title V of the Social Security Act to improve maternal and child health. Another federal funding opportunity includes a formula grant under the Individuals with Disabilities Education Act to enhance services for children with special needs.

School-based telehealth programs have demonstrated value and been shown to be effective. Ohio and Virginia Medicaid programs have covered school-based speech-language therapy delivered via telehealth since 2011.[14] Students receive remote therapy services in their schools from a licensed speech-language pathologist via an interactive audio-video connection. Hawaii Medicaid updated their telehealth coverage under Medicaid Fee-For-Service and Managed Care in 2016. Enacted legislation removed geographic and patient setting barriers and now permits access in both university- and school-based health centers.

Research shows that patients who receive care in their home are more likely to have better health outcomes and are less likely to be admitted, or readmitted, to the hospital, resulting in significant cost savings.[15] States may enact legislation or leverage waiver authority to offer telehealth to address specific populations or health conditions such as home-based remote patient monitoring for those with chronic conditions. Like school-based telehealth, states have numerous options to include Medicaid coverage of home-based remote patient monitoring. States may seek a federal waiver, such as a home- and community-based service waiver under Social Security Act section 1915(c), or health home option for chronic care under the Affordable Care Act section 1945. States may also apply for federal demonstration programs such as "Money Follows the Person" (MFP), authorized by the American Recovery and Reinvestment Act, which allocates federal funding for transitioning Medicaid beneficiaries from institutions to the community.

Kansas Medicaid covers home-based remote patient monitoring through a "Money Follows the Person" waiver to manage chronic illnesses of beneficiaries 65 years or older.[16] Louisiana and Pennsylvania have CMS-approved 1915(c), which allows Medicaid coverage of home-based telecare activity, sensor, health status, and medication monitoring for the elderly or adults with disabilities.[17]

Impressively, state telehealth private insurance parity laws have included provisions ensuring comprehensive service coverage and statewide access. In 1995, Louisiana was the first state to pass a telehealth parity law thereby prohibiting their private insurers from denying coverage or payment for services provided via telehealth compared to those provided in-person.[18] The state with the largest land mass in the country, Alaska, and those with the smallest land mass—Connecticut, Delaware, Rhode Island—have all enacted telehealth private insurance parity laws. Over the course of two decades 33 states and the District of Columbia have enacted similar laws.

Colorado enacted a parity law in 2001 that included rural restrictions. At the time, Colorado was the only state in the nation with statutorily enforced geographic restrictions for telehealth coverage under private insurance. In 2015, lawmakers amended the parity law to remove the rural-only restrictions and promote statewide access to telehealth.[19]

There are other opportunities to enhance telehealth coverage for state-regulated plans. Modernized network adequacy standards for managed care plans is another vehicle to promote access and availability to telehealth. Revised in 2015, the network adequacy model now includes a definition for telemedicine and telehealth and advises plans to describe ways in which they will use telehealth in their network access plans. Telehealth coverage under self-funded state employee health plans are affected by telehealth parity laws. These health plans purchase insurance through a state-regulated third party. Twenty-six states with telehealth parity laws also include coverage for state employee health plans.[20]

LICENSURE PORTABILITY

Issuing and determining criteria for health professional licensure is the right of each state. Within their capacity, a state determines and enforces clinical standards, qualifications, and parameters for each health professional practicing within the state border. Telehealth enables a licensed health care provider to remotely assess, diagnose, or treat a patient without needing to physically be in the same state, more less the same room, as the patient. However, if the provider is lacking a license in the state where the patient is located at the time of the health care encounter, then they risk violating state law and receiving sanctions imposed by the state licensing board. As such, state licensure policies that impede or encourage interstate collaboration greatly affect telehealth utilization and health care access overall.

The impact of state-by-state licensure laws goes beyond the health care professions. Patients and caregivers lead mobile lives. They travel out of state for personal reasons, including work, leisure, and education and to make purchases. Therefore, they may receive services from more than one health professional, including providers across state lines. Large health care systems have responded to this need for more accessible care by establishing provider networks across multiple states. Alternatively, health professional groups have created numerous licensure and exemption models to facilitate interstate practice and collaboration, alleviate workforce shortages, and accommodate patient choice.

Nine states offer a special telehealth license or registration process to enable out-of-state providers to use telehealth in their states.[21] The conditions of this special telehealth credential grant permission to the provider to only practice remotely and typically prohibit the out-of-state provider from physically practicing in the state. Maine and New Mexico require out-of-state providers to apply for a telehealth registration in addition to their respective board licensure requirements.

Some states have created policies that allow reciprocal agreement like a driver's license. Licensing boards in the District of Columbia, Maryland, and Virginia may establish standards for reciprocity for providers working in adjoining states. The nursing profession uses a model based on mutual recognition, which requires an agreement to join a compact by more than one state. In order for the compact to go into effect, a threshold must be met. The Nurse Licensure Compact (NLC) has existed for 15 years and has 25 participating states. The NLC promotes interstate practice for registered nurses, licensed practical nurses, and licensed vocational nurses. The NLC was enhanced in 2015 to include requirements for criminal background checks and is referred to as the Enhanced Nurse Licensure Compact. Arizona, Arkansas, Florida, Georgia, Idaho, Iowa, Kentucky, Mississippi, Missouri, Nebraksa, New Hampshire, North Dakota, Oklahoma, South Carolina, South Dakota, Tennessee, Utah, Virginia, West Virginia, and Wyoming joined the Enhanced NLC. The National Council of State Boards of Nursing also approved the creation of a new interstate compact for advance practice nurses (APRNs). Idaho and Wyoming are the first states to join the APRN Compact.

The Association of State and Provincial Psychology Boards (ASPPB) created their own interstate licensure compact called PSYPACT in 2016. Licensed psychologists can navigate numerous licensure alternatives to use telehealth, including ASPPB reciprocity agreements, other reciprocity agreements with jurisdictions, Certificate of Professional Qualification (CPQ) to expedite licensure, and full unrestricted licenses. States who join the PSYPACT will enable psychologists to practice telepsychology without the need for multiple licenses. Seven states are required to join for the compact to become active. Arizona, Nevada, and Utah are the first states to join the PSYPACT.

In 2015, the Federation of State Boards of Physical Therapy created a licensure compact to enable a licensure process to promote interstate physical therapy practice in-person and using telehealth. Ten states are required to join for the compact to become active. Arizona, Colorado, Kentucky, Mississippi, Missouri, Montana. North Dakota, Oregon, Tennessee, Utah, and Washington are the first states to join the now activated compact.

The Federation of State Medical Boards created the Interstate Medical Licensure Compact to enable an expedited licensure process to promote interstate practice, including telehealth. Physicians are still expected to have a full and unrestricted license in every state where they intend to practice. Eighteen states have joined the compact, and it is now active having reached its membership threshold.

Other conditions may be considered when formulating exemptions for out-of-state practice. Some states will waive the licensure process if one of the following conditions are met: the governor declares a state of emergency or natural disaster, the health professional is a military spouse, the health professional is an employee of a federal government agency or correctional facility, the health professional is engaging in temporary and infrequent consultation with a patient, or the health professional is consulting with another peer.

CLINICAL PRACTICE

Telehealth is a tool to facilitate the delivery of care. Just like health care delivered in person, the range of service needs and care circumstances for telehealth varies too widely for a "one size fits all" model. Some states have established different clinical practice rules for telehealth compared to in-person practice. Examples of some areas that yield dissimilar policies include patient setting, established patient–provider relationship and/or in-person examination, provider type, applicable technology, and patient consent. These rules may be prescriptive and provide no consideration for professional clinical discretion, provider shortages, or patient limitations.

The nature of any clinical encounter can differ between episodic urgent care, ongoing primary care, infrequent biometric monitoring, or medical emergencies requiring a specialist. As such, some uses of telehealth are very short term in nature, such as the involvement of a specialist or multidisciplinary care team, whereas other uses involve repeated remote engagement between mental health professionals and patients.

Given the array of different state regulatory bodies and the broad applications of telehealth affecting different health professions, states may choose to review and adapt their policies and procedures to address the needs of patients wishing to access care from an array of health care professionals providing services via telehealth.

Medical boards in Massachusetts and Minnesota have demonstrated the importance of streamlining medical practice standards for telemedicine providers. The boards broadly define telemedicine and provide no distinct rules, protocols, or standards for telemedicine providers to follow. In contrast, licensed physicians in Texas were formerly required to follow a separate standard of practice when using telemedicine, oddly practicing under two different standards of care for patients in the same state. As a result of 2017 legislation, physicians in this state are no longer required to consider scheduled in-person follow-up visits, patient locations, unique patient informed consents, or the presence of another health care provider; thereby holding physicians to the same standard of care. State policies in Arkansas and Colorado, however, recommend an in-person visit for licensed psychologists practicing using telehealth in their states.

Regarding Internet prescribing, some states have specific telehealth clinical practice proposals that require a health professional to obtain a medical or drug history, perform a physical exam, or see the patient in person to fulfill the provider–patient relationship. Other states simply require that the provider "personally know" the patient. A physician may also use a video connection to remotely supervise another health professional, such as a nurse practitioner or physician assistant, while they dispense a medication per physician's orders. Seventeen states have developed policies that prevent a health professional from remotely prescribing or dispensing abortion-inducing medication via telehealth.

Telehealth, when used appropriately, can be an appropriate method of prescribing and dispensing medication to patients. Some boards allow those health professionals with prescriptive authority to, at a minimum, use interactive audio-video encounters as a means of gathering clinical information and establishing a provider–patient relationship necessary to prescribe certain pharmaceuticals. In these instances, some states authorize a physician, nurse practitioner, or psychologist to use a video connection to properly assess a patient and prescribe medication per their treatment plan.

State legislative and regulatory entities are working within their capacity to integrate innovative health care delivery models into the health care, professional, and business fibers of their states. Health care innovation encourages states to think creatively and strategically about the permeability of state borders and, as a result, leverage federal resources and regional and national partnerships to foster a broader and more collaborative health ecosystem. Thus, their willingness to review and amend key state policies has allowed telehealth to grow and spread nationwide.

REFERENCES

1. The Federalist Papers 45. *The Alleged Danger From the Powers of the Union to the State Governments Considered.* https://www.congress.gov/resources/display/content/The+Federalist+Papers.

2. *Telemedicine for CSHCN: A State-by-State Comparison of Medicaid Reimbursement Policies and Title V Activities; Institute for Child Health Policy University of Florida.* July 2005. http://ichp.ufl.edu/files/2011/11/Telemedicine-in-Medicaid-and-Title-V-Report.pdf.

3. Thomas L, Capistrant G. State Telemedicine Gaps Analysis: Coverage & Reimbursement. Washington (DC): American Telemedicine Association. February 2017. http://www.americantelemed.org/policy-page/state-telemedicine-gaps-reports.

4. 42 U.S.C. § 1834(m).

5. 42 CFR 410.78. Telehealth services.

6. Centers for Medicare & Medicaid Services (CMS). *Telemedicine.* https://www.medicaid.gov/Medicaid-CHIP-Program-Information/By-Topics/Delivery-Systems/Telemedicine.html.

7. Pennsylvania Department of Public Welfare Medical Assistance Bulletin 09-07-15, et al. *Medical Assistance Program Fee Schedule: Addition of Telehealth Technology Code and Informational Modifier for Consultations Performed Using Telecommunication Technology.* November 30, 2007. http://www.dhs.pa.gov/cs/groups/webcontent/documents/bulletin_admin/d_004800.pdf

8. Birnie E, Monincx WM, Zondervan HA, et al. Cost-minimization analysis of domiciliary antenatal fetal monitoring in high-risk pregnancies. *Obstet Gynecol* 1997;89(6):925–929.

9. Ferrara A, Hedderson MM, Ching J, et al. Referral to telephonic nurse management improves outcomes in women with gestational diabetes. *Am J Obstet Gynecol* 2012;206(6):491.e1–e5.

10. Wood D. STORC helps deliver healthy babies: the telemedicine program that serves rural women with high-risk pregnancies. *Telemed J E Health* 2011;17(1):2–4. Doi:10.1089/tmj.2011.9996.

11. Pennsylvania Department of Public Welfare Medical Assistance Bulletin 09-12-31, et al. *Medical Assistance Program Fee Schedule: Consultations Performed Using Telemedicine.* May 23, 2012. http://www.dhs.pa.gov/cs/groups/webcontent/documents/bulletin_admin/d_005993.pdf

12. Pennsylvania Department of Public Welfare Office of Mental Health and Substance Abuse Services Bulletin OMHSAS-14-01. *OMHSAS Guidelines for the Approval of Telepsych Services in Health Choices*. March 18, 2014. http://www.dhs.pa.gov/cs/groups/webcontent/documents/bulletin_admin/c_075601.pdf

13. Centers for Medicare and Medicaid Services. *State Waivers List, 1915(c) Waiver Authority PA HCBW for Individuals Aged 60 & Over (0279.R04.00)*. https://www.medicaid.gov/medicaid/section-1115-demo/demonstration-and-waiver-list/waivers_faceted.html.

14. American Telemedicine Association. State Medicaid Best Practice: School-Based Telehealth. July 2013. http://www.americantelemed.org/main/policy-page/state-policy-resource-center/state-medicaid-best-practices

15. Baker LC, Johnson SJ, Macaulay D, Birnbaum H. Strategies to cut costs: integrated telehealth and care management. program for medicare beneficiaries with chronic disease linked to savings. *Health Aff (Millwood)* 2011;30(9):1689–1697.

16. Department of Health and Environment. Kansas Medical Assistance Program, Provider Manual, Home Health Agency, p. 33, January. 2013.

17. *Community Choices Waiver Billing Codes and Rates*. http://www.dhh.louisiana.gov/assets/docs/OAAS/publications/CommChoWaiverBillingCodesRates.pdf.

18. La. Stat. Ann. § 22:1821.

19. Colo. Rev. Stat. § 10-16-123.

20. Thomas L, Capistrant G. State Telemedicine Gaps Analysis: Coverage & Reimbursement. Washington (DC): American Telemedicine Association. January 2016. http://www.americantelemed.org/policy-page/state-telemedicine-gaps-reports.

21. Blackman K. Telehealth and licensing interstate providers. *NCSL Legisbrief* 2016;24(25):1–2.

Medicare Coverage and Reimbursement Policies

Gary Capistrant, MA

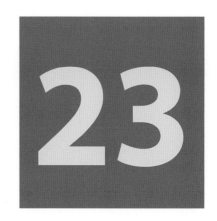

Medicare is the nation's largest payor for health care services—and often a leader in using the power of the purse to pursue innovations. However, with regard to telehealth (the term Medicare uses), Medicare greatly lags behind most payors in terms of coverage and openness. Medicare spending for telehealth in 2015 was merely *0.00003%* of total outlays.

Medicare is really two programs in one with roughly two-thirds of its beneficiaries in traditional volume-based or fee-for-service reimbursement and one-third in some variation of a value-based payment innovation. This is an important distinction for present telehealth because its coverage is often less restricted for value-based plans.

The shift is on, with the U.S. Department of Health and Human Services goals to have 50% of Medicare payments by value-based models and to adjust 90% of fee-for-service payments for quality or value, both by the end of 2018. This is an important trend for future telehealth because the shift to dramatically different provalue, antivolume incentives can provide a safer platform for telehealth use and innovation.

This area of Medicare and telehealth policy is expected to be much more dynamic than these HHS thresold percentages. Furthermore, momentum has been building in Congress for more fundamental and faster change, notably with a variety of legislative proposals on coverage and reimbursement.

COVERAGE

The terms coverage and reimbursement are often used interchangeably, in large part because both are often relatively comprehensive, consistent, and widespread. For telehealth, in contrast, Medicare coverage is relatively restrictive, and reimbursement has some oddities. This situation is largely because Medicare telehealth provisions reflect a snapshot of late 1990s best-use cases, when they were last significantly updated. There have been major increases, nevertheless, in the use of Medicare's essentially static coverage as reported recently by the Medicare Payment Advisory Commission[1] and shown in Figure 23-1.

The core provision in Medicare law about telehealth is Social Security Act section 1834(m)—also known as 42 U.S.C. 1395m(m)—and in regulation is 42 CFR 410.78 and 414.65.

The U.S. Centers for Medicare and Medicaid Services (CMS) defines telehealth services to include those services that require a face-to-face meeting with the patient via an interactive audio and video telecommunications system.[2]

Unfortunately, the hallmark of Medicare telehealth is how restrictive its coverage essentially is:

- No coverage for video-based services for about 80% of beneficiaries in metropolitan areas

- No coverage for video-based services to a beneficiary at home or locations other than a designated type of health establishment

- No coverage for some types of providers otherwise covered for in-person services, such as rehabilitation therapists

- No coverage of remote biometric monitoring of a beneficiary with one or more chronic conditions

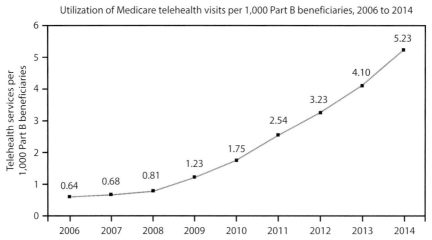

Utilization of Medicare telehealth visits per 1,000 Part B beneficiaries, 2006 to 2014

▲ **Figure 23-1.** Utilization of Medicare telehealth visits per 1,000 Part B beneficiaries, 2006 to 2014. (Source: MedPAC analysis of Medicare carrier file claims data. From Medicare Payment Advisory Commission. *June 2016 Report to the Congress: Medicare and the Health Care Delivery System*; 2016:240.)

- No coverage for "asynchronous" interpretations of visual medical information, such as an annual retinal scan of a beneficiary with diabetes or dermatological images
- Coverage is limited to Current Procedural Terminology (CPT) or Healthcare Common Procedure Coding System (HCPCS) procedure codes specified by the CMS and updated annually

On the positive side, CMS defines many of the most common uses of distant physicians as "physician services," not as telehealth. In part, the CMS definition includes services when a physician "is able to visualize some aspect of the patient's condition without the interposition of a third person's judgment." This is important for most of the remote interpretations of radiologists and clinical pathologists. This distinction is followed by most other payors.

These remote services are *not* considered "telehealth" or "telemedicine" by CMS. Rather, they are considered the same as services delivered in-person and are to be coded and will be paid in the same way. There are no geographic or facility limitations on these services.

Special CPT codes are used for the remote assessment of pacemakers as well as the collection and assessment of data from cardiac event recorders.

► Locations

For telehealth coverage, a beneficiary must be in a "rural" area and at a designated health facility (a so-called originating site). A rural area is basically a county outside of a standard metropolitan statistical area (MSA) or in a medically underserved census tract in the low-population-density fringes of a metropolitan area.

The originating site must be one of the following:

- The office of a physician or practitioner
- A hospital, including a critical access hospital
- A rural health clinic
- A federally qualified health center
- A skilled nursing facility
- A hospital-based dialysis center
- A community mental health center

It is important to note that for coverage purposes, the beneficiary may not be at their home or other common nonhealth locations.

There is no limitation on the location of the health professional delivering the medical service (the so-called distant site).

Services

Medicare telehealth coverage is further limited by provider and procedure.

The following health professionals may claim reimbursement for some telehealth services:

- Physician
- Nurse practitioner
- Physician assistant
- Nurse midwife
- Clinical nurse specialist
- Clinical psychologist
- Clinical social worker
- Registered dietitian or nutrition professional

The major health professional categories otherwise covered for in-person services but not telehealth services are rehabilitation therapists (physical, occupational, speech and hearing, and respiratory).

Medicare law has been a long-standing role model for payors in not requiring a "telepresenter" (a second provider) to be with the patient. (Having a telepresenter is left to the professional judgement of the remote treating provider.)

Medicare is one of the shrinking number of payors who limits coverage by procedure code (the CPT codes established by the American Medical Association of the HCPCS codes established by CMS). For 2016, Medicare covers 82 CPT or HCPCS codes for telehealth.

The use of telehealth is concentrated in a few codes. The Medicare Payment Advisory Commission recently reported, "The most common types of telehealth services in 2014 were evaluation and management (E&M) or other outpatient visits and psychiatric visits (individual psychotherapy and psychiatric diagnostic interview examinations)."[3] More detailed MedPAC analysis of utilization by type of service is shown in Table 23-1.

Cardiac Monitoring

Medicare also covers two types of cardiac monitoring:

- Transtelephonic monitoring of cardiac pacemakers (CPT code 93293) is for identifying early signs of possible pacemaker failure, thus reducing the number of sudden pacemaker failures requiring emergency replacement.

- Ambulatory electrocardiography (AECG) refers to services rendered in an outpatient setting over a

Table 23-1. Frequency of Telehealth Visits at Distant Sites by Service Type, 2014

Type of service	Number of visits	Share of visits
Evaluation and management visits	115,430	66.0%
Individual psychotherapy	19,914	11.4
Psychiatric diagnostic interview examination	12,952	7.4
Follow-up inpatient telehealth consultations	7,642	4.4
Telehealth consultations, emergency department or initial outpatient	7,626	4.4
Subsequent hospital care services	4,902	2.8
Subsequent nursing care services	3,341	1.9
Pharmacological management	1,766	1.0
End-stage renal disease–related services	1,078	0.6
Other	347	0.2
Total	174,998	100.0

Note: Components may not sum to totals due to rounding.

Source: CMS carrier file. From Medicare Payment Advisory Commission. *June 2016 Report to the Congress: Medicare and the Health Care Delivery System*; 2016:241.

specified period, generally while a patient is engaged in daily activities. AECG devices are intended to provide the physician with documented episodes of arrhythmia, which may not be detected using a standard ECG. AECG is most typically used to evaluate symptoms that may correlate with intermittent cardiac arrhythmias and/or myocardial ischemia. The AECG are both patient/event-activated and continuous recorders and use CPT codes 93271 and 93012. These services are performed by independent diagnostic testing facilities (IDTFs).

▶ National and Local Coverage Determinations

In addition, national and local coverage determinations may alter or expand the services that are eligible for reimbursement. Certain national coverage determinations by CMS have further expanded and explained coverage, such as the cardiac monitoring just discussed. Local intermediaries are allowed to make their own local determinations regarding covered services which may further expand coverage. For example, the Arkansas Blue Cross Blue Shield – Rhode Island intermediary has a ruling titled "Transtelephonic Spirometry," where patient-initiated spirometric recordings per 30-day period of time, including reinforced education, transmission of spirometric tracing, data capture, analysis of transmitted data, periodic recalibration, and physician review and interpretation, are covered.

▶ Claims Submission

Claims for professional consultations, office visits, individual psychotherapy, and pharmacologic management provided via a telecommunications system are submitted to the carrier that processes claims for the performing physician/practitioner's service area. Physicians/practitioners submit the appropriate CPT procedure code for covered professional telehealth services along with the 95 (formerly GT) modifier ("via interactive audio and video telecommunications system"). By coding and billing the 95 modifier with a covered telehealth procedure code, the distant site physician/practitioner certifies that the beneficiary was present at an eligible originating site when the telehealth service was furnished.

Physicians and practitioners at the distant site bill their local Medicare carrier for covered telehealth services, for example, 99245 GT. CMS has also established that the "place of service" code to be used for all telehealth services is now "02." Of more consequence for telehealth providers, CMS recently decided to pay all using the "practice expense" factors for facilities, which are lower or equal to the factors for non-facility providers.

Physicians' and practitioners' offices serving as a telehealth originating site bill their local Medicare carrier for the originating site facility fee. To claim an originating site fee, physicians/practitioners bill HCPCS code "Q3014, telehealth originating site facility fee"—short description "telehealth facility fee." The type of service for the telehealth originating site facility fee is "9, other items and services." For carrier-processed claims, the "office" place of service (code 11) is the only payable setting for code Q3014. There is no participation payment differential for code Q3014, and it is not priced off of the Medicare Physician Fee Schedule Database file. Deductible and coinsurance rules apply to Q3014. By submitting HCPCS code "Q3014," the biller certifies that the originating site is located in either a rural health professional shortage area (HPSA) or a non-MSA county.

REIMBURSEMENT

With two sites involved in a telehealth encounter, under fee-for-service reimbursement Medicare pays the remote treating physician or practitioner according to the Part B fee schedule (in other words, the same reimbursement as for the in-person way). Same service, same standards, same pay. To compensate the patient ("originating") site for their related costs, a nationwide flat fee—an "originating site facility fee"—is paid. To get paid, both sites must file.

Far-reaching changes be from implementation of the Medicare Access and CHIP Reauthorization Act of 2015 (MACRA)—the law replacing the "sustainable growth rate" limit on physician and practitioner spending under Part B. MACRA creates two major paths for reimbursement:

- Merit-Based Incentive Payment System (MIPS)
- Alternative Payment Models (APMs)

Merit-Based Incentive Payment System

MIPS is the traditional fee-for-service method combined with parts of several incentive programs in which physicians and practitioners will be measured based on:

- Quality
- Resource use
- Clinical practice improvement
- Meaningful use of certified electronic health record (EHR) technology

Physicians and practitioners will engage in new performance reporting, beginning as early as January 2017, to establish their payment adjustment for 2019. It will be important to allow telehealth-provided services as a patient-facing encounter for MIPS calculations and to consider added incentives for the use of telehealth to meet the Clinical Practice Improvement Activity goals.

Alternative Payment Models

APM is the new category label for what has been a variety of value-based payment innovations. Accountable care organizations (ACOs) and bundled payment models are some examples of APMs. Annually, CMS will identify models qualifying for APM and advanced APM incentives.

Next Generation Accountable Care Organizations

The Affordable Care Act created a Medicare shared savings program that "promotes accountability for a patient population and coordinates items and services under parts A and B, and encourages investment in infrastructure and redesigned care processes for high quality and efficient service delivery" for the beneficiaries in a selected geographic area. The overseeing group of providers and suppliers is known as an ACO.

CMS allows several ACO models, including next-generation telehealth coverage for all Medicare beneficiaries, and the patient may originate a telehealth-provided service from any patient setting, including their home. As of June 2017, 45 Next Generation ACOs were in service. Another round of applicants is under review.

Bundled Payment for Episodes of Care

Another Affordable Care Act provision is for a bundled payment for integrated hospitalization and post-acute care for an episode. The Center for Medicare and Medicaid Innovation (CMMI) began implementation of an Affordable Care Act provision for bundled payment innovation with four models. For Model 3: Retrospective Post-Acute Care Only, CMMI waived the telehealth restriction to serve only rural beneficiaries.

In April 2016, CMS began an expanded bundled program for knee or hip replacement episodes. (In 2014, more than 400,000 Medicare beneficiaries had a hip or knee replacement.) For this Comprehensive Care for Joint Replacement (CJR) model, CMS allows telehealth coverage for all Medicare beneficiaries, and the patient may originate their telehealth-provided service from any location, including their home. CMS has implemented the CJR model in 67 geographic areas, defined by MSAs.

On July 2016, CMS proposed a bundled program for heart attack, cardiac bypass surgery, and surgical hip/femur fracture episodes with similar opportunities for telehealth. For the new cardiac bundles, hospitals in 98 randomly selected MSAs would be required to participate in the bundled care model.

MEDICARE ADVANTAGE

By far, the largest Medicare value-based payment arrangement is its managed care program under Part C, called Medicare Advantage, with over 17 million beneficiaries. An even more concentrated opportunity for creating value using telehealth is for the over 1 million in "special needs plans," serving specific high-acuity beneficiaries.

In keeping with the financial incentives of a fully risk-based per member, per month payment method, Medicare Advantage plans have full authority to offer extra telehealth coverage as a "supplemental" benefit. Some plans have chosen to add telehealth supplemental benefits, and other plans find that the CMS provisions about costs and payments for supplemental benefits act as a deterrent.

In February 2016, President Obama proposed in his federal budget that Congress legislate to expand the ability of Medicare Advantage organizations to deliver medical services via telehealth by eliminating otherwise applicable Part B requirements that certain covered services be provided exclusively through face-to-face encounters.

In August 2016, CMS announced some opportunities for telehealth with an expansion of the Medicare Advantage Value-Based Insurance Design (MA-VBID) model. The MA-VBID model is an opportunity for some Medicare Advantage plans to offer "clinically nuanced" benefit packages only to targeted populations. Such benefits may include any service currently permitted under existing Medicare Advantage rules for supplemental benefits, such as physician consultations via audio and video technologies for people with diabetes or supplemental tobacco cessation assistance for enrollees with chronic obstructive pulmonary disease (COPD).

REFERENCES

1. Medicare Payment Advisory Commission. *June 2016 Report to the Congress: Medicare and the Health Care Delivery System, Chapter 8: Telehealth services and the Medicare program.* http://www.medpac.gov/docs/default-source/reports/chapter-8-telehealth-services-and-the-medicare-program-june-2016-report-.pdf.

2. Centers for Medicare and Medicaid Services. *Telehealth Services, ICN 901705.* December 2015. https://www.cms.gov/Outreach-and-Education/Medicare-Learning-Network-MLN/MLNProducts/downloads/telehealthsrvcsfctsht.pdf.

3. Medicare Payment Advisory Commission. op. cit., p. 240.

Legal and Regulatory Issues

Nathaniel M. Lacktman, JD, CCEP

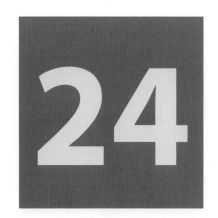

INTRODUCTION

▶ The Practice of Medicine via Telehealth Technologies

The practice of medicine via telehealth carries with it myriad opportunities as well as unique challenges. One area of particular attention is legal and regulatory compliance. No longer may health care providers follow only the law of their single "home" state as they expand to offer services to patients located across the country and the world. Just as telehealth requires its own tailored clinical approaches, so, too, does it require specific legal solutions and business structures designed to fully harness the promise of telehealth while remaining compliant with the complex universe of state and federal laws. This chapter addresses some of the key legal and regulatory issues in telehealth.

Telehealth and State Licensing

It is widely understood and accepted that in order to practice medicine, an individual must have a license. Licensing is a state law issue, and medical boards have jurisdiction over physician licensing. For telehealth services, licensing rules and applicable state medical practice laws are based not on the location of the physician, but rather the location of the patient at the time of the consult. For example, a physician licensed in New York and providing telehealth services to a patient located in Florida must have a license to practice medicine in Florida (or otherwise meet a licensure exception).

With the development of telehealth practices sweeping across geographic boundaries, licensure has become more of an impediment than it has been in the past. Patients want access to the best specialists, regardless of where they are located. They already have the technology to receive those consults. However, licensure remains a requirement and, for many, an administrative burden (although not insurmountable).

Attempts are underway to help streamline medical licensing. The most notable is the Federation of State Medical Board's Interstate Licensing Compact. This offers a uniform, fast-track option for a physician to obtain multiple licenses in the participating compact states. Thus far (October 2016), 17 states have passed laws to join the compact. States also offer a number of exceptions to licensure, allowing a doctor licensed in one state to deliver care (typically on a limited basis) to patients in the state where the doctor is not licensed. Some exceptions include medical emergencies and disasters, neighboring/border states, follow-up care, free "curbside" informal consults, and peer-to-peer consultations. Although certain exceptions exist in every state, they vary significantly, and providers should carefully understand the requirements or else risk unlicensed practice of medicine.

Telehealth and the Standard of Care

Fundamental to the practice of medicine, whether in person or via telehealth, is to meet the standard of care and deliver high-quality services. To that end, providers should adhere to the same standard of care in telehealth settings as they would when delivering care in person. Thus, labs, vitals, physicals, and any other information obtained in the in-person setting should be obtained when delivering care via telehealth.

Indeed, nearly every state expressly or implicitly holds that treatment recommendations made via telehealth, including issuing a prescription via electronic means, are held to the same standards of appropriate practice as those in traditional in-person settings. Although not every state requires real-time audio-video telehealth, the majority have laws stating that issuing a prescription based solely on an online questionnaire does not constitute an acceptable standard of care.

Telehealth Practice Standards

A number of states have promulgated telehealth practice standards. Not to be confused with the standard of care or scope of practice, telehealth practice standards are largely arbitrary rules and requirements providers must follow when practicing medicine via telehealth and often do not apply to in-person care. Examples of practice standards include patient informed consent to telehealth services, specific disclosures on the provider's website, mandatory forwarding of the patient's medical records to the patient's other caregivers, restrictions on the type of telehealth technology/modality that can be used, and requirements for in-person examinations. These practice standards may be well intended, but they often restrict the ability of providers to innovate in health care delivery. Moreover, it is entirely possible to meet every telehealth practice standard, yet fail to deliver services in accordance with the standard of care (and vice versa). Nonetheless, providers must understand and adhere to state practice standards, as failing to do so can expose them to board of medicine sanctions.

Remote Prescribing of Drugs and Controlled Substances

State Laws

The majority of states permit a physician to prescribe medication following a telehealth examination (also known as remote prescribing). In general, prescribing must occur in connection with a valid doctor–patient relationship, although some states offer narrow exceptions for situations such as cross-coverage and emergencies. There is always a risk that a board of medicine could sanction a physician for prescribing drugs without conducting an appropriate examination (in-person or otherwise), but that risk is based primarily on the clinical situation of the specific patient and whether or not the physician conducted an examination sufficient to meet the standard of care. All prescribing must be done for a legitimate medical purpose by a practitioner acting in the usual course of his or her professional practice. An arrangement where a provider conducts a real-time audio-video exam after reviewing the patient's lab results and medical records is widely considered a gold-standard approach to telehealth.[1] It might also involve an initial in-person exam of the patient, as appropriate, but a preference (or long-term approach) is to eliminate the need for an arbitrary in-person exam under state law.

Significant policy headway for remote prescribing has been achieved over the past five years, and the next frontier is remote prescribing of controlled substances. This is a more complex legal issue, as state laws tend to be more restrictive regarding controlled substances compared to other medications, and providers must navigate overlapping state medical practice laws, pharmacy board laws, state controlled substance diversion laws, and federal laws and regulations under the Drug Enforcement Agency (DEA). In some states, an in-person examination is not necessarily a prerequisite to prescribe controlled substances. In those states, a physician may create a valid doctor–patient relationship, conduct an examination of the patient via telehealth, and issue a prescription. A prescribing physician must review and comply with both state and federal laws, and federal laws supersede state law unless state law is more restrictive.

Federal Laws and the Federal Ryan Haight Act

The current federal regulations on remote prescribing of controlled substances are more restrictive than many state laws. The Ryan Haight Online Pharmacy Consumer Protection Act of 2008 (Ryan Haight Act) amended the federal Controlled Substances Act by adding a series of new regulatory requirements and criminal provisions designed to combat the proliferation of so-called "rogue Internet sites" that unlawfully dispensed controlled substances by means of the Internet. The act was enacted on

October 15, 2008, and became effective April 13, 2009. The DEA issued regulations effective that same date.[2]

The Ryan Haight Act prohibits distributing, dispensing, or delivery of controlled substances by means of the "Internet" (a broadly defined term) without a valid prescription.[3] The act, for the first time, imposed a federal in-person physical examination requirement by the prescribing practitioner, to be conducted prior to the first prescription. The act essentially constitutes a nationwide prohibition on form-only online prescribing (medical records–based prescribing) for controlled substances. Although the act was intended to target "rogue" Internet pharmacies, the broad language requires legitimate telehealth providers who engage in remote prescribing of controlled substances to review the regulations to ensure compliance. The provisions of the act do not apply to remote prescribing of any and all prescription drugs—only controlled substances.

A prescription for a controlled substance is not valid or effective unless it is issued for a legitimate medical purpose by an individual practitioner acting in the usual course of his professional practice.[4] Federal regulations require the physician to have a license to practice medicine in the state where the patient is located at the time of the consult. The responsibility for the proper prescribing and dispensing of controlled substances is on the prescribing practitioner. A physician who engages in the unauthorized practice of medicine under state law is not acting in the usual course of his or her professional practice and thus violates federal law.[5]

With respect to telehealth practices and remote prescribing, no controlled substance may be delivered, distributed, or dispensed by means of the Internet without a valid prescription.[6] The term "valid prescription" means a prescription that is issued for a legitimate medical purpose in the usual course of professional practice by 1) a practitioner who has conducted at least one in-person medical evaluation of the patient or 2) a covering practitioner.[7] The term "in-person medical evaluation" means a medical evaluation that is conducted with the patient in the physical presence of the practitioner, without regard to whether portions of the evaluation are conducted by other health professionals.[8] Once the prescribing practitioner has conducted an in-person medical evaluation, the regulation does not set an expiration period or a requirement for subsequent annual examinations.

The regulations offer seven "telemedicine" exceptions to the in-person exam requirement, but they are very narrow and do not reflect contemporary accepted clinical telehealth remote prescribing practices.[9] They are:

1. The patient is being treated in a DEA-registered hospital or clinic.

2. The patient is being treated in the physical presence of a DEA-registered practitioner.

3. The telemedicine consult is conducted by a DEA-registered practitioner for the Indian Health Service and who is designated as an Internet Eligible Controlled Substances Provider by the DEA.

4. The telemedicine consult is conducted during a public health emergency declared by the Secretary of the U.S. Department of Health and Human Services (HHS).

5. The telemedicine consult is conducted by a practitioner who has obtained a DEA special registration for telemedicine.

6. The telemedicine consult is conducted by a Veterans Health Administration (VHA) practitioner during a medical emergency recognized by the VHA.

7. The telemedicine consult is conducted under other circumstances specified by future DEA regulations.

Some of the exceptions, on their face, are of limited use to most providers (eg, VHA, public health emergency, Indian tribal organization). One exception requires a patient-side telepresenter also registered with the DEA (and presumably independently able to prescribe controlled substances for the patient). Another exception allows the physician to prescribe controlled substances without an in-person evaluation if (1) the patient is treated by and physically located in a hospital or clinic that has a valid DEA registration and (2) the telemedicine practitioner is treating the patient in the usual course of professional practice, in accordance with state law, and with a valid DEA registration (this registration must also be in the state where the patient is located). The DEA announced plans to draft a proposed rule that will create a special registration process allowing physicians to remotely prescribe controlled substances without an in-person exam. The proposed rule is expected to be published in January 2017.[10]

Managing Telehealth Tort Liability

Tort liability for telehealth is rooted in negligence (a breach of duty in the doctor–patient relationship) and is generally a state-law issue. As a general rule, states allow a patient to bring a malpractice claim in the courts of their resident state against a nonresident provider who practices telehealth in the patient's state. Although malpractice claims have been brought against providers for many years, much less is known of telehealth lawsuits compared to those arising in an in-person setting because only a fraction of the total malpractice claims involve telehealth. Moreover, the majority of malpractice claims (telehealth or otherwise) are resolved via confidential settlement agreements and are not reported in public court records.

A direct-to-patient model for telehealth services would need to create a valid doctor–patient relationship as a predicate for the medical services provided to the patient. To that end, telehealth providers should take steps to clarify and document the scope of services and the doctor–patient relationship. Providers should also consider including disclaimers and acknowledgements in the terms of use agreement signed by the patient when utilizing the telehealth services. Other steps taken by some telehealth companies to manage tort liability are as follows:

- Regularly poll patients to assess their satisfaction levels with the telehealth services, including the level of responsiveness and attention provided by the medical professionals. If a particular professional receives more than his or her share of complaints, it could be an indication of risk, as professionals who leave patients dissatisfied may be more frequent targets of malpractice complaints.

- A provider might require in its contracts/employment agreements with its professionals that each professional notify the provider group within three days of any complaints or requests for records from a patient or their legal representative.

- Providers should take the time to understand and follow the applicable laws and guidance (including but not limited to licensing, scope of practice, and fraud and abuse) in each state where the provider group offers telehealth services.

- Provide services only in states where the group's professionals are licensed/registered.

- Providers should understand and incorporate industry practice guidelines and standards as appropriate, such as the practice guidelines published by the American Telemedicine Association.

- Providers should allow sufficient information, resources, etc., for telehealth consults to be provided in accordance with accepted standards of care and clinical practice.

- Providers should document patient understanding of terms of use, limitations, and associated conditions.

- Providers should understand and follow the requirements and rules for telehealth informed consent in each state where the provider offers services.

Telehealth Malpractice Insurance Coverage

Many malpractice insurers have provisions in their agreements that provide malpractice coverage for telehealth services. Others expressly exclude it unless the covered entity affirmatively requests it be added. Some insurers retain the right to selectively deny coverage. Common reasons for selective denial of coverage include 1) the patient or service provided is not located in a state where the insurance company is licensed; 2) the provider/exposure presents an above-average risk; or 3) the coverage disallows telehealth direct patient care, but does allow peer-to-peer consultations. Ultimately, malpractice insurance is regulated at the state level, and this is not always compatible with multistate telehealth practices.

Some malpractice policies only cover encounters within the state in which the provider practices and is licensed. Consequently, providers who offer telehealth services to patients in states in which they are unlicensed risk uninsured claims under the terms of the carrier's policy. Moreover, some carriers assert they are only required to cover claims against providers when the provider is performing health care services in the state where the carrier contractually agreed to cover the provider. Some carriers also offer separate policies (or add-ons) if the telehealth service is only interpretive (eg, telepathology, teleradiology) in a peer-to-peer consultation setting and not a direct-to-patient model.

A provider can take certain steps to better guarantee it will have meaningful malpractice insurance coverage for its telehealth-based physician services:

- Select a carrier that offers a well-defined and thoughtful telehealth malpractice coverage product.

- Verify the malpractice carrier is licensed as an insurer in all the states where the provider group wants to provide telehealth services (ie, where the patients are located).

- Verify the malpractice policy itself extends coverage to all the states (and countries, if international) where the provider group wants to provide services.

- Obtain written assurances from the carrier that the malpractice liability insurance policy covers telehealth malpractice lawsuits.

- Verify the policy includes coverage for claims brought by a patient's estate.

- Verify the policy includes coverage for claims brought by a state licensing board or state department of health against the provider for standard of care and regulatory compliance issues.

- Determine if the policy is occurrence based rather than claims made, so tail coverage is included in the policy premium (if that is desired).

- In general, many providers are experiencing premiums for telehealth services at far lower costs than premiums for in-person services. The incidence of claims filed has been low, and the insurance premium price reflects that. Providers should be able to negotiate competitive rates for telehealth coverage.

▶ Other Laws and Regulations for Telehealth Providers

Corporate Law Issues and the Practice of Medicine

When building a direct-to-consumer telehealth service, one of the fundamental areas to address is the planned geographic footprint of the offering. Many practitioners are comfortable and experienced in creating a provider group within their home state, but telehealth providers routinely seek to avail themselves of the advantage that their patient base can be nationwide or even global. No longer is the provider's patient footprint limited to the zip codes surrounding their brick-and-mortar location. However, this means the provider will be subject to, and must comply with, the laws of all states in which it delivers services.

When preparing the provider's corporate documents, an initial issue to address is the prohibition on the corporate practice of medicine. Generally, the prohibition on the corporate practice of medicine prevents an entity from delivering medical services or employing physicians if the entity is owned by lay persons (ie, nonphysicians). This is a state law issue, and some states have no prohibition on the corporate practice of medicine. Some states with a notable enforcement history regarding the prohibition on the corporate practice of medicine include California, Colorado, New Jersey, New York, Tennessee, and Texas. Some states offer certain exemptions from this rule for hospitals, charitable foundations, and the like. For example, Florida law allows a lay person to own a medical group if the group successfully completes a site survey and obtains a Health Care Clinic license.[11]

When deploying a national direct-to-consumer telehealth offering, scalability is key. Maximizing the homogeneity of the provider's operations, processes, and corporate functions enables the provider to realize efficiencies and cost savings.

One approach gaining traction among telehealth provider groups is the use of a "friendly PC" arrangement. This is a particularly attractive option for telehealth providers founded by nonphysicians or that plan to seek external capital funding resulting in lay ownership. The friendly PC model frequently involves two entities: an investor-owned management services organization (MSO) and a professional corporation owned by a single physician owner (the PC or medical group). The MSO and the PC have a management services agreement under which the MSO provides certain services to the PC, and the PC in turn compensates the MSO. The compensation methodology under the management services agreement must also comply with state law on fee splitting, all payor antikickback statutes, and patient brokering laws.

Simply because a physician owner is licensed to practice medicine in one state does not mean that the physician can own a medical group in another state. Indeed, more than half the states require the owner of a medical group to hold a license to practice medicine in that state. Thus, a direct-to-consumer medical group seeking to provide services across all 50 states will need to have a physician owner licensed in many of those states or use an otherwise legally compliant approach.

In addition to medical board rules regarding physician ownership and corporate practice of medicine, legal counsel must know the corporate law and entity creation rules of every state where the telehealth provider plans to do business. Whereas some states allow a foreign PC to qualify to do business as a foreign corporation, other states do not.

Federal Fraud and Abuse Laws

Telehealth arrangements involving any federal health care program dollars (eg, Medicare, Medicaid) must comply with applicable federal fraud and abuse laws, including the Stark Law and the Anti-Kickback Statute.[12]

The Stark Law prohibits a physician (or immediate family member) from referring Medicare/Medicaid patients for certain designated health services (DHS) to entities with which the physician (or immediate family member) has a financial relationship, unless the arrangement meets a specific exception under the law.[13] If a telehealth arrangement or contract is subject to the Stark Law, it must meet an exception, as the Stark Law is a strict liability statute.

The federal Anti-Kickback Statute makes it a criminal offense to knowingly and willfully offer, pay, solicit, or receive any remuneration to induce referrals of items or services reimbursable by federal health care programs.[14] The term "remuneration" includes the transfer of anything of value, in cash or in kind, directly or indirectly, covertly or overtly.[15] The Anti-Kickback Statute has been interpreted to cover any arrangement where one purpose of the remuneration was to obtain money for the referral of services or to induce further referrals.[16] Violation of the Anti-Kickback Statute can also trigger false claims liability for the purposes of the federal False Claims Act. The statute ascribes criminal liability to parties on both sides of an impermissible "kickback" transaction. Violation of the Anti-Kickback Statute constitutes a felony punishable by a maximum fine of $25,000, imprisonment up to five years, or both. Conviction will also lead to automatic exclusion from federal health care programs, including Medicare and Medicaid.

If a telehealth arrangement potentially implicates the Anti-Kickback Statute, the parties should see if the contract can be structured to fit within an applicable safe harbor. The safe harbor regulations define practices that are not subject to the Anti-Kickback Statute because such practices would be unlikely to result in fraud or abuse.[17] The safe harbors include specific conditions that, if met, assure the parties will not be prosecuted or sanctioned for the arrangement. Safe harbor protection is afforded only to those arrangements that precisely meet all of the conditions in the specific safe harbor.

An arrangement that does not meet a safe harbor is not necessarily unlawful or illegal. Such arrangements require a detailed examination of the surrounding factual background and intent of the parties. Generally, the closer an arrangement can be structured to mirror as many possible elements of a safe harbor, the better. In addition, parties oftentimes build additional safeguards into the arrangement, designed to reduce the risk of fraud and abuse and the likelihood of an enforcement action.[18]

State Antikickback, Fee Splitting, and Patient Brokering Laws

As of October 2016, 29 states have all-payor antikickback statutes (sometimes known as "patient brokering statutes"), which function like the federal Anti-Kickback Statute but apply no matter the source of payment (eg, commercial insurance, self-pay, cash). Four additional states have such statutes applicable to commercial insurers but not cash payment. The primary purpose of these statutes is to prohibit payments for referrals of patients or health care items or services. This means a telehealth provider cannot simply avoid antikickback issues by not accepting Medicare or Medicaid dollars.

For example, the Florida Patient Brokering Act prohibits "any person, including any health care provider or health care facility to offer or pay any commission, bonus, rebate, kickback, or bribe, directly or indirectly, in cash or in kind, or engage in any split-fee arrangement, in any form whatsoever, to induce the referral of patients or patronage to or from a health care provider or health care facility." Similarly, the act prohibits anyone from "[s]olicit[ing] or receive[ing] any commission, bonus, rebate, kickback, or bribe, directly or indirectly, in cash or in kind, or engag[ing] in any split-fee arrangement, in any form whatsoever, in return for referring patients or patronage to or from a health care provider or health care facility." Unlike its federal counterpart, the Patient Brokering Act applies no matter the source of payment. This means that even if no federal health care program dollars are involved, the Patient Brokering Act can still apply. However, if a discount, payment, waiver of payment, or payment practice is not prohibited under the federal Anti-Kickback Statute, the practice does not violate the Patient Brokering Act.

Compared to the Office of Inspector General's (OIG) enforcement of the federal Anti-Kickback Statute, state all-payor antikickback statutes are not as frequently enforced by state regulators and attorneys general. However, despite the relative lack of state government enforcement of these laws, a trend is gaining traction wherein commercial health plans are using these laws as grounds to file commercial unfair trade practices suits against providers who have been paid claims by the insurer when those claims have been generated by practices or arrangements violating state patient brokering laws.

Privacy and Security

Whether delivering care in person or via telehealth, health care providers must adhere to federal and state laws regarding privacy and security of patient health care information. Complying with these laws can present a set of challenges when much of the care is electronic and data are stored in the cloud. Providers should have policies and procedures to comply with Health Insurance Portability and Accountability Act (HIPAA), state law, and potential cybersecurity threats. These issues are not unique to telehealth providers, and there are solutions and legal approaches to better ensure compliance in multistate or international medical practices.

Online Telehealth Services and Federal Communications Commission Rules

Telehealth providers using online platforms and apps to communicate directly with patients must also be cognizant of and comply with laws regarding phone communications and online services. Among these are the need to use properly structured patient consents and agreements with valid e-sign capability, appropriate terms of use (for patients and providers using the telehealth platform), and an online privacy policy properly tailored to the provider's actual privacy practices. With the proliferation of patient direct communications, alerts, and pings, the Federal Communications Commission (FCC) and the Telephone Consumer Protection Act (TCPA) comes into play for online medical service companies.[19]

The TCPA not only restricts telemarketing calls, automatic telephone dialing systems, and prerecorded voice messages, but restricts text messages as well. The law was implemented in 1992, but was revised in 2012 to create additional customer protections, including the requirement to obtain express written consent from the customer.

The good news for telehealth providers is the TCPA contains a health care exception. Health care providers can send prerecorded voice and text messages, without the patient's prior express consent, in order to convey important "health care messages." These exemptions include health care messages relating to appointments and exams, confirmations and reminders, wellness checkups, hospital pre-registration instructions, preoperative instructions, lab results, postdischarge follow-up intended to prevent readmission, prescription notifications, and home health care instructions. However, even when delivering the exempt health care messages, providers must still abide by various technical requirements in order to comply with the TCPA. For example, calls and messages are strictly limited to the purposes permitted earlier; must not include any telemarketing, solicitation, or advertising; may not include accounting, billing, debt collection, or other financial content; and must comply with HIPAA privacy rules.

Subscription Fee Models and Insurance Laws

An emerging area of interest among direct-to-consumer telehealth offerings is the use of a subscription model. Under this model, the patient pays a monthly fee (eg, $99/month) in exchange for unlimited telehealth consults. This is an alternative to the traditional fee-for-service or encounter-based payment. The subscription can cover an individual or a family. A subscription offering can be quite attractive to patients and constitute a source of recurring revenue for the provider. However, it is not without its own legal and regulatory issues.

One issue for subscription models is the risk the telehealth provider would be deemed to be offering health insurance by state insurance regulators. The business of insurance is broadly defined under state laws and typically means the assumption of risk from a number of consumers and the distribution of risk across those consumers. One type of risk is "utilization risk"—the risk that consumers will use more telehealth consults than their $99/month subscription fee actually pays for. This is the primary risk insured against by traditional health insurance (and the reason insurance companies have monetary capitalization requirements based on their number of members). State insurance regulators police businesses that could be providing insurance without appropriate licensure, both in response to consumer or competitor complaints and on their own initiative. A subscription model for telehealth services should be assessed to avoid the risk of it being deemed a small-scale health insurance offering.

For example, Florida Statutes Section 624.02 defines "insurance" as "a contract whereby one undertakes to indemnify another or pay or allow a specified amount or a determinable benefit upon determinable contingencies." The case, *Liberty Care Plan v. Dep't of Insurance* (710 So.2d 202 (Fla. App. 1998)), addressed the question of whether Liberty's product met the definition of insurance under Florida law. Liberty sold a membership that entitled members to purchase home health care services at a discount of approximately 50% from the market price for such services in Florida at the time. The court found that the membership was insurance, writing: "The Plan is a contract whereby appellant undertakes to allow a determinable benefit (i.e., home health care services at discount rates) upon a determinable contingency (i.e., the member's exercise of the option to purchase these home health care services at discount rates)."

Compare Florida's statute to Texas law, which enacted a "direct primary care" statute in 2015 expressly permitting such subscription arrangements and holding them outside the definition of insurance.[20] The provisions of this law exempt direct primary care (including maintenance of mental health) from regulation as insurance. Although the law specifically applies to physicians, it is silent regarding other health care professionals. Other states have enacted these "direct primary care" statutes, including, for example, Kansas, Washington, and Utah.

▶ Hospital Telehealth Credentialing and Privileging

Centers for Medicare & Medicaid Services (CMS) Conditions of Participation and Joint Commission Standards require hospitals to have a credentialing and privileging process for physicians and practitioners providing services to the hospital's patients, including those who provide services via telehealth. Federal regulations offer a process for streamlined credentialing of telehealth practitioners.[21] This process is commonly referred to as "credentialing by proxy." It permits the hospital receiving the telehealth services (known as the "originating site" hospital) to rely on the privileging and credentialing decisions made by the hospital or entity providing the telehealth services (known as the "distant site" hospital or "distant site telemedicine entity," respectively), provided certain requirements are met.

The originating site hospital can use credentialing by proxy when the telemedicine services are provided by a practitioner located at 1) a Medicare-participating distant site hospital or 2) another entity providing telemedicine services (a "distant site telemedicine entity" or "DSTE"). A DSTE is an entity that 1) provides telehealth services; 2) is not a Medicare-participating hospital; and 3) provides contracted services in a manner that enables the originating site hospital to meet all applicable Conditions of Participation, particularly those requirements related to the credentialing and privileging of telehealth practitioners.[22] A DSTE may be a physician group, a non–Medicare-participating hospital, or other nonhospital telehealth provider.[23] The DSTE rules are used when the provider of telehealth services is not a hospital.

In order to utilize credentialing by proxy, the originating site hospital must enter into a contract with the distant site hospital or DSTE, reflecting and confirming certain requirements (noted later).[24] The governing body of the originating site hospital always retains ultimate authority over privileging decisions regarding telehealth practitioners. The medical staff bylaws must include provisions for credentialing by proxy, and hospitals can consider using the opportunity to create a separate telemedicine staff classification if desired (with accompanying limits on telemedicine staff responsibilities and rights).

1. The distant site hospital or DSTE uses a credentialing and privileging program that meets or exceeds the Medicare standards hospitals have traditionally been required to use.

2. The individual practitioners providing services via telemedicine to the originating site hospital have been privileged at the distant site hospital or DSTE.

3. The distant site hospital or DSTE provides the originating site hospital with a list of the current privileges for the telemedicine practitioners.

4. The individual practitioners providing telemedicine services are licensed to practice in the state where the originating site hospital is located.

5. The originating site hospital periodically reviews the services provided to its patients by the telemedicine practitioners and reports this information to the distant site hospital or DSTE for use in performance evaluations. At a minimum, these reports must include all adverse events or complaints related to each telemedicine practitioner's services provided at the originating site hospital.

6. For contracts with DSTEs only, the agreement must also state the DSTE is a contractor of services to the originating site hospital, which furnishes contracted telemedicine services in a manner that permits the originating site hospital to comply with all applicable Conditions of Participation.

Credentialing by proxy requires the parties to share information regarding credentialing decisions, as well as periodic updates of practitioner reviews and assessments. Providers should be cognizant of state laws regarding peer review decisions, confidentiality, and practitioner disciplinary actions, as well as professional review activities under the federal Health Care Quality Improvement Act.[25] Even if a hospital enters into a credentialing by proxy agreement, it is not required to use that process for all (or any) telehealth practitioners. It retains the option to use the traditional credentialing process if desired. Moreover, depending on the nature of the telehealth service and the originating site hospital's bylaws, the distant site practitioner need not be credentialed at the originating site, as CMS recognizes there are certain situations when credentialing is not required. Providers should conduct a thoughtful assessment of any proposed telehealth arrangement to determine whether or not credentialing is necessary.

▶ Telehealth Payment Policy and Reimbursement

Medicare Coverage of Telehealth Services

Medicare does cover telehealth services, but is currently very limited, and the definitions and restrictions are established in statute by Congress.[26] For eligible telehealth services, the use of a telecommunications system is a substitute for an in-person encounter.

In general, Medicare imposes five conditions of coverage on telehealth services:

1. The beneficiary is located in a qualifying rural area at the time of the consult.

2. The beneficiary is located at one of eight qualifying facilities ("originating sites") at the time of the consult.

3. The telehealth services are provided by one of ten professionals eligible to furnish and receive Medicare payment for telehealth services ("distant site practitioners").

4. The beneficiary and distant site practitioner communicate via an interactive audio and video telecommunications system that permits real-time communication between the beneficiary and the distant site provider.

5. The CPT/HCPCS (Current Procedural Terminology/Healthcare Common Procedure Coding System) code for the service itself is named on the CY2016 (or current year) list of covered Medicare telehealth services.

In order to bill Medicare for telehealth services, the provider must fully comply with *each* of the telehealth requirements. If the telehealth arrangement does not meet each of these requirements, the service is statutorily noncovered, and the Medicare program will not pay for the service.[27] To certify each of these elements have been met, the distant site practitioner must add the GT modifier when billing the claim (the practitioner adds the GQ modifier for asynchronous services in Alaska and Hawaii).

Rural Geographic Restrictions

Under the Medicare conditions of payment for telehealth services, the patient must be located at a qualifying originating site (in a rural health care professional shortage area [HPSA] outside a metropolitan statistical area [MSA], or in a rural census tract, or a county outside of an MSA). This effectively renders facilities located in urban areas unable to qualify as an originating site and therefore ineligible for Medicare coverage of services to beneficiaries via telehealth. Entities participating in a federal telehealth demonstration project approved by or receiving funding from the Secretary of HHS as of December 31, 2000, qualify as originating sites regardless of geographic location. Such entities are not required to be in a rural HPSA or non-MSA. Recognizing the confusion and limitation this restriction has generated, HHS created a website where a beneficiary or provider can enter a zip code and determine whether or not the geographic location is potentially eligible for Medicare coverage of telehealth services. It is called the "Medicare Telehealth Payment Eligibility Analyzer" and is available at http://datawarehouse.hrsa.gov/tools/analyzers/geo/Telehealth.aspx.

Originating Site Restrictions

Not only must the beneficiary be located in a qualifying rural area at the time of the consult, the beneficiary must be located at one of eight qualifying originating sites. Eligible originating sites are:

- Offices of a physician or practitioner
- Hospitals
- Critical access hospitals
- Community mental health centers
- Skilled nursing facilities
- Rural health clinics
- Federally qualified health centers
- Hospital-based or critical access hospital (CAH)–based renal dialysis centers (including satellites)[28]

If a beneficiary receives telehealth services while at his or her home (Place of Service [POS] 12), those telehealth services are not covered by Medicare.[29] Many patients choose telehealth services for the convenience and access they offer as an alternative to driving to a practitioner's office and sitting in the waiting room. Accordingly, many telehealth offerings are built around making the services available to patients "on demand" at their home, workplace, or in the evenings. These services would not be covered by Medicare because a beneficiary located at home is not at one of the eight qualifying originating sites.

Eligible Distant Site Practitioners

Even if the first two requirements are met and the beneficiary is located at an eligible rural area and a qualifying originating site, the services themselves must be provided by a qualified distant site practitioner eligible to furnish and receive Medicare payment for telehealth services. Eligible distant site practitioners are:

- Physicians
- Nurse practitioners (NPs)
- Physician assistants (PAs)
- Nurse-midwives
- Clinical nurse specialists (CNSs)
- Certified registered nurse anesthetists
- Clinical psychologists (CPs) and clinical social workers (CSWs) (although CPs and CSWs cannot bill for psychiatric diagnostic interview examinations with medical services or medical evaluation and management services under Medicare)
- Registered dietitians or nutrition professionals[30]

This list of 10 eligible practitioners is defined by statute.[31] If a beneficiary receives telehealth services from a practitioner other than those listed here, the service is not covered by Medicare. Many patients enjoy telehealth services from other practitioners or specialty providers (eg, RNs, occupational therapists, physical therapists). Currently, services provided by such professionals would not be covered by Medicare because that distant site practitioner is not among the 10 listed types.

Eligible Telecommunications Technology

The Medicare coverage rules require the beneficiary and distant site practitioner to communicate via an interactive audio and video telecommunications system that permits real-time communication between the beneficiary and the distant site provider.[32] This means the practitioner may not use audio-only, store-and-forward, or other message-based communications if the services are to be covered by Medicare. There is a minor exception allowing asynchronous store-and-forward technology in federal telehealth demonstration programs in Alaska or Hawaii.

Eligible CPT/HCPCS Codes

Finally, the service itself must be listed among the eligible CPT/HCPCS codes CMS publishes each year as covered telehealth services. In CY2016, there are approximately 37 covered services (with approximately 50 associated codes). Unless a service is listed among the approved service codes for telehealth services, Medicare will not cover the service if provided via telehealth.[33]

The result of Medicare's restrictive telehealth law has been narrow coverage and few claims submitted. For example, in CY2015, Medicare paid a total of $17.6 million for telehealth service claims, compared to an overall $600 billion Medicare program budget. At the same time, patient demand for the convenience and access to care offered by telehealth services has created a willingness for patients (including Medicare beneficiaries) to self-pay out of pocket to enjoy the benefits of these new technologies.[34]

Medicaid Coverage of Telehealth Services

Medicaid coverage of telehealth services varies significantly across states, but almost every state Medicaid program offers some coverage of telehealth services. Highlights include the following:

- Forty-eight state Medicaid programs offer coverage for interactive live video telehealth services.

- Nine state Medicaid programs offer coverage of asynchronous (store-and-forward) telehealth services, not including states that only cover teleradiology.

- Sixteen state Medicaid programs offer coverage for remote patient monitoring.

- Thirty state Medicaid programs pay an additional transmission or facility fee when telehealth is used.

- Ten states impose some form of geographic requirement, restricting telehealth coverage to rural or underserved areas, or require a certain amount of distance between the originating site and the distant site.

- Twenty-three states impose originating site restrictions limiting coverage to when the patient is located at a specific list of facilities.[35]

Commercial Health Insurance Coverage of Telehealth Services

Currently, 31 states and the District of Columbia have enacted telehealth commercial insurance coverage laws, and bills are under development in several other states. These laws are generally referred to as "telehealth commercial payer statutes" or "telehealth parity statutes." They are designed to promote patient access to care via telehealth, whether the patient is in a rural area without specialist care or a busy metropolitan city without the time to leave work or the home and devote three or more hours to an in-person check-up in a crowded waiting room. There are significant variances across the 31 states, but two related but distinct concepts have emerged: telehealth coverage and telehealth payment parity.

Telehealth Commercial Coverage Laws

Telehealth coverage laws require health plans to cover services provided via telehealth to the same extent the plan already covers the services if provided through an in-person visit. The laws do not mandate the health plan provide entirely new service lines or specialties, and the scope of services in the enrollee's member benefit package remains unchanged. The only difference is that the patient can elect to see his or her doctor via telehealth rather than be compelled to drive to the doctor's waiting room for an in-person consult.

Telehealth coverage laws also frequently include language to protect patients from cost-shifting. They disallow health plans from imposing different deductibles, copayments, or maximum benefit caps for services provided via telehealth. Any deductibles, copayments, and benefit caps apply equally and identically whether the patient receives the care in-person or via telehealth. Such language prevents the patient from being saddled with higher copayments to access care via telehealth.

Some states, particularly those that have enacted telehealth coverage laws in the last few years, have elected to expand on telehealth coverage by also requiring health plans to cover remote patient monitoring. Remote patient monitoring includes a variety of patient oversight and communications devices, software, and processes to allow providers a greater ability to monitor patient care needs and immediately respond. States have taken this step because remote patient monitoring, by definition, is a virtual distance-based service and does not have an in-person equivalent that would likely already be found in a member's benefit package.

States that have enacted telehealth commercial insurance coverage laws as of October 2016 are:

1. Alaska
2. Arizona
3. Arkansas
4. California
5. Colorado
6. Connecticut
7. District of Columbia
8. Delaware
9. Georgia
10. Hawaii
11. Indiana
12. Kentucky
13. Louisiana
14. Maine
15. Missouri
16. Michigan
17. Minnesota
18. Mississippi
19. Missouri
20. Montana
21. Nevada
22. New Hampshire
23. New Mexico
24. New York
25. Oklahoma
26. Oregon
27. Rhode Island (effective Jan. 1, 2018)
28. Tennessee
29. Texas
30. Vermont
31. Virginia
32. Washington (effective Jan. 1, 2017)

Telehealth Payment Parity Laws

Telehealth payment parity enables providers for telehealth services to be reimbursed at the same or equivalent rate the health plan pays the provider when the service is provided in person. For example, assume a doctor's participation agreement with a health plan reimburses the doctor $100 for a patient exam. With a payment parity law, the health plan pays the doctor $100 whether he provides the service in person or via telehealth, so long as the doctor does not agree to accept a lower rate (or alternative payment model) for services provided via telehealth under the provider agreement. If the agreed-upon contract rate is $30 for the in-person service, it is also typically $30 for telehealth. Payment parity does not change the plan's existing utilization review processes. The doctor's services (whether in person or via telehealth) must still be of high quality, appropriately documented, and medically necessary in order to be paid.

Payment parity is, in part, a response to avoid the problem of health plans paying for telehealth services at only a percentage of the in-person rate or imposing restrictive conditions on telehealth. This situation currently exists in many states that enacted a telehealth coverage statute but failed to include payment parity language, including New York in 2016. The result: a telehealth payment statute that is largely useless after the fanfare of the legislation's signing ceremony. Payment parity is intended to level the field for providers to enter into meaningful negotiations with health plans as to how telehealth services are covered and paid.

Minnesota's telehealth insurance law includes both coverage and payment parity.[36] It states, in pertinent part, as follows:

- A health plan [...] **shall include** coverage for telemedicine benefits in the same manner as any other benefits covered under the policy, plan, or contract, and shall comply with the regulations of this section.

- A health carrier **shall not exclude** a service for coverage solely because the service is provided via telemedicine and is not provided through in-person consultation or contact between a licensed health care provider and a patient.

- A health carrier shall reimburse the distant site licensed health care provider for covered services delivered via telemedicine **on the same basis and at the same rate** as the health carrier would apply to those services if the services had been delivered in person by the distant site licensed health care provider.

- It is not a violation of this subdivision for a health carrier to include a deductible, co-payment, or coinsurance requirement for a health care service provided via telemedicine, provided that the deductible, co-payment, or coinsurance is not in addition to, and does not exceed, the deductible, co-payment, or coinsurance applicable if the same services were provided through in-person contact.

CONCLUSION

The multitude of federal and state laws and regulations can often intimidate new (and existing!) telehealth providers. However, scalable, efficient solutions are out there. A compliant telehealth arrangement frequently requires legal counsel with specific experience and expertise developing and creating these new arrangements and business models.

REFERENCES

1. Federation of State Medical Boards SMART Guidelines for Telehealth (2014).

2. See 21 CFR Part 1300, 1301, 1304, *et al.; see also* 74 FR 15596 (April 6, 2009).

3. 21 U.S.C. §829.

4. See 21 CFR 1306.04(a); 21 CFR 1306.03(a)(1) ("A prescription for a controlled substance may be issued only by an individual practitioner who is . . . authorized to prescribe controlled substances by the jurisdiction in which he is licensed to practice his profession.").

5. See, for example, *United States v. Moore*, 423 U.S. 122, 140-41 (1975).

6. 21 CFR 1306.09(a).

7. 21 CFR 1300.04(l)(1); 21 USC 829(e)(2)(A). The term "covering practitioner" means a practitioner who conducts a medical evaluation (other than an in-person medical evaluation) of the patient at the request of a practitioner who 1) has conducted at least one in-person medical evaluation of the patient or an evaluation of the patient through the practice of telemedicine, within the previous 24 months and 2) is temporarily unavailable to conduct the evaluation of the patient. *Id.* at 1300.04(b); 21 USC 829(e)(2)(C).

8. 21 CFR 1300.04(f); 21 USC 829(e)(2)(B).

9. 21 CFR 1300.04(i).

10. http://www.reginfo.gov/public/do/eAgendaViewRule?pubId=201604&RIN=1117-AB40.

11. See Florida Statutes Chapter 400, Part X.

12. Another related federal law is the Civil Monetary Penalties Law, which prohibits a provider from offering Medicare/Medicaid patients inducements to purchase or use that provider's services. 42 U.S.C. § 1320a-7a(a)(5).

13. 42 U.S.C. § 1395nn.

14. Section 1128B(b) of the Social Security Act. Violation of the federal Anti-Kickback Statute constitutes a felony punishable by a maximum fine of $25,000, imprisonment up to five years, or both. Conviction will also lead to automatic exclusion from federal health care programs, including Medicare and Medicaid. Where a party commits an act described in section 1128B(b) of the Social Security Act, OIG may initiate administrative proceedings to impose civil monetary penalties on such party under section 1128A(a)(7) of the Social Security Act. OIG may also initiate administrative proceedings to exclude such party from the federal health care programs under section 1128(b)(7) of the Social Security Act.

15. The federal Anti-Kickback Statute was amended by Section 6402(f) of the Patient Protection and Affordable Care Act ("ACA") enacted in March 2010 to provide that a person need not have actual knowledge of the statute or a specific intent to commit a violation thereof. Section 6402(f) of PPACA also amended the statute to provide that items or services resulting from a violation thereof constitute false claims for the purposes of the False Claims Act.

16. See, for example, *United States v. Borrasi*, 639 F.3d 774 (7th Cir. 2011); *United States v. McClatchey*, 217 F.3d 823 (10th Cir. 2000); *United States v. Davis*, 132 F.3d 1092 (5th Cir. 1998); *United States v. Kats*, 871 F.2d 105 (9th Cir. 1989); *United States v. Greber*, 760 F.2d 68 (3d Cir. 1985), *cert. denied*, 474 U.S. 988 (1985).

17. See 42 C.F.R. § 1001.952.

18. See, for example, OIG Advisory Opinions No. 98-18, 99-14, 04-07, and 11-12.

19. 47 U.S.C. § 227.

20. See Tex. Occ. Code § 162.251 *et seq*.

21. 76 FR 25550 (May 5, 2011) (regulations became effective July 5, 2011); see also 75 FR 29479 (May 26, 2010) (proposed rule).

22. See 76 FR 2550, 25551.

23. For critical access hospitals ("CAH"), the regulations contain an exception to the requirement that CAH agreements for clinical services may only be with a Medicare-participating provider or supplier, because DSTEs do not necessarily participate in Medicare. See 42 C.F.R. § 485.635(c)(5).

24. 42 C.F.R. §§ 482.12(a)(8), (9); 42 C.F.R. § 482.22(a); 42 C.F.R. § 485.616(c); 42 C.F.R. § 485.635; TJC LD.04.03.09; TJC MS.13.01.01; see also Medicare State Operations Manual, App. A and W, CMS Pub. 100-07

(containing survey standards regarding credentialing by proxy); see also CMS S&C Letter 11-32-Hospital/CAH (July 15, 2011).

25. See 42 U.S.C. § 1101 *et seq.*

26. Section 1834(m)(4) of the Social Security Act.

27. See Section 1834(m)(4)(F) of the Social Security Act; 42 CFR 410.78(f); CMS Pub. 100-02, Medicare Benefit Policy Manual, Ch. 15 section 270.2; CMS Pub. 100-04, Medicare Claims Processing Manual, Ch. 12 section 190.3.

28. See CMS' MLN "Telehealth Services" for CY 2016 (Dec 2015).

29. *Id.*; see also, for example, Noridian Telehealth Services Q&A No. 6 (rev. May 29, 2015) (noting that POS Code 12: home is ineligible for payment).

30. See CMS' MLN "Telehealth Services" for CY 2016 (Dec 2015).

31. See Section 1834(m)(4)(E) of the Social Security Act.

32. See 42 CFR 410.78(a)(3).

33. See Section 1834(m)(4)(F) of the Social Security Act; 42 CFR 410.78(f); CMS Pub. 100-02, Medicare Benefit Policy Manual, Ch. 15 section 270.2; Medicare Claims Processing Manual, Ch. 12 section 190.3.

34. Note: Coverage rules for Medicare Advantage plans and Medicaid Managed Care organizations are notably more flexible than traditional Medicare. These plans are encouraged to develop new and innovative ways to provide care and are generally subject to fewer restrictions on coverage of telehealth services.

35. Center for Connected Health Policy. *State Telehealth Laws and Medicaid Program Policies.* April 2016. www.cchpca.org.

36. MN Stat. 62A.672 (emph. added).

Index

Note: Page numbers followed by *f* and *t* indicate figures and tables, respectively.